THE BIOLOGY AND CHEMISTRY
OF ACTIVE OXYGEN

DEVELOPMENTS IN BIOCHEMISTRY

THE BIOLOGY AND CHEMISTRY
OF ACTIVE OXYGEN

Editors:

J. V. BANNISTER
Inorganic Chemistry Department, University of Oxford, Oxford, England

and

W. H. BANNISTER
*Nuffield Department of Clinical Biochemistry, University of Oxford,
Radcliffe Infirmary, Oxford, England*

ELSEVIER
New York • Amsterdam • Oxford

©1984 by Elsevier Science Publishing Co., Inc.
All rights reserved.

Published by:

Elsevier Science Publishing Co., Inc.
52 Vanderbilt Avenue, New York, New York 10017

Sole distributors outside the United States and Canada:

Elsevier Science Publishers B.V.
P.O. Box 211, 1000 AE Amsterdam, The Netherlands

Library of Congress Cataloging in Publication Data

The Biology and chemistry of active oxygen.

    Includes index.
    1. Active oxygen. 2. Active oxygen in the body.
    I. Bannister, J. V. (Joe V.), 1945-   II. Bannister, W. H.
QP535.01B58   1984   591.19'214   84-1503
ISBN 0-444-00924-8

Manufactured in the United States of America

This book is dedicated to Professor Alessandro Rossi-Fanelli

TABLE OF CONTENTS

PREFACE

Prefaces to volumes of this sort tend to be of two kinds. Some prefaces do
the work of an Introduction. We have been spared this task because R.J.P.
Williams has written an Introduction (Chapter 1) with the express purpose of
drawing together the threads of the various Chapters "so that the overall biology
of oxygen can be seen readily." Other prefaces go briefly over the ground
covered by the various authors doing a sort of "Who wrote what." We have seen
no need for this kind of exercise because the Chapter titles in the Contents
are sufficiently informative in this respect.

This book is founded on the theme "Oxygen in Biology." "Oxygen and Life"
might seem a good way of expressing this theme but we do not think it fully con-
veys the uneasy relationship that exists between life and oxygen. The utilization of oxygen in biology is fraught with problems of toxicity which are a major
concern of this book (Chapters 4-11). The term "Active Oxygen," used in the
title of the book, is (hopefully) close to the paradoxical idea of an agent
which is both harmful and beneficial to life. Oxygen has been of immense interest
to chemists and biologists since it was discovered some two hundred years ago
and it is not surprising that the term "Active Oxygen" is not new. To Lavoisier
we owe the name oxygen ("principe oxygine") for the gas discovered by Priestley
(in 1774) and Scheele (about 1772). The term "Active Oxygen" does not have such
a precise history as "principle oxygine." It arose in stages in chemical and
biological studies. The idea of activation before "the air which Nature has
provided for us" is utilized in cellular respiration became current in the 19th
century when Lavoisier's concept of direct oxidation of foodstuffs was dropped.
In *The History of Cell Respiration and Cytochrome*, David Keilin has attributed
the demise of Lavoisier's direct oxidation to E.F.W. Pflüger who "demonstrated
that cellular combustion is to a very great extent independent of the partial
pressure of ordinary 'inactive' oxygen." Historically, the concept of "active
oxygen arose in chemical studies of slow auto-oxidation processes in the presence
of water with formation of hydrogen peroxide. The oxygen consumed in the formation of hydrogen peroxide was called "active oxygen" and said to be "activated"
or "rendered active" during the oxidation process. These studies furnished
purely chemical models for biological oxidations until the conjecture of bio-
catalysis, due to Berzelius, and the rise of the enzymatic theory of metabolism
provided the impetus for the idea of "oxygen-activating enzymes." In the 1890s
in studies of what he called the "oxidase" of laccase G. Bertrand originated the

idea of catalysis of biological oxidation by metal ions even though he was wrong in two respects: he did not regard oxygen as the (hydrogen) acceptor and regarded manganese as the functional metal of his laccase. Of course we now regard biological oxidations as dehydrogenations and the dehydrogenases that utilize (molecular) oxygen as hydrogen acceptor are our "oxidases" (Chapter 3). In modern language Lavoisier's theory of biological oxidation postulated the incorporation of molecular oxygen into the substrate. Subsequent theories (theorists) demanded the addition of "activated" oxygen to the substrate. The theory of enzymatic dehydrogenation, due to Wieland, disposed of this concept of biological oxidation but left the hiatus filled by monooxygenases and diooxygenases (Chapter 4).

C.F. Schönbein, who discovered ozone in 1840, is said to have regarded oxygen as "omnipotent." Less extravagantly Irwin Fridovich has remarked that oxygen, like James, has two faces, the benign and the malignant. The problem of oxygen toxicity, the malignant face of oxygen, is discussed at several levels in Chapters 5-11 of this book. Oxygen poisoning was described by Paul Bert in 1878 who speculated that it might be due to inhibition of "fermentative" reactions in the cell. Some enzymes are inactivated during hyperoxia (particularly dihydroxy acid dehydratase in $E. coli$) and natural selection has not evolved oxygen-resistant forms. The hazards of oxygen utilization as electron acceptor in living cells are more probably associated with the intermediates from oxygen to water than with dioxygen itself. If these intermediates were not toxic, singly or jointly, it is reasonable to suppose that living cells would not have evolved a variety of strategies against them. The constant battle between living cells and oxygen free radicals is a recurring theme in this book. Sherrington wrote: "The scientific journey has no end. It has only halting places at which the traveller can look around and survey." It is in the spirit of need to "look around and survey" the field of oxygen in biology, with its continuing debates, that this book has been written.

J.V. Bannister
W.H. Bannister
Oxford, England

ACKNOWLEDGMENTS

The chapters published in this book were written during 1981 and 1982. The cooperation of the various authors in putting this volume together is grate- fully acknowledged. Dr. J.V. Bannister and Professor W.H. Bannister thank the Wellcome Trust, London, England for Research Fellowships.

THE BIOLOGY AND CHEMISTRY
OF ACTIVE OXYGEN

CHAPTER 1   AN INTRODUCTION TO THE BIOLOGICAL CHEMISTRY OF OXYGEN

R.J.P. WILLIAMS
University of Oxford, Inorganic Chemistry Laboratory,
South Parks Road, Oxford OX1 3QR, England

The purpose of this introduction is to draw together the threads of the chapters in this volume so that the overall biology of oxygen can be seen readily.

The chemistry of oxygen is described in a recent book (ref. 1). Oxygen is a relatively inert molecule. Its activation is brought about by reduction in complexes. While it is a basic molecule in that it can form complexes by making weak σ-donor bonds it is also a π-acid, accepting electrons in its complexes. Its π-acid strength means that when it forms a complex $O_2.X$ the oxygen becomes partially reduced and activated. It is a series of subsequent complete steps of electron transfer to O_2,

$$X + O_2 \leftrightarrows X.O_2 \xrightarrow{e} X.O_2^{\cdot -} \xrightarrow{e} X(H_2O_2) \xrightarrow{e} (X).OH^{\cdot} \xrightarrow{e} H_2O \qquad (1)$$

which interests us most strongly and which includes the production of $O_2^{\cdot -}$, H_2O_2 and $OH^{\cdot}$. One primary concern will be the source of reducing equivalents in this chain since it can be X itself, a cofactor, some substrate, or some complicated electron transfer pathway in a gross biological organization, Table 1. A second concern is the nature of X, the group which binds O_2, $O_2^{\cdot -}$, H_2O_2 (and $OH^{\cdot}$), Table 2. A further concern is the positioning in space of the group X within biological compartments and its timed activation, regulations. Biological catalysts have controlled syntheses, positions and catalytic activities. We return to these points later.

TABLE 1

Classification of Reactions of Oxygen

Reaction	Example
$O_2 \rightarrow H_2O$	(a) Energy Capture, Cytochrome Oxidase (Cytochrome chain reduction) (b) One Electron Reduction, Laccase (Copper chain reduction)
$O_2 \rightarrow O_2^{\cdot -}$	Reduction by NADH, Flavo-Enzyme
$O_2^{\cdot -} \rightarrow H_2O_2 \rightarrow OH^{\cdot}$	Reduction by Metal Ions, Superoxide Dismutases (no other components)
$O_2 \rightarrow RO_2H$	Dioxygen Insertion, Dioxygenase
$O_2 \rightarrow ROH$	Hydroxylation, e.g., Cytochrome P-450, Mono-oxygenase (Requires subsidiary reductant such as NADH or α-ketoglutarate)

TABLE 2

Reaction Centres for Dioxygen[a]

Reaction Centre (X)	Example
Iron (a) Heme	Many: Cytochrome oxidase, Cytochrome P-450, Myoglobin
Iron (b) Non-heme	Many: Mono- and Dioxygenases, Hemerythrin, Superoxide Dismutase
Copper (a) Dimeric	Many: Oxidases, Laccase Hemocyanin, Superoxide Dismutase
(b) Monomeric	Amine Oxidases
Flavin (Pterin)	Oxygenases Superoxide production
Manganese	Oxygen release in chloroplasts Superoxide Dismutase

---

[a]Note: A very different list of centers activate $O_2^{\cdot -}$ and H_2O_2.

The most pressing point about oxygen in biology is of course its value. Generated together with reduced carbon by plants in the reaction, catalyzed uniquely by Mn

$$h\nu + 2\ H_2O + CO_2 \rightarrow CH_4 + 2\ O_2 \qquad (2)$$

it is used by many forms of life in two ways (a) as a source of energy, reversing equation (2), and (b) as a metabolite for incorporation into organic molecules. Energy production lies largely with the reactions of cytochrome oxidase, Chapter 3. Oxygen metabolism is covered in Chapters 4 and 5. These activities require that oxygen should be distributed to very many cells and there are therefore O_2-carriers such as hemoglobins and storage compounds for oxygen such as myoglobins, see Chapter 2. All these are positive features of oxygen biology. The groups X which are involved in these functions are described in Table 2. We see that with the exception of the heterocyclic ring systems, pteridine and flavin, X is a "trace" element and usually a π-donor metal ion. The reactions of oxygen are not catalyzed directly by the side-chains of proteins. We return to this point later.

In the course of transport of oxygen and its reduction to water there is either the risk of, or the deliberate involvement of, production of the free intermediate reduced species $O_2^{\cdot -}$, H_2O_2 and $OH^{\cdot}$. The risk arises since X the carrier or catalyst is always an electron donor and although it might have retained these intermediates in all cases there is always some probability (and sometimes a deliberate need) for them to be released. Free $O_2^{\cdot -}$, H_2O_2 and $OH^{\cdot}$ are more reactive than O_2 and as freely diffusing reagents are a hazard. They have also the advantageous possible use as reagents in syntheses or as reagents in defense mechanisms usually on a degradative path. In other words when these reagents are free they are potentially either useful or harmful to all biological systems but the harm can be done to others (defense) or to one's self (accident). It is a matter of *where* and *when* the intermediates are made and used. The same problem arises in the release of for example proteases for digestion. Thus the controlled release in special compartments of these reduced oxygen species is a part of health and their unfortunate accidental release generates disease. Clearly genetic and species differences are also involved. To prevent random damage (disease) biological systems have a fall-back clearance system (compare protease inhibitors) which can remove free $O_2^{\cdot -}$, H_2O_2 or $OH^{\cdot}$ should they appear at the wrong time or in the wrong place, Table 3. These matters are dealt with in Chapters 6 - 10. An overview of the uses of $O_2^{\cdot -}$, H_2O_2 and $OH^{\cdot}$ in protection is given in Table 4. Notice that the use of oxygen in defense includes chemical detoxification (cytochrome P-450, involving bound $OH^{\cdot}$, see later), biological detoxication or attack on biological enemies (a flavin oxidase and superoxide dismutase (to give $OH^{\cdot}$)), and preparative synthesis of protective polymers such as a lignins (laccase and peroxidase) and even collagen (lysine and proline hydroxylases and lysine oxidase).

TABLE 3

Removal of Dioxygen Reduction Products[a]

Product	Removal System
$O_2^{\cdot -}$	CuSOD in cytoplasm (eukaryotes) MnSOD in cytoplasm (prokaryotes) FeSOD and MnSOD in various organelles
H_2O_2 (RO_2H)	Catalase in vesicles Peroxidases in vesicles Glutathione Peroxidase in cytoplasm Vitamin E in membranes
$OH^{\cdot}$	Almost impossible to eliminate once formed but compounds such as metal complexes and vitamin E react very rapidly with it.

[a]See Chapters 6 - 10

TABLE 4

Protective Value of $O_2^{\cdot -}$, H_2O_2 and $OH^{\cdot}$ [a]

Leukocytes $\longrightarrow O_2^{\cdot -} \longrightarrow$	H_2O_2 $OH^{\cdot}$ ClO^-	} Attack bacteria
Peroxyzomes + H_2O_2 $\longrightarrow$	Phenol Oxidation	} Protective polymers on plant surfaces
P-450 + O_2 → FeO(V) FeO(IV)	$\longrightarrow$	Chemical detoxication
Amine oxidation	$\longrightarrow$	Removes transmitters and hormones

[a]See Chapters 4 and 5

Finally it must not be thought that oxygen metabolism is just degradative. Oxygen is used in the deliberate syntheses of such molecules as adrenalin, hydroxylated sterols and in modified amino-acids for incorporation into proteins, e.g., tyrosine. Of course oxygen atoms are more frequently introduced from water. All these are useful features of O_2 chemistry.

Many of the reactions of O_2 are now seen to be in a flow system:

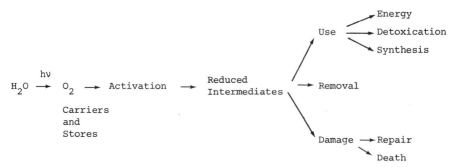

Carbon dioxide and water are the end products (of O_2 metabolism) and oxygen is recycled using manganese in the reaction $H_2O \rightarrow O_2$. There is no permanent steady state of this flow but rather a set of possible states which can be switched at any stage after activation. The levels of each of the reduced species depends upon the exact position in space in an organism and the exact time of observation. We leave these complicated matters to look first at some chemical points regarding the nature of X.

The Nature of X - The Binding Group for Dioxygen

The first peculiarity of X, the activator center for oxygen, is that it can be one of the metals, iron (most common), copper or possibly manganese or an organic molecule, flavin or pteridine. Why is there a multiplicity of activators? Again the intermediates $O_2^{\cdot-}$, H_2O_2 and $OH^{\cdot}$ are handled by Fe, Cu or Mn or certain organic molecules, Table 2. Why is this so?

Already we have stressed the nature of the group X which activates oxygen·in all the reactions. Before examining X more closely we must notice again the combined intermediate forms of reduced oxygen. It is conventional to write the combined forms of (reduced) oxygen in particular ways $X.O_2$, $X.O_2^{\cdot-}$, $X.O_2H^-$, XO, etc. Unfortunately in this form the equivalences of certain combinations with X in terms of oxidizing capacity and the differences in oxidizing power in terms of potentials cannot easily be recognized since they depend on the oxidation state stability of the compounds of X. Table 5 attempts to rectify this use of convention. Note that FeO(IV) is also written as a complex of Fe^{3+} and $OH^{\cdot}$ and has nearly the same oxidizing power as this formulation implies. $MO_2^{\cdot-}$ can be equal in oxidizing capacity to $M^-.O_2$ or MO^+. Such apparently similar species as MoO, R_2SeO and FeO may have

TABLE 5

Some Combined States of Oxygen Moieties[a]

	O_2	$O_2^{\cdot\,-}$	O_2^{2-}	$O^{\cdot\,-}$	O^{2-}
H^+		$HO_2^{\cdot}$	HO_2^{-}, H_2O_2	$OH^{\cdot}$	H_2O, OH^-
Flavin or Pteridine	$(Fl^{2-}.O_2)$	$[FlO_2]^{3-}H^+$	FlO_2H	$(Fl^{\cdot})$	
M^{2+}	$M^{2+}.O_2$	$M^{2+}.O_2^{\cdot\,-}$	$M^{2+}.O_2H^-$	$MO(III)$	$M^{2+}(H_2O)$
	$M^{3+}.O_2^{\cdot\,-}$	$M^{3+}.O_2^{2-}$	$[MO(IV)]^{2+}$	$M^{3+}OH^-$	$M^{2+}(OH^-)$
		$[MO(V)]^{3+}$		$[MO(III)]^{+}$	$[MOH]^{+}$
					$[MO]$
$[M_2]^{4+}$	$[M_2].^{4+}O_2$	$[M_2].^{4+}O_2^{\cdot\,-}$	$[M_2].^{4+}O_2^{2-}$	$[M_2].^{4+}O^{\cdot\,-}$	
	$[M_2].^{2+}O_2^{2-}$	$[M_2].^{5+}O_2^{2-}$	$[M_2].^{4+}O_2H^-$	$[M_2].^{5+}O^{2-}$	
	$[M_2].^{3+}O_2^{\cdot\,-}$	$[M_2].^{5+}(O_2H)^{-}$	$[M_2].^{6+}(OH^-)$	$[M_2].^{5+}OH^-$	
	$[(MO)_2]^{4+}$	$[M_2O]^{5+}$	$[M_2O]^{4+}$		
Se			SeO		

[a]Note: That best representation of a complex is not necessarily given by a single formula. Again for different metals M = Mn, Fe, Co, Cu or Mo the best representation is not the same even for the same species M_xO_y.

the same redox capacity but have very different redox powers. The full formulae give the maximum possible capacity for oxidation relative to the elementary state of X and to H_2O, but it is not useful unless we also know the thermodynamic (and kinetic) properties of the states. MoO is not like FeO except in formula. The thermodynamic properties of concern are therefore the acid/base properties of the state of X(O) in the complex and its redox potential. The kinetic properties are the ease of bond breaking in the units of Table 5, not forgetting that homolytic and heterolytic fission are possible. Note that metals form more ionic intermediates than flavin. The properties of $X.O_2$ intermediates decide their functional value.

Before exploring the different possibilities briefly we note that proteins will play a major role in the control of the reaction intermediates. Not only does the protein have the binding groups which hold X but it also controls the bio-energetics and kinetics of X complexes to a large degree through strain, stereochemical restriction and dynamic facets. It also controls the part of space in which X is placed. However it cannot override completely the idiosyncratic nature of X itself.

The Thermodynamics of X

Consider hemoglobin. The $Fe.O_2$ complex, written as $Fe(II).O_2$ or $Fe(III).O_2^{\cdot\,-}$, holds, potentially, the capacity of four oxidizing equivalents relative to Fe(II) and its redox potential $Fe(O_2)/Fe(H_2O)_2$ must be close to that of O_2 itself $\sim+0.8$ volts. However the complex does not act as a redox reactant. Thus kinetic barriers must stop reaction. Now the first barrier is the high energy of the reduced intermediates such as FeO(IV) (redox capacity 2). We can estimate the stability of this state from the known redox potential of Fe(II)/Fe(III) in hemoglobin (+0.2 volts) and the general statement that FeO(IV) will only be stabilized in complexes which stabilize Fe(III) relative to Fe(II). It is a feature of oxo-cation chemistry (ref. 2), MO, that where this group has a formal charge of n+, it behaves as if it had a charge of approximately (n+1)+. VO(II) for example is more like V(III) than V(II) in binding to ligands. Thus FeO(IV) in hemoglobin will not be very greatly stabilized relative to Fe(III) but both are stabilized relative to Fe(II). Knowing that Fe(II)/Fe(III) potentials and some potentials of model Fe(III)/Fe(IV) complexes we can estimate that the redox potential of Fe(III)/FeO(IV) in hemoglobin is >1.0 volt. Oxygen will not readily raise Fe(II) to FeO(IV) in hemoglobin. Moreover hemoglobin has no sites for the binding of reducing substrates and for subsequent one-electron reaction with them, contrast peroxidase and cytochrome P-450 below. Thus the reaction $Fe(II)O_2 \rightarrow Fe(III) + O_2^{\bullet-}$ (or any further change) does not occur easily although some superoxide is formed, and the red cell has to clear this and reduce Fe(III) back to Fe(II). We begin to see the essential complicated design of hemoglobin needed to perform its carrier function but the subtle nature of the heme-binding to the protein is much greater than regulation of redox potential and access for substrates would imply. In fact the iron binding of O_2 relays itself through protein changes so that the energetics of O_2-binding are protein energetics. One part is the stress in the Fe-histidine (F8) bond, another the shape changes of heme itself, and another the exact disposition of side-chains, H-bonds, and even the dispositions of helices, Chapter 2. Now we have shown clearly in cytochrome-c that even changes of oxidation state of haem iron from Fe(II) to Fe(III) run from the iron to the surface of this monomeric protein (ref. 3) and that certain single changes of amino-acid in many parts of the sequence change the iron redox potential. Thus changes at the iron in proteins create running cooperative changes (signals) over wide regions of a protein. O_2-binding in hemoglobin involves an equally great change--a spin-state change. Because of the deep involvement of many amino acids and the geometry of the spin-state change, the function of the heme, oxygen-carrying, is a property of the whole amino-acid sequence. Cooperativity and the Bohr effect, i.e., acid/base reactions, are included within the potential of this set of running interactions. We expect the same possibilities to arise in all other protein.X complexes of O_2, $O_2^{\bullet-}$ or H_2O_2. We must always look very carefully at the peculiarities of each protein since often an organism will use a family of them, say several hemoglobins, to supply its different parts in different ways, see Chapter 2.

Other hemo binding centers for O_2 are similar to that of hemoglobin, e.g., in
P-450, but they are not the same. This can be clearly seen in the ratio of
intensities of bands in the absorption spectrum, e.g., of the $\alpha:\beta$ bands. Now in
turn this ratio correlates with the redox potential of the haem, which depends on
the binding of Fe to the protein, the distal protein environment, and strain in
these units in the different oxidation states. For hemoglobin, an O_2 carrier,
FeO_2 is the best state with oxygen minimally activated by electron transfer within
the FeO_2 bond. As stated above this is best achieved if the redox potentials of
Fe are high. Any electron transfer or reaction with organic molecules is further
prevented by placing all oxidizable groups far from the iron. Increasing activation
of FeO_2 is brought about by lowering simultaneously the redox potentials of the
Fe(II)/Fe(III) and Fe(III)/Fe(IV) couples, e.g., in peroxidases and cytochrome P-450,
and by allowing closer approach of oxidizable compounds such as the phenol substrates
in peroxidases (substrate binding site 10Å away) and the camphor in P-450 (substrate
binding site 4Å away). Thus there are two general distinctions between hemoglobin
and these enzymes. In P-450 these are accentuated by the change of iron ligand,
histidine (imidazole) in hemoglobin and cysteine (thiolate) in P-450. The latter
permits the O of FeO in P-450 to become extremely activated, perhaps the accessible
excited state is -S˙FeO˙⁻, when H-atom abstraction from the *adjacent* substrate
becomes possible. In all the proteins the role of the amino-acid sequence in
adjusting the properties of the intermediates and in providing rapid fluctuations,
so that the flow of reaction is fast, is crucial. In P-450 the heme pocket must
close around the substrates. In the heme iron oxidation catalysts we begin to
understand these functions. Note that just as every man has many hemoglobins,
he has many P-450 enzymes and each plant has many peroxidases, so that very fine
control can be exerted over the exact oxygen tension or the exact compounds oxidized.
Different isoenzymes are produced in different places and at different times. For
further details see Chapters 2 to 4 and note in Chapter 5 the use of a heme protein
in the formation of prostaglandins.

A heme enzyme which is used in energy capture, cytochrome oxidase, has a different
aspect. Here O_2 is not strongly activated (high iron redox potential) but a ready
source of electrons is supplied by adjacently positioned external cytochrome c,
which needs little or no activation energy. Here however the redox potential of
the oxo-cation Fe(III)/Fe(IV) is lowered relative to Fe(II)/Fe(III) by the presence
of an adjacent metal to give FeOCu. A similar intermediate is found in laccase
CuOCu but in neither is the oxygen atom activated for attack on organic molecules
in any oxidation state since the second metal stabilizes and protects the
intermediates. At the same time the protein acts as an electron capacitor
controlling the reduction of O_2 directly to H_2O via this bis-metal complex by
retaining these intermediates. Complexes which pick up O_2 between two metal ions
do not appear to activate O_2. Interestingly the properties of cytochrome oxidase

in the membrane generates H^+-flow as well as electron flow. Energy is largely
conserved although the reaction is irreversible. Effectively the energy captured
is due to the diffusional (now directional) uptake of protons by O_2. The full
significance of the total reduction reaction including the proton uptake

$$O_2 + 4e + 4H^+ \rightarrow 2H_2O$$

can now be seen. Whereas in normal enzyme reactions H^+ is isotropically buffered
so that O_2 reduction need only be related to electron flow between chemicals and
no spatial regulation is generated, here it is connected to charge and proton
gradients *within the spatial structure of the membrane protein.* The two ends of
the protein and then the two sides of the membrane are at different proton chemical
potentials. The hub of energy capture lies in directional diffusion control (ref. 4).
How does the protein do this? Chapter 3 offers some insights.

Through the work of especially Chance and his collaborators using EXAFS the
different states of cytochrome oxidases during redox cycles are much clearer. The
involvement of the proton in the cycle clearly involves bound proton states, i.e.,
changes of pK_a associated with oxidation on one side of the membrane. The energy
conversion is then not simply chemi-osmotic but is constrained by local control
of proton diffusion pathways. Whether these local paths extend to the ATP-synthetic
machinery is not yet known.

All the above heme-enzymes bind O_2 and many activate it yet there is one heme
enzyme which does not function in this way. Catalase has such a low redox potential
and the low-spin state of Fe(II) is so inaccessible that not only does it not take
up O_2 but it releases it in the disproportionation of H_2O_2 to H_2O and O_2. The fifth
ligand to iron, is here a phenolate group. Catalase iron has then some features
in common with the manganese which releases O_2 in photosynthesis and the iron,
copper and manganese which release O_2 in the superoxide dismutases. In all these
cases the chemistry of the metal must be such that O_2 is not bound. Manganese is
peculiarly inept at binding O_2 since Mn(II) complexes are all poor π-donors (high-
spin) but the problem is more acute in Fe(II) and Cu(I) chemistry which are π-donors
and can bind and activate O_2.

Nonheme Iron Proteins

We shall not describe the Fe_nS_n proteins since they are either electron transfer
proteins or activators of hydrogen. Oxygen activation rests with two types of
nonheme iron protein one of which is permanently in the Fe(III) state apparently
and the other of which is a (dissociable) Fe(II) complex, Chapter 4. Amongst them
there are probably both thiolate and phenolate complexes and the binding of iron
will be through these reducible anions, carboxylates, and imidazoles. There is
already a known representative structure in hemerythrin, Fig. 1. Except for
hemerythrin, an oxygen carrier, and superoxide dismutase the redox potentials,
Fe(II)/Fe(III), are expected to be below +0.3 volts. The potentials will be the

lower the more anionic the complexes, either through the ligands themselves or the surrounding protein side chains. By analogy with heme proteins we expect the complexes with higher potentials to act as O_2 carriers, those with lower potentials to act as O_2 activators, and those connected to secondary sources of electrons and of a low Fe(II)/Fe(III) redox potential and especially those with a thiolate ligand to act as hydroxylating agents of the most active kind. In the class of enzymes which are permanently in the Fe(III) state attack of the metal is on the substrate and O_2 attacks the Fe(III) substrate complex, while those enzymes which cycle through Fe(II)O_2 activate O_2 to attack substrates.

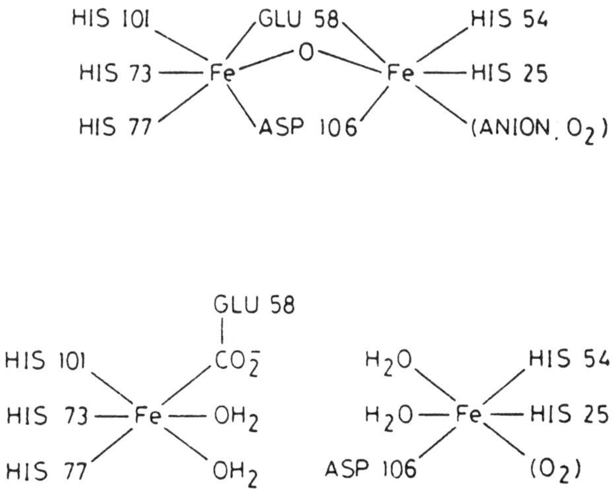

Fig. 1. The active site of hemerythrin in the Fe(III) state (above) and a possible structure of the Fe(II) state (below) (ref. 6).

Co-Reductants

The P-450 cytochromes require NADH or NADPH to supply two electrons to activate O_2 in FeO_2. A more curious situation arises in the specific requirements for ascorbate and especially of α-ketoglutarate in a number of coupled oxidations for nonheme iron enzymes:

α-ketoglutarate + SH + O_2 → succinate + CO_2 + SOH

Chapter 4 describes the reactions in detail. Such a requirement suggests that the pathway of oxidation of SH is deliberately coupled to the pathway of reactions of α-ketoglutarate which is a key substrate in both the citric acid cycle and in (NH$_3$) nitrogen fixation. In other words SH is not oxidized unless the cell has a good acetate supply. The compounds, SH, which are so controlled include lysyl and prolyl oxidation in higher organisms.

It is a feature of many of these nonheme iron proteins that in the Fe(II) state they dissociate. They may well be involved therefore in controlling cell metabolism, e.g., the citric acid cycle, following the cytoplasmic concentration of Fe(II) rather than just being true metallo-enzymes. One way in which the control may operate is that when iron is low the enzymes dissociate and the intermediates which then accumulate are ion scavengers, (ref. 2). Other possibilities are discussed in (ref. 1).

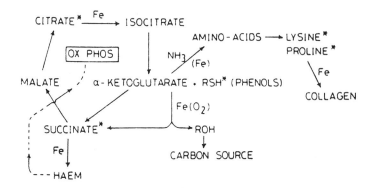

Fig. 2. The citric acid cycle (top left) and its relationship to iron scavengers (precursors shown *) and to iron-dependent enzymes including several oxidases, Chapter 4.

Copper and Oxygen in Biology

Turning away from iron to copper the most obvious question is: Why do both copper and iron redox catalysts occur in biology? One reason undoubtedly is that the very different stability of their complex ions allows them to be used very differently in biological space, compare Table 6, copper and Table 7, iron.

TABLE 6

Some Extracellular and Vesicular Copper Enzymes

Enzyme	Situation
Caeruloplasmin	Extracellular (plasma)
Lysine Oxidase	Extracellular (aorta)
Galactose Oxidase	Extracellular (bacterial)
Laccase	Extracellular (plant sap)
Tyrosinase	Extracellular (plant sap)
Ascorbate Oxidase	Extracellular (and intracellular?)
Cytochrome Oxidase	Vesicular (mitochondria)
Amine Oxidase	Plasma
Dopamine β-Hydroxylase	Vesicular (chromaffin granules)
Hemocyanin	Oxygen carrier in hemolymph

TABLE 7

The Iron Proteins Associated with Oxygen and Their Spatial Distribution[a]

Protein	Function	Spatial Position
Heme Proteins,[b] P-450, etc.	O_2-carriers O_2-enzymes	In cell cytoplasm or in cell membranes
Lysine and Proline Hydroxylases	Hydroxylation	Cytoplasm
Nonheme Mono-oxygenases Nonheme Dioxygenases Lignin Oxidase	Oxidative degradation Oxidative degradation Oxidative degradation	Prokaryote cytoplasm Prokaryote cytoplasm Outside cells?
Peroxidases and Catalases	Oxidation using H_2O_2	Vesicles
Hemerythrin	O_2-carrier	Plasma (rare)

[a] Electron-transfer proteins are not included. They are usually in membranes. Iron transport proteins and enzymes which are extracellular are Fe(III) proteins and do not carry out redox reactions.
[b] There is one exception in this huge group of enzymes. The hemoglobin of certain worms is a free extracellular protein.

Copper can be used anywhere in principle since it is very stable in proteins but it seems that its use is very restricted in biology not only in space, mainly outside the cell, but in the redox potential range which it covers. In fact in biology it functions between +400 and +800 millivolts. This is just the redox range in which it is very difficult to make *stable* Fe(II)/Fe(III) or Fe(III)/Fe(IV) couples. Fig. 3 shows schematically the redox potentials of many transition metal ions in water at pH = 0 whereas Fig. 4 shows the redox potentials of the same couples in biology. Nearly all redox couples fall substantially from water to biological complexes but that of Cu(I)/Cu(II) rises. Whereas Fe(II)/Fe(III) and Fe(III)/Fe(IV) couples drop more or less together, the Co(I)/Co(II) and Co(II)/Co(III) couples become more equal. Both the Mn(II)/Mn(III) and Mn(III)/Mn(IV) couples come into the biological range but probably become more separated, i.e., Mn(III) is stabilized. It is seen immediately that these changes made mononuclear Fe, Co and Mn into two-electron capacity reagents within the biological range of potentials, +0.8, to -0.5 volts, while mononuclear copper remains as a one-electron capacity atom of great use inside the cell at special redox potential. The capacity of copper can only be increased in dimers where following Malström we must suppose that the Cu O Cu state of formal oxidation state Cu(III) can exist as an intermediate and as such it is frequently used outside cells. Given these restrictions the major uses of copper in oxygenases are outside the cell, where other metal/protein complexes are unstable, and in one-electron reactions of special redox potential inside cells.

12

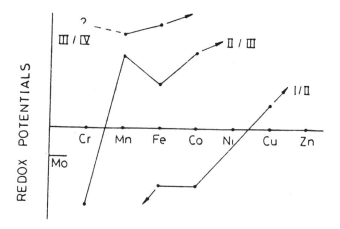

Fig. 3. An outline of the variation of the redox potentials of simple aqueous
ion couples (pH = 0) (refs. 1, 2). The horizontal line is the H^+/H_2 potential.
Mo indicates that all three Mo(III)/Mo(VI) couples have about the same potential.

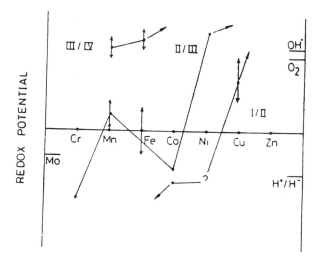

Fig. 4. An outline of the redox couples of metal ions in proteins at pH = 7.
Arrows indicate ranges of potentials. The horizontal line is the H_2/H^+ potential
at pH = 0. Note the relative changes compared with Fig. 3.

The two functions come together in the complex oxidases such as laccase.

The dominance of hemocyanin as the second most useful O_2 carrier also springs
from the stabilities of copper complexes outside cells and the redox properties
of the Cu(I)/Cu(II) couple. Hemerythrin is much less valuable as the iron in it

in the reduced state is much more likely to dissociate. Heme-proteins only became
the dominant form of oxygen transport and storage when they had gained the intracellular protection of reductases since although they are stable to dissociation
in both oxidation states the oxidized form, Fe(III), is vulnerable to porphyrin
degradation. It is also the case that heme synthesis needs a high concentration
of free Fe(II) to be supplied to the chelatase and that this is made available to
the inside of cells through special Fe(III) transport systems. The unique role
of copper is seen again in the superoxide dismutases.

Superoxide Dismutases (Chapters 6-10)

In superoxide dismutases the two redox reactions, $O_2^{\bar{\cdot}} \rightarrow O_2 + \underline{e}$ and $O_2^{\bar{\cdot}} + \underline{e} \rightarrow H_2O_2$,
must occur in order to keep the catalyst cycle. The redox potentials of the two
steps are -200 and +800 millivolts so that an intermediate potential of about 300
millivolts is best for the catalyst. In fact all three types of enzymes have the
same redox potential +300 millivolts (ref. 5). Given the available protein ligands
and the need to achieve this redox potential it is almost impossible to conceive
of a really stable mononuclear Mn(II) or Fe(II) protein. Now prokaryotic cells
and mitochondria pump in Fe(II) and Mn(II) so that the Mn(II) and Fe(II) dissociable
enzymes are protected in these regions of space. This applies to the oxygenases
of Chapter 4, and to many other manganese and iron enzymes of mitochondria and
prokaryotes other than superoxide dismutases. If this analysis is correct it was
necessary for the stability and protection of the cytoplasm of eukaryotes and
especially for the long-lived cells of multicellular organisms that a stable (copper)
dismutase should evolve to replace the iron or manganese enzyme. Copper proteins
are preferred over iron enzymes for their stability (and over a limited redox
potential range) but they are not so generally useful since they do not provide a
simple way of generating controlled O-atom or O_2-insertion. Moreover the dissociation
of iron generates a potential control mechanism over metabolism.

Flavins

We now turn to the example where flavin is the group X, Table 8. It is noteworthy
that a flavin complex is the major deliberate source of $O_2^{\bar{\cdot}}$, Chapter 9. Flavins
also activate O_2 in dioxygen and mono-oxygen insertion reactions but here they use
covalent intermediates and their aggressive strength is then very different from,
and less than, the more ionic intermediates where X is a metal ion. There is no
equivalent in flavin chemistry to the oxo-cations, e.g., FeO which have a very high
redox potential and can be highly aggressive, e.g., in P-450. Flavin then acts as
a mild hydroxylating agent.

$$\text{Flavin } O_2 \rightarrow \text{Flavin } O_2^{\bar{\cdot}} \rightarrow \text{Flavin } O_2H \rightarrow \text{Flavin}$$

$$Fe^{2+}O_2 \rightarrow Fe^{3+}O_2^{\bar{\cdot}-} \rightarrow FeO \rightarrow Fe^{3+}$$

In addition to the curious character of the oxo-cation the metal ions have the
kinetic advantage of *retaining* anions in *ionic* intermediates. In fact the use of

14

TABLE 8

Some Flavin Oxidases (Chapter 4)

Enzyme	Location
Amine Oxidase	Mitochondria
Superoxide Formation	Neutrophil membrane
Oxidative Decarboxylase (e.g., lysine or lactate	Bacteria
Hydroxylases (e.g., salicylate)	Bacteria
Dioxygenases (e.g., 2-NO_2 propane)	Bacteria

flavin in O_2-reactions always presents a hazard, e.g., the loss of $O_2^{\cdot -}$, which can only be weakly retained since flavin in any oxidation states binds the *anions* such as $O_2^{\cdot -}$ and HO_2^- very poorly. The correct reaction pathway is then best achieved by using a compulsory order mechanism in which substrate binds before O_2 is bound and converted to $O_2^{\cdot -}$ say for dioxygen insertion. This compulsory path is also seen in iron dioxygenases and in P-450 enzymes, Chapter 4. Given the flexibility of the reactions of iron in different coordination spheres and at different redox potentials it still remains something of a mystery that flavin should be used at all. One possible explanation lies in the instability of the simple Fe(II) protein complexes since flavin does not dissociate from its enzymes. Note that flavin is the only possible substitute for iron in many redox reactions since it is a two-electron couple like iron, contrast the one-electron reactions of copper and cobalt couples and the inability of Mn(II) to bind O_2. Since flavin intermediates are much less aggressive than those of iron it may be that they can be used so much more selectively in attack on sensitive molecules.

Molybdenum

Brief mention only will be made of molybdenum since it would not appear to activat oxygen in any enzyme although it is involved in oxidases. In fact it seems to act in chains of reactants connected to oxygen by flavin. The feature of Mo chemistry is its ability to function easily in atom-transfer reactions giving good leaving-group chemistry coupled to redox changes. Examples are $(SO_4^{2-})NO_3^- + Mo \rightleftarrows MoO + (SO_3^{2-})NO_2^-$; $CH_3COOH + Mo \rightleftarrows MoO + CH_3CHO$. Thus it acts as a multi-electron oxidant which may at times involve hydride or hydrogen atom transfer intermediates.

Conclusion

This introduction was put together after reading the chapters which follow. The references to any detailed point is in the chapters and I do not give such references here. I hope it allows the book to be seen as a unity rather than as a collection of essays, since the biological systems we are attempting to describe are built together to attain functional advantages. The overall involvement of oxygen in cellular activity is clearly very complex. An example of the complexity is given in Fig. 5 which shows the way in which the two metal ions Mn^{2+} and Fe^{2+} are related to O_2 release and absorption in organelles and are also related to the production of extracellular protective polymers.

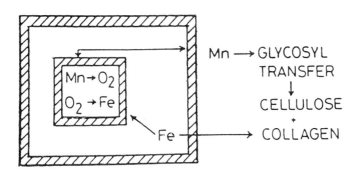

Fig. 5. An illustrative diagram showing that Mn(II) (and its enzymes) are to be found in vesicles and outside the cytoplasm of eukaryote cells while Fe(II) (and its enzymes) are largely in mitochondria. Heme enzymes occur in many compartments but not outside cells. In prokaryotes iron enzymes are in the cytoplasm. The location of copper enzymes is discussed in the text.

Finally while we have concentrated on the distribution in space of the various oxygen reactions we have not referred to time control. This is particularly important in defense, see Chapters 6 to 10. The activating enzymes are usually held in membranes or in vesicles. How they are activated is not known, but there is a strong suggestion that calcium ions are involved.

REFERENCES

1 Oxygen and Life, Chem. Soc. Special Publ. No. 39, Royal Soc. Chem. (London), 1981.
2 C.S.G. Phillips and R.J.P. Williams, (1966) Inorganic Chemistry, Oxford University Press, Oxford.
3 G.R. Moore and R.J.P. Williams, (1981) Eur. J. Biochem. 103, 503-543.
4 R.J.P. Williams, (1961) J. Theor. Biol. 1, 1-13.
5 G.D. Lawrence and D.T. Sawyer, (1979) Biochemistry, 14, 3045-3050 and personal communication.
6 R.E. Stenkamp, L.C. Sieker and L.H. Jensen, (1981) Nature, 291, 263-264.

CHAPTER 2   THE REACTION OF HEMOGLOBIN WITH OXYGEN

MAURIZIO BRUNORI[1], GIORGIO M. GIACOMETTI[2], and BRUNO GIARDINA[3]
[1]Institute of Chemistry, CNR Centre for Molecular Biology, Faculty of Medicine, University of Rome, 00100 Rome, Italy; [2]Istituto di Biologia Animale, Via Loredan 10, Padova, Italy; [3]Institute of Biochemistry, Faculty of Science, University of Cagliari Cagliari, Italy.

1. General Introduction (Refs. 1,2)

Myoglobin and hemoglobin are the oxygen carriers of vertebrates. Myoglobin is a component of the striated muscles, where it fulfills the role of an oxygen reserve and facilitates oxygen diffusion from the blood to the mitochondrion. Hemoglobin, contained in the red blood cells is the oxygen carrier from the environment to the tissues.

In both proteins the oxygen binding site is a prosthetic group, the heme, which consists of an organic moiety and an iron atom. The organic part, the protoporphyrin IX, is made up of four pyrrole rings linked by methene bridges to form a tetrapyrrole macrocycle. Four methyl, two vinyl and two propionate side chains are attached to the pyrrole rings at specific positions.

The iron atom at the center of the porphyrin ring forms four bonds with the pyrrol nitrogens. One of the axial coordination sites of the metal (the "fifth" coordi- nation position) makes a covalent bond (the "proximal" bond) with the polypeptide chain. The residue involved in this bond (the "proximal" residue), in both myoglobin and hemoglobin, is a histidyl side chain occupying the position F8 (i.e., position 8 in the Helix F) along the polypeptide chain. The opposite axial coordination site ("sixth" coordination position) is the oxygen-binding site. The heme iron can assume the ferrous (2^+) or the ferric (3^+) oxidation state; only ferrous hemoglobin binds reversibly dioxygen.

In the native state, both proteins are globular in shape, the heme group being located in a crevice formed by the polypeptide chain near its surface (hydrophobic pocket). This nonpolar environment represents one of the structural features which ensures protection against autoxidation of the metal.

The gross features of the three-dimensional structure such as the basic fold, are similar in myoglobin and hemoglobin, although myoglobin is a monomer (MW ~16250) containing a single heme group, whereas hemoglobin is a tetramer (MW ~64,000) built up of two types of chains (two α and two β chains), each one carrying its own heme group.

Hemoglobin is not only structurally, but also functionally much more complex than myoglobin: it is devoted to the transport of H^+ and CO_2 in addition to O_2, and its affinity for these molecules is a complex function of the concentration of all these

species. In what follows we shall examine the general features and the structural
basis of the O_2 binding properties to hemoglobins.

2. Ligand Binding to Hemoglobin (Refs. 1,3,4)

The saturation with a ligand ($\overline{Y}$) is defined as the fractional occupancy of the
oxygen-binding sites; its value ranges from 0 (all sites empty) to 1 (all sites occupied). A plot of $\overline{Y}$ versus the partial pressure of oxygen in the gas phase, p, is
referred to as the oxygen dissociation curve. The oxygen dissociation curves of
myoglobin and hemoglobin differ in two respectes: i) for any given value of p, $\overline{Y}$ is
higher for myoglobin than for hemoglobin (i.e., myoglobin has higher affinity for O_2),
Thus the oxygen pressure at which half of the sites are occupied, P_{50}, is typically
1 mm Hg for myoglobin and 26 mm Hg for hemoglobin under physiological conditions (at
37°C and pH 7.4); ii) the oxygen dissociation curve of myoglobin has a hyperbolic
shape, whereas that of hemoglobin is sigmoidal. It was reported long ago that the
shape of the oxygen dissociation curve of hemoglobin is particularly suited to its
physiological role as an oxygen carrier, and it implies a complex mechanism as
discussed below.

In the case of myoglobin the hyperbolic shape of the oxygen dissociation curve is
just as expected for a simple binding process:

$$Mb + O_2 \rightleftharpoons MbO_2; \quad K = \frac{[MbO_2]}{[Mb][O_2]} = \frac{[MbO_2]}{[Mb] \cdot p} \tag{1}$$

which yields

$$\frac{\overline{Y}}{1 - \overline{Y}} = K \cdot p \quad \text{or} \quad \overline{Y} = \frac{K \cdot p}{1 + K \cdot p} \tag{2}$$

The sigmoidal character of the O_2 dissociation curve of hemoglobin is the preeminent
phenomenological manifestation of cooperativity. Other physiologically significant
effects of third components (such as protons and organic phosphates) are considered,
in the modern description of allosteric regulation, as regulatory effects linked to
the basic phenomenon.

2.1 Early Studies (Ref. 5)

The first explanation of the sigmoidal character of the hemoglobin-oxygen equilibrium curve was presented by A. V. Hill at a time in which the actual aggregation
state of hemoglobin in solution was still uncertain. Hill postulated that the oxygenation of hemoglobin proceded through a multimolecular reaction, which was
represented by the equation

$$Hb + n\, O_2 \rightleftharpoons Hb(O_2)_n \tag{3}$$

The application of the law of mass action to this process yields

$$\frac{\overline{Y}}{1-\overline{Y}} = Kp^n \quad \text{or} \quad \overline{Y} = \frac{K \cdot p^n}{1 + Kp^n} \tag{4}$$

where $\overline{Y}$, referred to as fractional saturation, represents the average number of occupied sites divided by the total number of sites; p is the oxygen partial pressure and K is the equilibrium constant (see also above).

The oxygenation curve of hemoglobin can be satisfactorily described by Hill's equation in the range $0.1 < \overline{Y} < 0.9$, with a value of Hill's coefficient n = 2.8. This equation, in its original formulation is still in use in the modern analysis of binding data on hemoglobin as a means to describe the oxygen dissociation curve with minimum number of parameters, the value of n being an index of the heme-heme inter-actions in the system. Although its applications in terms of reaction mechanism is not adequate, its meaning has been amply recognized after the theoretical work of Wyman (Ref. 4).

2.2 The Adair Scheme

Taking advantage of the determination of the molecular weight of hemoglobin, which was established to be a tetramer, Adair (Ref. 6) proposed a phenomenological equation characterized by four equilibrium constants, one for each stage of binding:

$$\text{Hb}(O_2)_{i-1} + O_2 \rightleftharpoons \text{Hb}(O_2)_i \tag{5}$$

$$K_i = \frac{[\text{Hb}(O_2)_i]}{[\text{Hb}(O_2)_{i-1}]} \quad (1 \le i \le 4) \tag{6}$$

The Adair scheme is a very general one, and as such describes the equilibrium curve of any macromolecule with n binding sites, even if they are not identical, provided the system is chemically homogenous and there is no dissociation into subunits. Under these conditions the fractional saturation may be calculated according to the equation

$$\overline{Y} = \frac{\sum\limits_{j=1}^{n} \prod\limits_{i=1}^{j} j \, K_i \, p^j}{n \left[1 + \sum\limits_{j=1}^{n} \prod\limits_{i=1}^{j} K_i \, p^j \right]} \tag{7}$$

Thus in the case of hemoglobin equation (7) yields

$$\overline{Y} = \frac{K_1 p + 2K_1 K_2 p^2 + 3K_1 K_2 K_3 p^3 + 4K_1 K_2 K_3 K_4 p^4}{4(1 + K_1 p + K_1 K_2 p^2 + K_1 K_2 K_3 p^3 + K_1 K_2 K_3 K_4 p^4)} \tag{8}$$

The four constants (K_1, K_2, K_3, K_4), referred to as the Adair constants, are pheno-menological parameters which are related to the affinity of the four individual sites (K_1', K_2', K_3', K_4') by a statistical factor, which may be calculated from the general relation:

$$K_i' = \frac{i}{n-i+1} K_i \qquad (9)$$

At a molecular level, the constant K_i' represents the affinity for the i h molecule of ligand when $(i-1)$ sites of the macromolecule are occupied. Application of the Adair's scheme to hemoglobin, principally by Roughton and co-workers (Ref. 7), revealed that cooperativity in O_2 binding results from a value of $K_4' \sim 200\ K_1'$. Generally speaking, the sigmoidal shape of the equilibrium curve implies that one or more equilibrium constant, corresponding to steps successive to the binding of the first ligand, exceed their statistical value. This, in turn, implies that the oxygen binding sites must be affected by the presence of oxygen at the other hemes in the same molecule.

Although this formulation contains no hypothesis about the molecular mechanism underlying heme-heme interactions, unequivocal thermodynamic information can be obtained from the analysis of hemoglobin's dissociation isotherm in terms of Adair's equations.

The free energy change on binding oxygen at each successive step is given by:

$$\Delta G_i = - RT \ln K_i'$$

and the average free energy of binding is:

$$\Delta G = - \frac{1}{4} RT \ln K' \qquad (10)$$

where $K' = K_1'K_2'K_3'K_4' \dfrac{[Hb(O_2)_4]}{[Hb] \cdot p^4}$, the product of the intrinsic Adair association constants (Equation 9), corresponds to the equilibrium constant in the Hill equation (Equation 4).

If the O_2 binding curve is symmetrical (see otherwise Ref. 4), the oxygen partial pressure at which $\overline{Y} = 0.5$ is related to K' by:

$$p_{50}^4 = \frac{1}{K'} \qquad (11)$$

and $\Delta G = RT \ln p_{50}$ \qquad (12)

A useful way of analyzing the experimental data is presented by the Hill plot, i.e., $\log \overline{Y}/(1-\overline{Y})$ versus $\log p$ (Fig. 1). In the case of a macromolecule with four sites

20

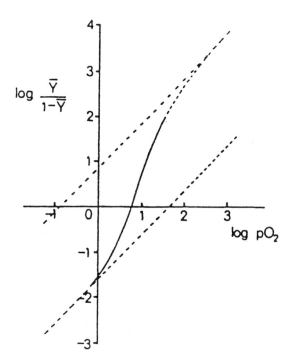

Fig. 1.   Hill plot of the O_2 dissociation curve of tetrametric hemoglobin.   The solid line covers the range over which experimental data are usually collected by conventional techniques.   Dashed lines are extrapolations obtained by fitting the data with the four Adair's constants.   Careful measurements at the extreme saturations (very low and/or very high) allow the experimental determination of the asymptotes and thus of the first and last Adair's constant (see also text).   The Hill plot for the isolated chains or myoglobin is almost coincident with the upper asymptote for hemoglobin.

the general expression may be derived from Eqs. (8) and (9) yielding:

$$\frac{\overline{Y}}{1 - \overline{Y}} = \frac{K_1'p + 3K_1'K_2'p^2 + 3K_1'K_2'K_3'p^3 + K_1'K_2'K_3'K_4'p^4}{1 + 3K_1'p + 3K_1'K_2'p^2 + K_1'K_2'K_3'p^3} \tag{13}$$

We may notice that if the association constants are all equal to K', Eq. (13) reduces to

$$\frac{\overline{Y}}{1 - \overline{Y}} = K' \cdot p \tag{2}$$

which corresponds to a straight line of slope 1, as expected for a monomeric or a non-cooperative macromolecule.   In the limits of very low and very high saturation, the

Hill plot would also be a straight line with unitary slope:

at low p $\qquad \log \dfrac{\overline{Y}}{1 - \overline{Y}} \rightarrow \log K_1' + \log p$

at high p $\qquad \log \dfrac{\overline{Y}}{1 - \overline{Y}} \rightarrow \log K_4' + \log p$

Extrapolation of the asymptotes to log p = 0 give the first and last Adair constants, as shown in Fig. 1. From the central part of the curve two parameters can be determined: the value of p required to give 50% saturation (p_{50}) and the Hill's constant n. In terms of the Adair's constants, p_{50} is obtained from Eq. (13) imposing $\overline{Y}/1-\overline{Y} = 1$:

$$2K_1'K_2'K_3'p_{50}^3 + K_1'K_2'K_3'K_4'p_{50}^4 = 1 \qquad (14)$$

2.3 Structural Models for Cooperativity

Deeper understanding of cooperative binding demands a molecular scheme of the interactions among the binding sites. In this direction a first model was proposed by Pauling in 1935 (Ref. 8). He proposed that cooperativity could be described in terms of an interaction constant, α, between adjacent oxygen-containing hemes. Thus for an arrangement of four identical subunits the phenomenological Adair constants can be expressed in terms of a single intrinsic constant, K', and a single interaction parameter:

$$K_i = f (K, \alpha)$$

The model may be applied to different topological situations for a tetrametric molecule, giving rise to different interaction patterns and hence to different functions of the two parameters. Moreover it can be further complicated by the introduction of a difference between α and β chains. A basic concept introduced by Pauling is that of "structural promotion," by which oxygen binding is facilitated by stronger structural interactions with successive binding steps yielding cooperativity.

The idea of "structural promotion" lead, through various developments, to the proposal of the so-called "induced fit" model by Koshland, Nemethy and Filmer (Ref. 9) In its simplest formulation, this model assumes that ligand binding to a subunit in a polymeric macromolecule induces, in that subunit, a conformational change which will affect the conformational stability, and hence the reactivity, of the neighboring subunits. The induced fit model, which has been successfully applied in dealing with functional interaction for a number of enzymes, is one of the limiting cases of a more general scheme describing the complex behavior of a multisubunit protein displaying conformational changes associated to ligand binding (Refs. 10,11). The other extreme case is the classical "two state concerted model," proposed by Monod, Wyman and Changeux (Ref. 12). An outline of the quantitative treatment for the application of these two models to hemoglobin will be given here.

The "induced fit" model (Ref. 9). This model assumes that each of the four sub-units of tetrameric hemoglobin may exist in two conformations, A and B, in equilibrium and that only the subunits in state B can bind the ligand X. Hence the following equilibria are defined:

$$A \xrightleftharpoons{L} B \; ; \; L = \frac{[B]}{[A]}$$

$$B + X \xrightleftharpoons{K} BX; \; K = \frac{[BX]}{[B][X]}$$

(15)

The possible interaction between subunits may be expressed by two equilibrium constants:

$$K_{AB} = K_{BA} = \frac{[AB][A]}{[AA][B]}$$

$$K_{BB} = \frac{[BB][A][A]}{[AA][B][B]}$$

(16)

where the concentration terms [AA], [AB], and [BB] indicate the concentration of interacting subunits, whereas [A] and [B] indicate the concentration of noninteracting subunits. Fig. 2 illustrates the interaction possibilities and the statistical factors associated to this description.

In the absence of interaction between subunits, the interaction constants K_{AA}, K_{AB}, K_{BB} will be equal to unity and the fractional saturation is given by

$$\overline{Y} = \frac{XL(X)}{1 + KL(X)}$$

which is the mass law expression for a single site with affinity constant $K' = KL$.

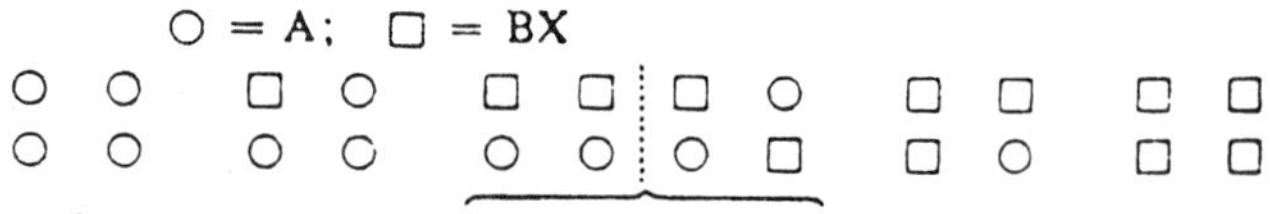

$$\bigcirc = A; \quad \square = BX$$

	0	1	2		3	4
Number of X bound	0	1	2		3	4
Number of ways of arranging X	0	4	4	2	4	1
Number of AB interactions	0	2	2	4	2	0
Number of BB interactions	0	0	1	0	2	4
Number of AA interactions	4	2	1	0	0	0

Fig. 2. Topological scheme of the possible interactions and statistical factors involved by the "induced fit model" applied to a tetrametric molecule.

In general the shape of the equilibrium curve will depend on the value of K_{AB} and K_{BB}, since values higher than 1 will stabilize the protein conformations containing AB or BB configuration, while the AA state would be stabilized by values lower than 1.

In the general case, the fractional saturation $\overline{Y}$ is given by

$$\overline{Y} = \frac{R_1(X) + 2\,R_2(X)^2 + 3\,R_3(X)^3 + 4\,R_4(X)^4}{R_0 + R_1(X) + R_2(X)^2 + R_3(X)^3 + R_4(X)^4} \tag{17}$$

where the values R_i are related to the various molecular species present at equilibrium (A_4, A_3, BX, $A_2B_2X_2$, AB_3X_3, B_4X_4) in different ways according to the different topologies of the particular scheme assumed. For a regular square situation, represented in Fig. 2, the values of R_i, taking into account the statistical factors, are given by

$$R_0 = 1; \quad R_1 = 4\,K_{AB}^2\,(KL): \quad R_2 = (2\,K_{AB}^4 + 4\,K_{AB}^2K_{BB})\,(XL)^2; \quad R_3 = 4\,K_{AB}^2K_{BB}^2(KL)^3;$$

$$R_4 = K_{BB}^4(KL)^4 \tag{18}$$

In the "induced fit" model stabilizing interactions between ligated and unligated subunits (K_{AB}) are taken into account, in addition to stabilization of the liganded subunits (K_{BB}) which is equivalent to the constant α of Pauling (Ref. 8).

The two state concerted model (Ref. 12). The basis of the two state allosteric model (often referred to as the MWC model) is the new idea that the intrinsic ligand affinity is determined by the quaternary state of the tetramer rather than by the number of ligand molecules already bound. The model assumes that only two quarternary states of the molecule, referred to as the low affinity T-state and high affinity R-state are populated (Refs. 12-14).

If K_R and K_T represent the intrinsic oxygen dissociation constants in each one of the two quarternary states, the respective fractional saturations are given by:

$$Y_R = \frac{[O_2]}{K_R + [O_2]} \quad ; \quad Y_T = \frac{[O_2]}{K_T + [O_2]} \tag{19}$$

Within this framework, five states of ligation can be defined for each quaternary state, as illustrated in Fig. 3. In the energy level diagram (Ref. 13,14) these states are equally spaced in free energy, K_T and K_R specifying the corresponding separation energy for the two quaternary states. The complete energy diagram requires one more parameter to specify the relative energy of R with rest to T. This parameter is defined as the equilibrium ratio between T_0 and R_0:

$$L_0 = \frac{[T_0]}{[T_0]} \tag{20}$$

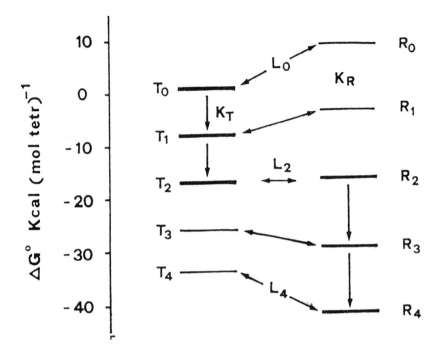

Fig. 3. Energy levels diagram for the "two state concerted model" applied to hemo-globin. T_i and R_i represent respectively the state in which i molecules of O_2 are bound to a tetramer in the low affinity T and in the high affinity R conformations. K_T and K_R represent the O_2 binding constants to the T and R quaternary states. L_i is the equilibrium constant for the interconversion of the quaternary state for a molecule having i O_2 molecules bound.

A value of $L_0 > 1$ implies therefore that the T quaternary state is more populated at low saturations.

Each of the other constants L_i, is related to L_0 (often referred to simply as L) by the simple equation

$$L_i = L \, c^i \qquad (21)$$

where

$$c \equiv \frac{K_R}{K_T} \qquad (22)$$

Within this model, characterized by two quaternary structures and four equivalent sites, the oxygen saturation is given by

$$\overline{Y} = \frac{(1 + \alpha)^3 + L \alpha C(1 + \alpha C)^3}{(1 + \alpha)^4 + L(1 + \alpha C)^4} \tag{23}$$

where $\alpha \equiv p/K_R$.

The Hill parameter n at $\overline{Y} = 0.5$, which is defined as

$$n = \left[\frac{\partial \ln (\overline{Y}/1 - \overline{Y})}{\partial \ln p} \right] \overline{Y} = 0.5 \tag{24}$$

may be expressed in terms of the allosteric constants as

$$n = 1 + 3 \frac{(1 - C \alpha_{50})(\alpha_{50} - 1)}{(1 + C \alpha_{50})(\alpha_{50} + 1)} \tag{25}$$

where $\alpha_{50} = \frac{P_{50}}{K_R}$ is the value of α at $\overline{Y} = 0.5$.

It is interesting to note that the "switch-over" point (i.e., the stage of ligation at which R and T have the same energy) can be simply calculated imposing $L_i = 1$ in Eq. (21):

$$i = \frac{\log L}{\log C} \tag{26}$$

The Adair constants for the binding of oxygen in four successive steps may be expressed in terms of the allosteric parameters as follows:

$$K_1' = \frac{LC + 1}{K_R(L+1)} \quad ; \quad K_2' = \frac{LC^2 + 1}{K_R(LC+1)} \quad ; \quad K_3' = \frac{LC^3 + 1}{K_R(LC^2+1)} \quad ; \quad K_4' = \frac{LC^4 + 1}{K_R(LC^3+1)} \tag{27}$$

It may be seen that if $C < 1$, the successive intrinsic Adair constants increase yielding cooperative binding.

A graphic interpretation of the allosteric parameters is shown in Fig. 4. K_R and K_T may be evaluated from the asymptotic values of the O_2 dissociation isotherm. Fig. 4 also shows the results of the computation where L takes several values from 1 to $1/C^4$. For $L = 1$ the system displays high affinity and low cooperativity; $L = 1/C^2$ gives the maximum cooperativity; and for $L = 1/C^4$, cooperativity is again lost, but the affinity is also low.

The best fit to hemoglobin experimental data at pH 7 and 20°C yields $n_{50} = 2.8$, $L = 3 \times 10^5$ and $C = 0.01$.

3. Regulation of Hemoglobin Function: Phenomenological Description

The position of the oxygenation curve in relation to oxygen pressure is of critical physiological importance, since it determines the amount of O_2 released at level of

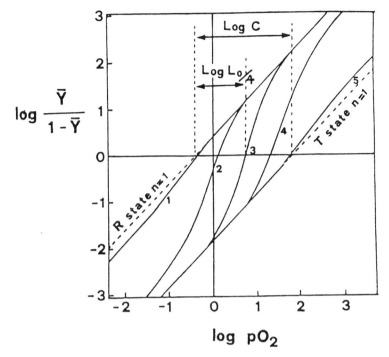

Fig. 4. O_2 dissociation curves for hemoglobin calculated on the basis of the MWC model assuming K_T = 71 mm Hg, K_R = 0.4 mm Hg and for increasing values of L_0 from L_0 = 1 (solid line number 1) to L_0 = 10^9 (solid line number 5). The dotted lines are the asymptotes obtained for $L_0 \to 0$ (upper) and $L \to \infty$ (lower). The graphical interpretation of $C \equiv K_R/K_T$ and of L_0 in one condition (line number 3) are indicated

---

tissues (and that taken up at level of the lungs). As reported above, the midpoint of the equilibrium curve (p_{50}) is the parameter generally used in most laboratories to describe the position of dissociation curve.

A number of factors, such as temperature and neutral salt, can affect p_{50} thereby acting as modulators of hemoglobin function (Ref. 1). The first recognized control mechanism for O_2 transport is the heterotropic linkage existing between O_2 and proton binding sites, which is well known as the Bohr effect. Thus, within the pH range 9 to 6, an increase in proton activity is accompanied by a decrease in the O_2 affinity of hemoglobin. This phenomenon is referred to as the alkaline Bohr effect, in opposition to the acid or reverse Bohr effect that is operative below pH 6 (where the oxygen affinity rises with decrease in pH).

The alkaline Bohr effect is of physiological relevance for two main reasons: first it contributes substantially to the neutralization of the protons produced by the CO_2 at the level of the venous blood, and secondly it causes an enhancement of the unloading of O_2 in response to a very narrow range of oxygen concentration change.

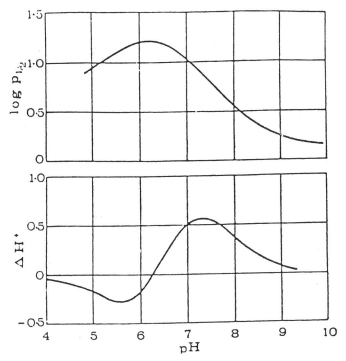

Fig. 5. The Bohr effect of hemoglobin illustrated as dependence on pH of the oxygen affinity (upper panel) and of the number of protons released or absorbed during O_2 binding (lower panel).

According to Wyman's theory of linked functions (Ref. 4), the effect of pH on the oxygen affinity of hemoglobin may be described by the following general expression, valid provided that linked effects due to other solvent components may be neglected under the conditions used:

$$\left(\frac{\partial \log p_{O_2}}{\partial \text{pH}} \right)_{\overline{Y}} = \left(\frac{\partial H^+}{\partial \overline{Y}} \right)_{\text{pH}} \tag{28}$$

This equation clearly indicates that: (a) the O_2 partial pressure necessary to obtain a given ligand saturation depends on pH; and (b) the effect is a reciprocal one, and at constant pH the number of protons bound by the protein depends on the fractional saturation with oxygen. Moreover, introducing the concept of the median oxygen pressure p_m (see Ref. 4), a simplified form may be used:

$$\frac{\partial \log p_m}{\partial \text{pH}} = \Delta H^+ \tag{29}$$

where $p_m = p_{50}$ if the binding curves are symmetrical.

This interrelationship is illustrated by Fig. 5, where the O_2 affinity (expressed as log p_{50}) and the number of protons released or taken up upon oxygenation are reported against pH. As shown in the figure, O_2 binding causes respectively a release of protons above pH 6 (alkaline Bohr effect) and an uptake of protons below pH 6 (acid or reverse Bohr effect). The molecular basis for this effect lies in perturbations of the ionization constant of certain α-amino and histidine residues (see below), perturbations determined by the ligand-linked conformational transition (Ref. 15).

TABLE 1

Values of the Adair constants[a]

| pH | K_i (mm Hg^{-1}) | | | |
	K_1	K_2	K_3	K_4
8.8	0.107	0.39	1.06	9.50
7.4	0.0292	0.061	0.16	7.42

[a] Heme concentration 60 µM; phosphate buffer 0.1 M; 20°C. (From Ref. 16)

Although several ionizable groups are involved in the Bohr effect of human hemoglobin, the experimental data appear compatible with the involvement of only one acid and one alkaline Bohr group per heme. Within this approximation the alkaline group has a pK value of 7.8 in deoxy and 6.8 in oxyhemoglobin, and the acid group a pK value of 5.25 in deoxy and 5.75 in oxyhemoglobin.

Analysis of the binding curves at different pH values according to the Adair scheme has indicated that the effect of pH is very small on the fourth Adair constant (K_4), while the first Adair constant (K_1) is strongly pH dependent (see Table 1) (Refs. 7,16)

The identification of specific amino acid residues of the α- and β-chains involved in the acid and the alkaline Bohr effect is complicated by differential interactions of other charged solution components (anions and cations) to deoxy and oxyhemoglobin. Thus a preferential binding of a given anion (i.e., Cl^- and/or 2,3 DPG) to deoxyhemoglobin involves the alteration of the pK of some cationic groups, thereby contributing to the overall observed Bohr effect. However, studies (Ref. 17) of the Bohr effect on hemoglobins from various species and of several abnormal hemoglobins have allowed to assign about half the acid Bohr effect to β143 His, which has an abnormally low pK in oxyhemoglobin, due to interaction with the cationic groups of two lysines residues, i.e., β82 and β144. As to the alkaline Bohr effect, the data up to now available indicate the involvement of several residues, reported in Table 2. Since, as outlined above, the relative contribution of some of these groups depends on the presence of anions (such as 2,3 DPG and/or Cl^-), Table 2 indicates if a particular ionizable ground is contributing to the Bohr effect through a differential binding of one (or both) of these species (see also Ref. 18).

TABLE 2

Groups of the alkaline Bohr effect for human hemoglobin (HbA$_0$)[a]

	DPG	Cl$^-$
(a) 0.1M NaCl + 2 mM DPG		
α1 (NA2) Val	no	yes
α122 (H5) His	no	?
β1 (NA1) Val	yes	$\pm$
β2 (NA2) His	yes	$\pm$
β143 (H21) His	yes	$\pm$
β146 (HC3) His	no	no
(b) 0.1M NaCl		
α1 (NA2) Val		Cl$^-$ linked
α122 (H5) His		
β82 (EF6) Lys		Cl$^-$ linked
β146 (HC3) His		

[a] (From Ref. 18, modified.)

Carbon dioxide transport (Ref. 19). The contributions of hemoglobin to the transport of carbon dioxide residues in two different mechanisms which may be summarized as follows:

(a)   Direct transport: Carbon dioxide binds to hemoglobin with the formation of carbamino compounds, involving the α-amino groups of both α and β chains. Since the N-terminal valine residues involved in this binding are partially protonated around neutral pH, the reaction can be described by the scheme:

$$p - NH_3^+ \rightleftharpoons p - NH_2 + H^+ \qquad (30)$$

$$p - NH_2 + CO_2 \rightleftharpoons p-NHCOO^- + H^+ \qquad (31)$$

Therefore, the overall binding constant, generally indicated as λ, is related to proton concentration by the following expression:

$$\lambda = \frac{K_c K_z}{K_z[H^+]+[H^+]^2} \qquad (32)$$

where K_c is the equilibrium constant of the carbamate reaction and K_z is the ionization constant of the N-terminal α-amino groups (Ref. 19).

The binding of CO_2 is oxygen-linked, i.e., deoxyhemoglobin binds more CO_2 than oxyhemoglobin. Once more the differential binding, whose physiological significance is obvious, finds its molecular basis in the ligand-linked conformational changes of the hemoglobin molecule which modify the structure and reactivity of the CO_2 binding sites.

Since carbamate formation is more pronounced in deoxy than in oxyhemoglobin, CO_2 affects the O_2 affinity by the same mechanism as hydrogen ions (in the alkaline part of the Bohr effect), favoring the deoxy conformational state and hence the unloading of oxygen at level of tissues.

(b)   Indirect transport: Carbon dioxide is hydrated by carbonic anhydrase to yield bicarbonate ions and protons. The protons produced in venous blood by this reaction are almost exactly neutralized by the absorption of protons arising from the decrease of hemoglobin oxygen saturation. Of course, in the lungs the reverse sequence takes place. Drastic pH changes are, therefore, avoided by coupling CO_2 and H^+ interactions.

Organic phosphates. Other ligands which bind to hemoglobin in the red cell are the organic phosphates, 2,3 DPG and ATP (Ref. 20).

2,3 DPG is present in human erythrocytes in equimolar concentrations with Hb ($\sim$5 mM) and its principal function is to maintain the O_2 affinity within the physiologically useful range. Thus, addition of 2,3 DPG progressively decreases the O_2 affinity indicating a higher binding constant of this effector for deoxyhemoglobin.

The molecular basis of this effect is now well understood: thus 2,3 DPG binds to hemoglobin in a ratio of 1 mole per hemoglobin tetramer the interaction being, at least under physiological conditions, nearly specific for deoxyhemoglobin. Hence, once again the relationship between O_2 and 2,3 DPG binding is a reciprocal one and if the 2,3 DPG concentration is increased the equilibrium curves will be progressively shifted toward decreasing affinities with unloading of oxygen. Conversely an increase in pO_2, i.e., an increase in O_2 fractional saturation of Hb, should lead to liberation of 2,3 DPG.

In the case of human hemoglobin, the binding site of 2,3 DPG has been identified along the dyal axis of the molecule, in the crevice existing between the two β chains (Ref. 21). The amino acid side chains involved in the electrostatic interactions with the negatively charged groups of 2,3 DPG have been identified, both by direct crystallographic observations and by a number of chemical studies (Ref. 22). The site is such that four pairs of basic groups: valine 1, histidine 2, histidine 143 and lysine 82 of both β chains may complement the acidic groups of 2,3 DPG by forming seven salt bridges.

The thermodynamics of this effect has its basis in the framework of the linkage theory (Ref. 4). Thus, the median O_2 pressure, p_m, provides a measure of the free energy required to fully oxygenate the tetrameric macromolecule ($\Delta G = RT \ln p_m$). A determination of p_m for a series of O_2 binding curves, each in the presence of a given concentration of organic phosphate (or in the general case of a given third component), provides a rigorous determination of the variation in total binding free energy induced by the phosphate effector (Ref. 20). The experimental data, obtained at different organic phosphates concentrations, can be quantitatively fitted by using the following relationship:

$$\log p_m = \log p_m^0 + \frac{1}{4} \log \frac{1 + K_d\,[\overline{Z}]}{1 + K_0\,[\overline{Z}]} \tag{33}$$

where p_m^0 and p_m are the median pressure of an oxygen binding curve respectively in the absence and in the presence of a given concentration of organic phosphate; $[\overline{Z}]$ is the concentration of free phosphate in equilibrium with the Hb at p_m; K_d is the association equilibrium constant of organic phosphate to the unliganded tetramer; and K_0 is the association equilibrium constant of the organic effector to fully oxygenated hemoglobin. The factor $1/4$ refers to the presence of four O_2 binding sites per molecule, and is appropriate only assuming that O_2 binding to hemoglobin is a concerted reaction and no appreciable amounts of intermediates exist.

A difficulty in applying this relationship lies in the fact that the concentration of free organic phosphate, $[\overline{Z}]$, is always unknown. For this reason the total concentration, $[Z_t]$, has generally been used on the ground that $[Z_t] \simeq [\overline{Z}]$ if the ratio of $[Z_t]$ to hemoglobin concentration, $[p_t]$, is sufficiently large. Numerical analyses of several sets of data have shown that in the case of 2,3 DPG the approximation described above is good over most of the range for variation of p_m. The equilibrium constants corresponding to the binding of 2,3 DPG by HbA under different conditions (Ref. 23) are reported in Table 3.

TABLE 3

pH Dependence of the binding of D-glycerate 2,3 Biphosphate (2,3 DPG) to deoxy and oxyhemoglobin[a]

pH	K_d (M^{-1})	K_d (M^{-1})
6.8	5.0×10^4	3.5×10^3
7.2	6.5×10^4	1.1×10^3
7.7	1.4×10^4	1.9×10^2

[a] K_d and K_0 are the association constants for the binding of deoxy and oxyhemoglobin respectively. Experimental conditions: 0.1M Bis tris, 0.1M Cl⁻ at 25°C (From Ref. 23.)

However, in some cases, such as that of IHP, it is of particular importance to conduct studies under conditions in which the above assumption ($[Z_t] \simeq [\overline{Z}]$) is inapplicable. In these cases a more rigorous analysis, such as that recently developed by Ackers, should be applied (24 and Refs. therein).

Since the 2,3 DPG binding site (central cavity between the two β chains) involves several positively charged groups, H^+ and 2,3 DPG influence each other. Thus at constant 2,3 DPG concentration, the observed Bohr effect may arise from the superimposition of the "intrinsic" Bohr effect and of an additional contribution due to the different amount of 2,3 DPG bound at various pH values. The physiological importance of the organic phosphate effect is outlined by the higher O_2 affinity of fetal (HbF) blood in relation to maternal blood. Thus, under stripped conditions, both hemoglobins behave identically, while in the presence of 2,3 DPG HbF has a higher affinity for oxygen; this fact has been explained on the basis of a perturbation of the 2,3 DPG binding site induced by an amino acid substitution which involves His 143, which in the γ chains is replaced by Ser (Ref. 20).

Binding of chloride and other small ions. The O_2 affinity of hemoglobin is also affected by the presence of chloride ions. The effect observed at concentrations below ~1 M implies that chloride ions bind preferentially to deoxyhemoglobin, as proven directly by Cl^--NMR measurements (Ref. 25). X-ray diffraction and solution studies of specifically carbamylated human hemoglobin A, as well as abnormal hemoglobins (Ref. 26), have demonstrated the existence of two Cl^- binding sites in deoxyhemoglobin, the first involving α1 Val and α141 Arg of the opposite chain, and the second involving α1 Val and α131 Ser of the same chain. In addition, the O_2-linked Cl^- binding site at the level of β82 Lys has been confirmed by a series of functional and spectroscopic data on abnormal or modified hemoglobins. The binding sites in oxyhemoglobin have not been identified unequivocally, but on the basis of studies on abnormal and enzymatically modified hemoglobins possible candidates are: α122 His, α103 His and β97 His.

A number of other small ionic components have similar effects on the O_2-binding properties of HbA (Ref. 1). A systematic investigation and analysis has been recently carried out (Ref. 27).

Effect of pH and temperature on the shape of the O_2 binding curve. For many years it has generally been accepted that the shape of the O_2 equilibrium curve does not change over a wide pH range (Refs. 3,4). This conclusion has been reached essentially on the basis of two experimental evidences: (a) the fractional number of released protons is essentially proportional to the fractional oxygen saturation; (b) the usually accessible saturation range (from 5 to 95%) does not show a significant sensitivity to pH changes.

However, precise oxygen equilibrium curves of human hemoglobin determined at different pH values (Refs. 7,16) have shown that the Adair constants depend on pH in nonuniform manner; in particular the pH dependence of K_4 is much smaller than that of K_1. As a consequence the contribution of each step of O_2 binding to the alkaline Bohr effect is not uniform. This gives rise to a pH dependence of the shape of the equilibrium curve which however is clearly evident only at the extreme ends of the curve.

Moreover, the linearity of the number of released protons with O_2 saturation is not incompatible with the observed pH dependence and could be attributed to the cooperative character of O_2 binding by hemoglobin, i.e., to instability of the intermediate species ($Hb(O_2)_2$ and $Hb(O_2)_3$), which appear during oxygenation. In other words facilitated successive oxygen binding makes the change of the $Hb(O_2)_4$ population approximately proportional to O_2 saturation, thereby originating a linear relation between proton release and O_2 binding.

As in the case of pH, very accurate oxygen equilibrium curves, performed under stripped condition in order to avoid complicating effects due to heterotropic interactions, have shown that the binding curve is not temperature independent (Refs. 1,7, 28). Thus ΔH_4 (-15 Kcal/mole of O_2 at pH 7.4) is significantly larger in absolute value than ΔH_1 (-10 Kcal/mole of O_2). The difference between ΔH_1 and ΔH_4 indicates that the shape of oxygen equilibrium curve is not completely invariant with temperature. A complete analysis indicates that the temperature dependence may be related to enthalpic contribution from heterotropic effects (such as differential Cl^- binding). Calorimetric measurements as a function of saturation have shown linearity over the range ~5 to 95% (Ref. 29). Therefore, the temperature invariance of the shape seems to hold in the middle region of the binding curve, but not in the lower and higher regions.

4. Molecular Basis of Cooperative Phenomena

Homotropic and heterotropic interaction effects in hemoglobin have been correlated, since a long time, to conformational changes of the macromolecule, which have been amply documented (Refs. 1,2,15). The experimental evidences for a difference in conformation between oxy and deoxyhemoglobin have formed the basis of the ideas on which the allosteric mechanism of cooperative O_2 binding has been based.

Comparison of structural information pertaining to deoxy and liganded hemoglobins led to establish unequivocally that, upon O_2 binding, a number of structural perturbations occur. These involve the macromolecule as a whole, and can be differentiated, for purely schematic reasons, into modifications (i) at the ligand binding site; (ii) at the tertiary level, within each subunit; and (iii) at the quaternary level. A wealth of quantitative information has been obtained through the use of several physical techniques applied to the study of the structure of the macromolecule; but without doubt fundamental information at every level of resolution has been obtained by X-ray crystallography. Over a number of years, the work of Perutz and collaborators (Refs. 2,30) has led to the refinement of the structure of a number of hemoglobin derivatives, both for normal, HbA, and for abnormal or chemically modified molecules. From these structural studies, an interpretation of the characteristic functional properties of hemoglobin has been attempted, leading predictions and new experiments.

A number of geometric properties of the heme in hemoglobin have been confronted to crystallographic results obtained on low-spin and high-spin metalloporphyrins and model compounds. Table 4 reports some of the relevant parameters for the high and low spin derivative of one model compound (2-methyl imidazole pivalamidophenylporphyrin) and for sperm whale Mb (Refs. 31,32). Among the important findings is definitely the out-of-plane geometry of the iron atom in deoxy Mb. The out-of-plane conformation of the high-spin metal has been confirmed since the initial proposal of Perutz (Ref. 15), and is thought to play a crucial role in the stereochemistry of ligand accessi-

TABLE 4

Stereochemistry of 2-methyl imidazole pivalamidophenylporphyrin (model
compound) and of the heme in oxy and deoxy myoglobin

Compound	Coordination number	Fe-N$_p$ [a]	Out-of-plane displacement
		($\mathring{A}$)	($\mathring{A}$)
2-Me-ImPiv PP Fe(II)	5	2.072	0.40
2-Me-ImPiv PP Fe(II)O$_2$	6	1.996	0.09
Mb deoxy	5	2.06	0.55
Mb oxy	6	2.05	0.26

[a] N_p = pyrrole nitrogens

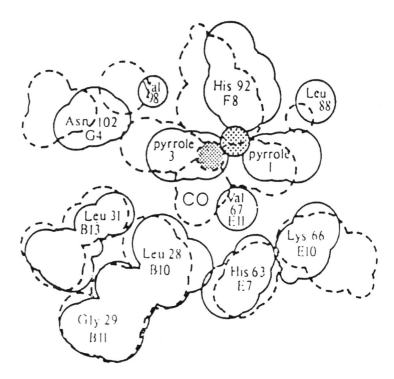

Fig. 6. Structural changes at level of the heme pocket of the β subunits in going
from deoxy (continuous lines) to carbonmonoxy (dashed lines) hemoglobin. The figure
represents a section through a space-filling model cut perpendicularly to the heme
plane and passing through the iron atom and the nitrogen atoms of pyrroles 1 and 3.

On ligand binding, a shift (1.5 $\mathring{A}$) and a rotation (9°) of the heme is observed. This
structural rearrangement makes room for the ligand (CO) by displacing the β67 (E11)
Val, which is not shown in the liganded state.

bility and binding to the heme iron.

In both the α and β chains, the number of atoms in contact with the heme is similar consisting of 75 contacts contributed by 16 amino acid residues. Thus the metallo-porphyrin is held into position by a number of weak interactions involving the periphery of the porphyrin, which have also an important role in determining the cooperative effects in O_2 binding (Ref. 1).

The residues at the axial position are critical. On the distal side, i.e., on the side where the ligand is bound, the distal imidazole of His (E7) plays a definite role. It has been recently shown by neutron diffraction of oxy Mb single crystal (Ref. 33) that the bound dioxygen forms an H-bond involving the first atom (i.e., the one bound to the metal) and the N-atom of the imidazole ring of His (E7). This is consistent with the small, but significant, Bohr effect reported in Mb at acid pH values, and if present also in Hb may be of significance in the mechanism of heme-heme interactions. In some abnormal hemoglobins the substitution of His (E7) may involve large alter-ations of the ligand reactivity; this was shown unequivocally in Hb Zürich (Ref. 34), where the distal residue of the β chains in Arg $(\alpha_2^A \ \beta_2^{His \ 63 \ \rightarrow \ Arg})$. On the distal side, Val (E11), an invariant residue, appears to block the entrance of the ligand to the pocket with its γ_2 methyl, particularly in the β chains (Refs. 14,15). This situ-ation, however, does not seem to impose any large constraint to the dynamics of ligand binding, as verified by kinetic data (Refs. 35,36).

The imidazole ring of the proximal His (His F8) which is directly coordinated to the metal, is in very close contact with the N-atom of the pyrrole rings. The orien-tation of the imidazole plane is such that its C_ϵ-atom is in Van der Waals contact with the N atom of pyrrole 1 in deoxy Hb (Refs. 37,38). The binding of a ligand (in this case CO) to a deoxy Hb in the T-state leads to a shift and reorientation of the whole porphyrin, as indicated in Fig. 6 (Ref. 37). This is demanded for by the pull exerted by the ligand on the metal which, in the absence of a structural rearrange-ment would lead to an unstable liganded complex, justifying qualitatively the low ligand affinity of a subunit in the T-state.

The hemes of both chains change their angle of tilt in going from deoxy to met (taken to be the same as oxy, to a first approximation). The movement is more pronounced in the β chains, whose heme moves slightly out of the pocket.

Large structural changes involve helices F and E, and the FG corner. The most marked differences are at the level of the C-terminal and the SH group of β93 Cys. Some of these critical residues are involved in deoxyhemoglobin in a number of weak interactions of electrostatic nature (salt bridges) which are schematically indicated in Fig. 7 (Ref. 30). The stabilization due to these bonds keeps into definite position the penultimate tyrosines (β145 Tyr); which on liganding become undefined in the crystallographic maps and therefore mobile. Once Tyr is out of the pocket formed in between helices F and H, the SH group of β93 Cys moves into position and forms an

H-bond with the main chain carbonyl of β89 Ser. Changes in the reactivity of the
SH group with ligation was a valuable documentation of the ligand-linked structural changes in Hb; in dynamic experiments this effect was used to probe the
structure of kinetic intermediates (Ref. 39).

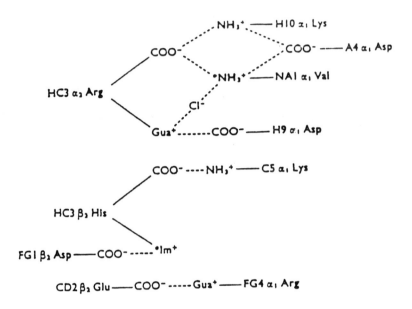

Fig. 7. Inter- and intra-chains salt bridges in deoxyhemoglobin indicated by
dotted lines. The groups marked by a star (HC3 β₂ His and NA1 α₁ Val) are
thought to account for about 60% of the alkaline Bohr effect.

The relative stability of the two states, which is such as to favor the T-state
in the unliganded derivative (i.e., T_0) depends on the preferential salt bridges
made in the deoxygenated Hb, as well as on the larger surface area of contact
between chains (Ref. 37).

The changes in quaternary structure between deoxy and oxy Hb are most dramatically reflected in the ligand linked dissociation into subunits (Ref. 1). It is
well proven that while liganded (CO, O_2 ...) Hb dissociates into noncooperative
dimers at micromolar concentrations, deoxy Hb is a stable tetramer down to nano-
molar concentrations. The linkage between assembly of the subunits and state of
ligation of the heme has been referred to as "Polysteric linkage" (Ref. 40).

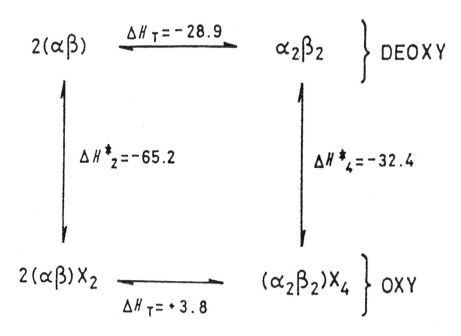

Fig. 8. Enthalpies of subunits aggregation in liganded and deoxyhemoglobin. The sign of the enthalpy changes is referred to the reactions from left to right and from top to bottom.

Fig. 8 summarizes the enthalpy changes associated to the formation of dimers in in deoxy and oxy HbA; the results have been summarized from Valdes and Ackers (Ref. 41), who carried out extensive equilibrium and calorimetric experiments ligand binding and subunit dissociation of HbA.

Crystallographically it is easily seen that all the subunit contacts, except the $\alpha_1\beta_1$ surfaces (see Fig. 9), undergo a large rearrangement (Refs. 14,15,30). Particularly marked and definite changes occur at the level of the $\alpha_1\beta_2$ contact, where in deoxy Hb α42 Tyr forms an H-bond with β99 Asp, and β37 Trp fits into a groove made by α93 Val. In met Hb there is a shift of the two surfaces, such that a new H-bond between α94 Asp and β102 Asn is formed, while the environment of β37 Trp is perturbated. The latter structural perturbation is clearly reflected in a change in the light absorption properties of this aromatic, which acts as a marker of a quaternary structural shift (Ref. 2). The crucial role of some of these residues in the surface is also indicated by the fact that they are found in all cooperative tetrametric hemoglobins, even from far-removed species (Ref. 42).

A very important subunit shift occurs along the dyad axis of the molecule. As shown by Arnone (Ref. 21), in deoxyhemoglobin several of the residues coating the surface of the cavity in between the two β chains are in perfect stereochemical

38

complementarity with 2,3 DPG, the physiological allosteric effector (see above).
Thus Val 1, His 2, Lys 82 and His 143 of the two β chains are involved in electrostatic interactions with DPG. Upon ligand binding this cluster of positive charges
is perturbed and, for example, the amino termini move away and the EF segments
close up, restricting accessibility to DPG. This stereochemical picture accounts
for the difference in the DPG-binding affinity as between oxy and deoxy Hb, and
it has been amply confirmed through structural and functional studies of abnormal
or chemically modified hemoglobins.

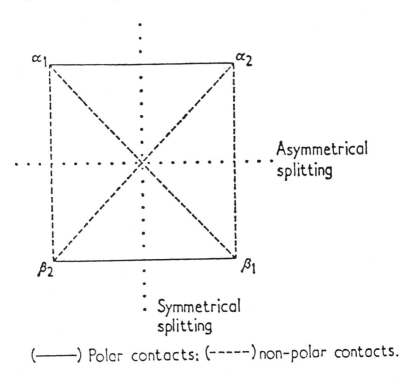

Fig. 9. Scheme of the polar (solid lines) and nonpolar (dashed lines) interactions
between the chains in hemoglobin as shown by the crystallographic work of Perutz
and collaborators. (Refs. as text.)

The free energy of homotropic interactions. The O_2 binding data provide information on the free energy of heme-heme interactions, which can be quantitatively
determined from the spacing of the asymptotic values of the ligand affinity in a
Hill plot (Ref. 4). This estimate varies somewhat with pH, temperature and type of
hemoglobin; however in human hemoglobin at physiological pH values it amounts to
approx. 3 Kcal/O_2 binding site, or 12 Kcal/tetramer. Thus the binding of O_2 to an
Hb molecule in the T-quaternary state is less favorable than binding to the R-
quaternary state by ∼3 K cal/site.

A problem of great interest is represented by the localization of this difference in free energy of O_2 binding between the two extreme states (Refs. 15,43,44). As to this, two alternative views have been advanced: (a) the energy of heme-heme interaction is stored largely at the heme and the bond between the N_ε of the proximal imidazole ring His (F8) and the iron atom plays a crucial role in this respect; (b) the energy of heme-heme interaction is diffused throughout the protein, and a large number of weak chemical bonds contribute to the overall difference. Relevant information has been obtained through analysis of the crystallographic data on the one hand, and through a number of spectroscopic techniques on the other.

High resolution resonance Raman spectroscopy has been recently applied to hemoglobin (Ref. 45). The Fe-O_2 stretching frequency in the fully liganded R_4 and T_4 states has been determined and shown to be the same (567 cm^{-1}). This result has been taken, in agreement with previous NMR data, to indicate that no strain of the iron-ligand bond is induced by the quaternary shift.

In deoxy Hb the Fe-N_ε (His F8) stretching mode has been assigned, and measured in both quaternary states. The line, at 216 cm^{-1}, displays a small change in going from T_0 to R_0, which according to a quantitative analysis is consistent with a change in strain energy of ~ 0.3 Kcal/site, i.e., approximately 1/10 of the total interaction free energy.

Thus although some of the strain energy is stored at the level of the heme, indicated also by resonance Raman (Ref. 46), a fraction (and possibly a large fraction) is stored elsewhere in the molecule.

It remains as a definite piece of information, substantiated by spectroscopy and crystallography, that the bond between the metal atom and the proximal His is involved in the spreading of the conformational change from the metal-ligand complex to the globin.

5. Comparative Aspects

Hemoglobins from different species, and sometimes different hemoglobin components in the same organism, may display special functional properties which are related to the particular demands which the animal is faced with. For this reason, comparative studies are of primary importance both as a test of the general validity of the molecular mechanisms underlying hemoglobin function, and as a means to understand the allosteric control mechanisms which have developed in different hemoglobins in the course of the evolutionary process.

In what follows we will present only few examples which, in our opinion, are representative of what can be learned from this type of approach.

The two different hemoglobin components from chicken erythrocytes have been studied in detail, both from the structural and functional point of view (Ref. 47). The functional behavior of these hemoglobins is essentially similar to that of normal human hemoglobin A. However the effect of organic phosphates (2,3 DPG and IHP) is remarkably lower. This finding should be considered in more detail and in connection with the type and number of amino acid residues which have been identified within the organic phosphate binding site (Ref. 21). As previously outlined, in the case of human hemoglobin A this site has 8 positively charged amino acid residues which may strongly interact with the negative charges carried by the 2,3 DPG molecule. On the basis of the stereochemical model these electrostatic interactions are reduced in oxyhemoglobin due to the quaternary conformational change associated to ligand binding. The amino acid sequences of the β chains of the chicken hemoglobins show that in the crevice which forms the organic phosphates binding site the number of positively charged residues is remarkably high (12 charged residues as compared to 8) This finding may suggest a stronger interaction with the organic phosphate molecules, although binding needs not be O_2 linked. The experiments show that the effect of 2,3 DPG is almost negligible and that of IHP ~ 8 times lower than that observed in HbA. The absence of a significant effect of 2,3 DPG indicates that the interaction energy of the effector with the two extremes conformational states, T.(deoxy) and R(oxy), is very similar, thereby abolishing preferential binding and thus an effect on O_2 affinity. Since steric constraints may be excluded on the basis of the bigger effect of IHP, the lower degree of differential binding should be ascribed to the presence of a larger number of positively charged residues. Likely the presence of 12 positive charges (versus 8) increases the number of possible electrostatic inter-actions in both quaternary states and 2,3 DPG loses its selective power with respect to these two conformational states. On this basis we may find a rationale for the fact that in avian erythrocytes the physiological effector is IPP (inositol penta-phosphate), whose molecule carries a larger number of negative charges. Thus an increase in the number of negative charges carried by the effector seems to be nec-essary to restore some differential binding with respect to the oxy and deoxy conformational states.

The importance of the organic phosphates effect in the regulation of hemoglobin function is strongly outlined by the results obtained on amphibian hemoglobins (Amphiuma means, Triturus cristatus). These hemoglobins show, in fact, an inversion of the Bohr effect depending on the absence or presence of organic phosphates (Refs. 48,49). Thus, their Bohr effect negative under stripped conditions becomes posi-tive in the presence of organic phosphates. In other words the heterogenic linkage existing between hemes and proton binding sites, is in these animals under strict control of anion binding. Hence organic phosphates may modulate not only the ampli-tude but also the sign of the Bohr effect. Whatever the molecular mechanism under-lying this peculiar feature may be, without any doubt, it represents a molecular adaptation to the particular environmental life conditions and for Amphiuma means it has been suggested to be related to the metabolic needs of the animal during hibernation.

An interesting system studied in detail during the last few years is represented by the two major hemoglobin components from trout (Salmo irideus) blood, i.e., Trout

Hb I and Trout Hb IV (Ref. 50).

The functional properties of Trout Hb I are outstanding insofar as the ligand binding isotherm displays strong homotropic interactions ($n_{1/2} \simeq 2.6$), but it is devoid of heterotropic effects. In addition the protein shows no tendency to dissociate into dimers, even at concentrations well below micromolar, and α-β functional heterogeneity may be neglected. The lack of Bohr effect is well proven being the shape and position of the binding curve essentially pH independent over a wide range (pH 6-8). Moreover a set of calorimetric experiments has shown convincingly that no Bohr protons are being liberated upon ligand binding.

The absence of ligand-linked ionization effects has been correlated with the structural information available on the groups involved in the Bohr effect of HbA (Ref. 17). In Trout Hb I β146 His is substituted by Phe and the α-NH_2 of αl Val is acetylated (Ref. 18). Thus the only residue which is not substituted or modified in Trout Hb I is α122 His. The complete lack of pH effect in this Hb constitutes therefore a negative evidence for the role of the latter residue in the alkaline Bohr effect of human hemoglobin A. Furthermore in Trout Hb I heme-heme interactions are strongly influenced by temperature. In the case of O_2 the apparent ΔH of oxygenation is approximately zero at very low saturation and increases as a function of fractional saturation reaching the value of $\sim$-10 Kcal/heme at 98% saturation (Ref. 51). This value is very similar to that normally observed for hemoglobins in the R conformational state. A key element which emerges from the analysis of the binding data for Hb I is that the allosteric quaternary transition is associated with a large positive enthalpy charge (ΔH_{L_0} = + 28 Kcal/mole tetramer), which implies that the population of the conformational states is strongly temperature dependent. It has been calculated that at a temperature of 75-80°C the two states (T_0 and R_0) should be equally populated, since the increase in temperature favors the high affinity state of the molecule over the low affinity state (ref. 52).

An opposite behavior is displayed by tuna hemoglobin whose cooperativity diminishes as temperature decreases, a fact which is considered advantageous for a warm bodied fish (Ref. 53).

The functional behavior of Trout Hb IV (Ref. 50) is characterized by a pronounced and parallel reduction of both ligand affinity and cooperativity ($n_{1/2}$ = 2.3 at pH 7.5 $n_{1/2} \leq$ 1 at pH 6.5), as the pH is brought towards acid values (< 7.5) (Root effect). Furthermore this hemoglobin at acid pH values is only partially saturated with O_2 up to a gas pressure of $\sim$20 atmospheres. This special behavior is a general characteristic of Hbs from teleost fishes (Ref. 54), and has been correlated to the function of the swim bladder which controls the buoyancy of the fish at various depths.

As to the mechanistic interpretation of the Root effect, analysis of the data has indicated the existence of two different and complementary phenomena:
(a) A progressive stabilization of a low affinity state of the molecule brought about by protons. In this respect the essential feature of the functional behavior of Trout Hb IV lies in a proton-induced shift of the allosteric equilibrium constant, as

indicated in the energy level diagram reported in Fig. 10. Thus at pH = 7.5, where the equilibrium curve is cooperative ($n_{1/2}$ = 2.3), the T state is preferentially populated in the deoxy form $T_0 \gg R_0$), while at saturating O_2 concentrations the reverse situation is observed (i.e., $R_4 \gg T_4$). At pH 6 where the equilibrium curve is noncooperative and the O_2 affinity is very low, the T state is significantly populated both in the presence and in the absence of the ligand.

(b) A functional intramolecular heterogeneity as between the two types of chain (α versus β), which becomes more and more pronounced as the H^+ concentration is increased. At pH 6 this phenomenon induces an O_2 equilibrium curve which is clearly biphasic and represents the successive saturation with O_2 of the two different types of chains (as shown by high pressure spectrophotometry) (Ref. 55)

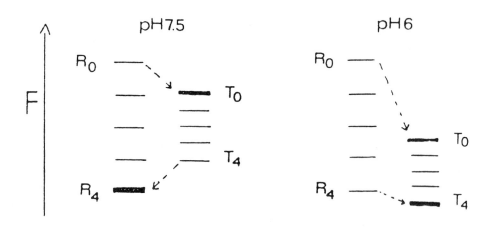

Fig. 10. Energy levels diagram for the "Root effect" in Trout Hb IV. At pH 7.5 the fully unligated (sub 0) protein is stable in the T state whereas the saturated molecule (sub 4) is stabilized in the R state (cooperative system). At pH 6 the T state is more stable independently of the degree of saturation and therefore the system is noncooperative.

In conclusion the overall functional behavior is a complex average of both quarternary (low affinity $\longleftrightarrow$ high affinity transition) and tertiary (intramolecular heterogeneity) effects. This last phenomenon plays an additional very important role in the physiological context. Thus it facilitates pumping O_2 into the swim bladder, even against very high gas pressure. This effect is achieved by coupling the concentration gradients of two ligands (O_2 and H^+), against which the macromolecule displays a negative linkage. Therefore the free energy necessary to transport O_2 in one direction is ensured by the flow of protons in the opposite direction, and the whole system may be considered as an energy transducer.

REFERENCES

1. Antonini, E. and Brunori, M. (1971) Hemoglobin and Myoglobin in Their Reactions with Ligands, North Holland, pp. 445.
2. Perutz, M. F. (1978) Scient. Am., 239, 92-125.
3. Wyman, J. (1948) Adv. Protein Chem., 4, 407-531.
4. Wyman, J. (1964) Adv. Protein Chem., 19, 223-286.
5. Edsall, J. T. (1972) Hist. Biol., 5, 205-220.
6. Adair, G. S. (1925) J. Biol. Chem., 63, 529-545.
7. Roughton, F. J. W. (1964) in Handbook of Physiology, Respiration, Vol. 1, Am. Physiol. Soc., Washington, DC, pp. 767-825.
8. Pauling, L. (1935) Proc. Natl. Acad. Sci. USA, 21, 186-191.
9. Koshland, D. E., Nemethy, G., and Filmer D. (1966) Biochemistry, 5, 365-385.
10. Eigen, M. (1968) Quart. Rev. Biophys., 1, 1-34.
11. Wyman, J. (1968) Quart. Rev. Biophys., 1, 35-80.
12. Monod, J., Wyman, J., and Changeux, J. P. (1965) J. Mol. Biol., 12, 88-118.
13. Shulman, R. G., Hopfield, J. J., and Ogawa, S. (1975) Quart. Rev. Biophys., 8, 325-420.
14. Baldwin, J. M. (1975) Prog. Biophys. Mol. Biol., 29, 225-320.
15. Perutz, M. F. (1970) Nature, 228, 726-739; Perutz, M. F. (1972) Nature, 237, 495-499.
16. Imai, K. and Yonetani, T. (1975) J. Biol. Chem., 250, 2227-2231.
17. Perutz, M. F., Kolmartin, J. V., Nishikura, K., Fogg, J. H., and Butler, P. J. G. (1980) J. Mol. Biol., 138, 649-670.
18. Brunori, M., Giardina, B., and Bannister, J. V. (1979) Inorg. Biochem., 1, 159-209; Brunori, M., Giardina, B., and Kuiper, H. A. (1982) Inorg. Biochem., 3, 126-182.
19. Kilmartin, J. V. and Rossi-Bernardi, L. (1973) Physiol. Rev., 53, 836-890.
20. Benesch, R., Benesch, R. E., and Bauer, C. (1975) Red Blood Cell, 2nd Ed., (Surgenor, D. M., ed.) Academic Press, N.Y., 2, 825-839.
21. Arnone, A. (1972) Nature, 237, 146-148.
22. Bonaventura, C. and Bonaventura, J. (1978) in Biochemical and Clinical Aspects of Hemoglobin Abnormalities, Caughey, W. S., ed., Academic Press, N.Y., pp. 647-664.
23. Van Beek, G. G. M. and De Bruin, S. H. (1979) Eur. J. Biochem., 100, 497-502.
24. Ackers, G. K. (1979) Biochemistry, 15, 3372-3380.
25. Chiancone, E., Norne, J. E., Forsen, S., Bonaventura, J., Brunori, M., Antonini, E., and Wyman, J. (1975) Eur. J. Biochem., 55, 385-390.
26. Poyart, C., Bursaux, E., Arnone, A., Bonaventura, J. and Bonaventura, C. (1980) J. Biol. Chem., 225, 9465-9469.
27. Amiconi, G., Antonini, E., Brunori, M., Wyman, J. and Zolla, L. (1981) J. Mol. Biol., 152, 111-115.
28. Imai, K. and Tyuma, I. (1973) Biochem. Biophys. Res. Comm., 51, 52-58.
29. Noll, L. A., Gaud, H. T., Gill, S. J., Gersonde, K. and Barisas, B. G. (1979) Biochem. Biophys. Res. Comm., 88, 1288-1293.
30. Perutz, M. F. (1976) Brit. Med. Bull., 32, 195-208.
31. Jameson, G. B., Molinaro, F. S., Ibers, J. A., Collman, J. P., Brauman, J. I., Rose, E., and Suslick, K. S. (1978) J. Am. Chem. Soc., 100, 6769-6770.
32. Takano, T. (1977) J. Mol. Biol., 110, 569-584.
33. Phillips, S. E. V. and Schoenborn, B. P. (1981) Nature, 292, 81-84.
34. Giacometti, G. M., Brunori, M., Antonini, E., Di. Iorio, E. E., and Winter-halter, K. H. (1980) J. Biol. Chem., 255, 6160-6165.

35. Moffat, K., Deatherage, J. F., and Seybert, D. W. (1979) Science, 206, 1035-1042.
36. Olson, J. S. and Gibson, Q. H. (1973) J. Biol. Chem., 248, 1623-1630.
37. Baldwin, J. M. and Chothia, C. (1979) J. Mol. Biol., 129, 175-220.
38. Gelin, B. R. and Karplus, M. (1977) Proc. Natl. Acad. Sci. USA, 74, 801-805.
39. Antonini, E. and Brunori, M. (1969) J. Biol. Chem., 244, 3909-3912.
40. Colosimo, A., Brunori, M., and Wyman, J. (1976) J. Mol. Biol., 100, 47-57.
41. Valdes, R., Jr. and Ackers, G. K. (1977) J. Biol. Chem., 252, 88-91.
42. Bossa, F., Barra, D., Coletta, M., Martini, F., Liverzani, A., Petruzzelli, R., Bonaventura, J., and Brunori, M. (1976) FEBS Lett., 64, 76-80.
43. Hopfield, J. J. (1973) J. Mol. Biol., 77, 207-222.
44. Weber, G. (1972) Biochemistry, 11, 864-878.
45. Nagai, K., Kitagawa, T., and Morimoto, M. (1980) J. Mol. Biol., 136, 271-289.
46. Shelnutt, J. A., Rousseau, D. L., Friedman, J. M., and Simon, S. R. (1979) Proc. Natl. Acad. Sci. USA, 76, 4409-4413.
47. Pau, C., Vandecasserie, C., Fraboni, A., Depreter, J., Leonis, J., and Schnek, A. G. (1977) Coloq. Inserm., 70, 183-200.
48. Bonaventura, C., Sullivan, B., Bonaventura, J., and Bourne, S. (1977) Nature, 265, 474-476.
49. Condo, S.G., Giardina, B., Lunadei, M., Ferracin, A., and Brunori, M. (1981) Eur. J. Biochem., 120, 323-327.
50. Brunori, M. (1975) Curr. Top. Cell. Reg., 9, 1-39.
51. Brunori, M., Giardina, B., Colosimo, A., Coletta, M., Falcioni, G., and Gill, S. J. (1980) in Interaction Between Iron and Proteins in Oxygen and Electron Transport, (Ho, Chien, ed.), Elsevier-North Holland, New York.
52. Brunori, M., Giardina, B., Colosimo, A., Falcioni, G., and Gill, S. J. (1980) J. Biol. Chem., 255, 3841-3843.
53. Carey, F. G. and Gibson, Q. H. (1977) Biochem. Biophys. Res. Comm., 78, 1376-1382.
54. Riggs, A. (1970) Fish Physiol., 4, 209-252.
55. Brunori, M., Coletta, M., Giardina, B., and Wyman, J. (1978) Proc. Natl. Acad. Sci., USA, 75, 4310-4312.

CHAPTER 3   OXIDASES

ALFREDO COLOSIMO AND ERALDO ANTONINI*
Istituto di Chimica, Facoltà di Medicina e Centro di Biologia Molecolare
del C.N.R., Città Universitaria, 00185 Roma, Italia.

1.1   Definition and general properties

The name "oxidases" is given for the group of enzymes catalyzing oxido-reductive reaction when molecular oxygen (dioxygen) is the electron acceptor and water is the product.

The reaction may be indicated as follows:

$$O_2 = 4\ e^- + 4\ H^+ \rightarrow 2\ H_2O$$

In this respect oxidases may be distinguished from other oxido-reductases such as oxygenases or other oxidative enzymes which use molecular oxygen but have hydrogen peroxide as a product.

The general features of the oxidases are as follows:

(1) They are metallo-proteins containing heme and/or copper; the functional unit contains four centers represented by metal ions;

(2) The electrons enter the unit at a definite site and are transferred within the protein to the oxygen binding site;

(3) The kinetic features of the various oxidases are similar in spite of large differences in structure of the redox sites and of the molecule as a whole, indicating a common basic mechanism.

1.2   Classification of oxidases

Oxidases may be classified into heme- and copper oxidases.

The most representative (also because most studied) enzymes of the two groups are, for heme-containing oxidases, the cytochrome c oxidase (which also contains copper), and for copper-oxidases, laccase.

In the framework of the enzyme nomenclature they can be classified as reported in Table 1.

Deceased 19 March 1983.

TABLE 1

Oxidases

Recommended name	Reaction	Other names	Systematic names	Comments
Cytochrome c oxidase (EC 1.9.3.1.)	4 Cyt c^2 + O_2 = 4 Cyt c^3 + $2H_2O$	Cytochrome a_3 Indophenolase Atmungsferment	Ferrocytochrome c:O_2 oxidoreductase	Cytochrome of the a type containing Cu
Pseudomonas cytochrome oxidase (EC 1.9.3.2.)	4 Cyt c^{2+}_{551} + O_2 = 4 Cyt c^{3+}_{551} + $2H_2O$	Cytochrome c d	Ferrocytochrome c:O_2 oxidoreductase	Cytochrome
Laccase (EC 1.10.3.2.)	4 Benzenediol + O_2 = 4 Benzosemiquinone + $2H_2O$	Phenolase Polyphenol oxidase	Benzenediol:O_2 oxidoreductase	A group of copper proteins of low specificity acting on both o- and p-quinones
Ascorbate oxidase (EC 1.10.3.3.)	2 L-Ascorbate + O_2 = 2 Dihydroascorbate + $2H_2O$	Ascorbase	L-Ascorbate:O_2 oxidoreductase	Copper protein
Catechol oxidase (EC 1.10.3.1.)	2 Catechol + O_2 = 2 1,2-Benzoquinone + $2H_2O$	Tyrosinase O-diphenolase	1,2-Benzenediol:O_2 oxidoreductase	A group of copper proteins acting also on a variety of substituted catechols
o-Aminophenol oxidase (EC 1.10.3.4.)	o-Aminophenol + $\frac{3}{2}$ O_2 = isophenoxazine + $3H_2O$	Isophenoxazine synthase	o-Aminophenol:O_2 oxidoreductase	Requires Mn^{2+} flavoprotein
Ceruloplasmin (EC 1.16.3.1.)	2 Fe^{2+} + O_2 + $4H^+$ = 2 Fe^{3+} + H_2O	Ferroxidase[a]	Iron(II):O_2 oxidoreductase	Copper protein

[a] Fe^{2+} substrate with highest V_{max} and lowest K_m (Frieden, E. and Hsieh, H.S. (1976) Adv. Exp. Biol. Med., 74, 505–529).

1.3   Thermodynamic and kinetic difficulties in electron addition to oxygen

Oxygen is known to fit best the role of final electron acceptor in the respiratory chain of aerobic organisms, having a strong oxidizing power together with
kinetic stability which prevents unspecific oxidation of organic molecules.

The sluggish reactivity of dioxygen in the absence of appropriate catalysts
is partly due to the adverse potential for the first-electron reduction.

A second factor which has been implicated, refers to the peculiar electronic
structure of molecular oxygen. Like most stable molecules it has an even number
of electrons, but still there are two unpaired electrons in the highest occupied
molecular orbital or, in other words, the molecule has a triplet ground state.
Its stable reduction products (H_2O_2, H_2O) have, on the other hand, no unpaired
electrons and any reaction leading to these products would consequently involve
a triplet-to-singlet conversion and be slow because of the spin restriction
imposed by the Pauli principle.

When oxygen is reduced in the presence of oxidases, the type of oxygen-reduction
may be classified into four categories: four-electron, two-electron, one-electron
and mixed mechanisms. The mechanism for each particular oxidase depends on the
environmental factors to the catalytic site at which oxygen is reduced, and the
ability of stabilizing intermediates which occur in the process of oxygen
reduction appears to have great influence on the mode of electron transfer.

1.4   The mechanism of catalysis in oxidases

Investigations on the catalytic mechanism of oxidases as of other enzymes,
aim to the identification of relevant enzyme intermediates which are present
during the turnover and to the direct measurements of individual reaction steps.
In such way the overall catalytic cycle may be reconstructed on the basis of a
definite reaction scheme. Such a task is facilitated in oxidases by the presence
of large optical or EPR signals arising from the metal redox centers.

Events occurring on the enzymes as a result of redox reactions or binding
of ligands may be directly followed by the use of rapid reaction techniques.

This approach involves three main types of experiments:

(1) Measurements of the reaction of the fully reduced enzyme with oxygen.

(2) Measurements of the reaction of the oxidized enzyme, in the absence of oxygen,
with the reducing substrates.

(3) Measurements of the changes occurring on the enzyme during the catalytic cycle.

Studies of this kind have been performed with all the oxidases described here
and allow some generalizations in spite of the widely different structure of the
various enzymes.

The reactions of the fully reduced enzymes with oxygen are very rapid and
oxygen-bound intermediates can only be observed under very special conditions

(i.e., very low temperatures).

Electrons from the reducing substrate enter the enzyme through a definite redox site in a rapid second-order reaction, and are progressively transferred to the other oxidized sites. This intramolecular electron transfer is relatively slow and represents the rate-limiting step in turnover.

2.1   Cytochrome oxidase

Cytochrome c oxidase (EC 1.9.3.1) is responsible for the uptake of more than 90% of the total oxygen consumption in the eukaryotic cells (Ref. 1). Although this enzyme is not the only one catalyzing oxygen activation, it is probably unique in providing the energy for the cell by coupling the electron transport through the cytochrome chain with the process of oxidative phosphorylation (Ref. 2).

Although the role of the cytochromes in cellular respiration was established in 1935 (Ref. 3), the nature of the final reaction with molecular oxygen and of the cytochrome oxidase that catalyzed it remained uncertain since the isolation of the autoxidable component of the respiratory chain seemed to be extremely difficult. In 1939 however, Keilin and Hartree with an improved preparation of submitochondrial particles could see the absorption spectrum of an apparently new component closely associated with the previously discovered cytochrome a, which they called cytochrome a_3 (See Fig. 1). Because the heme groups of cytochromes a and a_3 are the same, and because the two have never been separated, many workers refused to accept the separate existence of cytochrome a_3 attributing the spectroscopic effects observed by Keilin and Hartree to complicated interactions between cytochrome c and O_2. Nowadays everybond agrees that cytochrome oxidase is a lipoprotein containing two chemically identical heme groups which behave differently towards cytochrome c, oxygen and inhibitors (Ref. 4). They interact not only by intramolecular electron transfer but also by modifying each other's chemical behavior (see below). The binding of cyanide by cytochrome a_3 is affected by the oxidation state of cytochrome a, the redox potential of cytochrome a is affected by the oxidation state of cytochrome a_3, and even the spectrum of one component may be modified by the other. In addition, two copper atoms are present in the a a_3 system are also difficult from each other in their properties (Cu_α, Cu_β). Thus, the "functional unit" catalyzing the reaction between cytochrome c and oxygen is a four-electron acceptor and donor.

2.2   Distribution and cellular localization

Cytochrome c oxidase is present in the mitochondria, the respiratory organelles of the more highly developed cells, and, in the bacteria, in the cytoplasmic membranes, cytochrome oxidase of the a a_3 type has also been found in marine invertebrates. In some arthropod muscles it occurs in high concentration (up to 40 µmoles of heme a/kg) and with the a/a_3 ratio resembling that of mammalian tissue

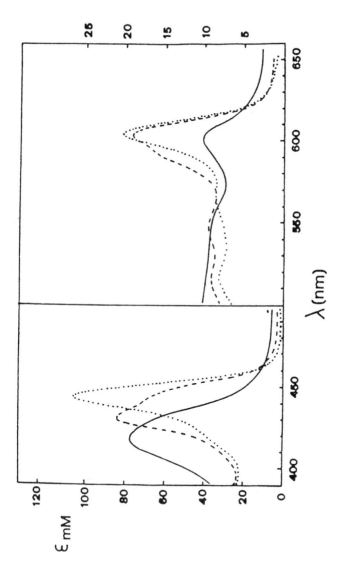

Fig. 1. Absorption spectra in the visible and Soret regions of the oxidized (————), dithionite-reduced (·····) and dithionite-reduced + CO (————) cytochrome c oxidase purified from beef heart and solubilized in 0.1M phosphate buffer, pH 7.4, containing 1% (w/v) Tween 80, at 25°C. The ordinate gives the absorbance in mM⁻¹ cm⁻¹ (per heme a).

($\sim$ 1).

Plants and bacteria have a great variety of oxidases. It has become increasingly clear that in plants cytochrome c oxidase is the major terminal oxidase and that copper-containing oxidases, such as ascorbate oxidase, play only a minor role. The position of the absorption bands of plant cytochrome $\underline{c}$ oxidase differs slightly from that of the mammalian oxidase, and the α band may be double. Cytochrome $\underline{a}$ without $\underline{a}_3$ is also found in algae, e.g., in Euglena, while the cytochrome oxidase of yeast is similar to mammalian oxidase (Ref. 2).

Aerobic bacteria also use cytochromes to transfer electrons to oxygen. The cytochrome $\underline{a}$ $\underline{a}_3$ is sometimes found as the terminal oxidase, but in addition, and often in the same organism, other cytochromes act as alternative oxidases for the reduction of inorganic salts (nitrate, nitrite, sulphate, etc.) which bacteria may use as electron acceptors in place of oxygen.

In mammals, cytochrome $\underline{c}$ oxidase is restricted to the mitochondria.

Studies with crude immune serum directed against cytochrome $\underline{c}$ oxidase as well as with the membrane-impermeant reagent p-diazonium benzene sulfonate, suggested that the enzyme is a transmembrane protein with cytochromes $\underline{a}$ and $\underline{a}_3$ exposed on opposite surfaces of the mitochondrial inner membrane (Fig. 2).

2.3   The redox sites and the basic functional unit

It is now generally accepted that there is only one kind of heme in cytochrome oxidase, the heme $\underline{a}$, which was earlier shown to have a formyl group, two carboxyls and one vinyl, and a large alkyl or fatty acid nonesterified side chain (see Fig. 2). It was suggested, without supporting evidence, that the long side chain may have an important role in electron transfer and/or coupled phosphorylation. EPR data of Van Gelder et al. (Ref. 5) revealed that only approximately 30% of the heme of the oxidized enzyme was represented in the signal, the other 70% being presumably rendered EPR nondetectable by heme-heme or heme-copper interaction.

Cytochrome oxidase contains copper in a 1:1 ratio to heme and it is accepted that the copper functions as an electron acceptor and donor. The most useful tool for studying the participation of copper in electron transfer has been EPR spectroscopy. However, the limitation is that only about 40% of the copper can be detected by this method. The view held by Beinert (Ref. 6) and supported by others, is that there is an exchange interaction between closely placed paramagnetic species (copper-copper and/or copper-heme) which decreases the paramagnetism of each.

The basic functional unit in cytochrome oxidase is a complex containing four metal centers. This is supported by the fact that other oxidases, such as laccase, contain four metal atoms per active unit, a fact which, as pointed out by Malmström (Ref. 1), cannot be a simple coincidence. On the other hand it has also been suggested that the dimeric structure of beef cytochrome oxidase, which in solution

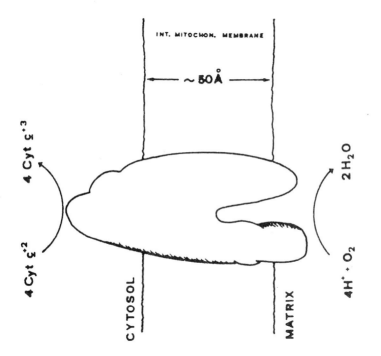

Fig. 2. Relationships between the internal mitochondrial membrane and the cytochrome c oxidase complex. The location of the active sites within the molecular structure is not yet clarified.

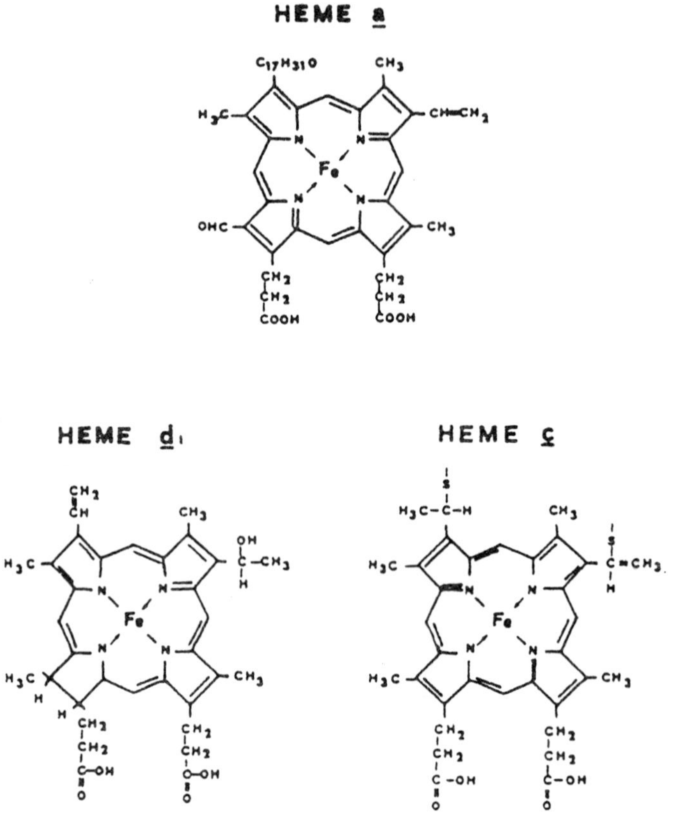

Fig. 3. Heme structures found in vertebrate and *Pseudomonas* cytochrome c oxidase.

is a complex containing eight metals, may have a functional and mechanistic significance.

2.4   Isolation and molecular properties

Cytochrome oxidase is water insoluble and its isolation in pure form from the mitochondrial membrane requires the use of surface-active reagents. All of the reported methods (for a review seen Wilson and Erecinska, (Ref. 7)) are based on the same principle: extraction of the oxidase by a detergent and its purification from the contaminating membrane fragments by repeated fractionation with salts in the presence of a detergent.

Purified cytochrome oxidase contains variable amounts of lipid. It has been found that cardiolipin is the most tightly bound phospholipid since, in the ratio one cardiolipin/one oxidase, it forms a stable lipoprotein complex necessary for the oxidase activity, additional phospholipid being then required for maximal activity. Some detergents can replace phospholipids insofar as their "dispersing" role is concerned, but cannot replace cardiolipin in the internal lipid-protein interaction.

Electron microscopy shows that cytochrome oxidase passes through the membranes, and recent studies on vesicles crystals have given information on the overall shape of the complex extracted from beef heart. The monomer has the general shape of a distorted Y, with the step protruding towards the cytosolic side and the arms, largely embedded into the membrane, sticking into the solvent on the matrix side. The number and nature of the constituent polypeptide chains of eukaryotic cytochrome oxidases has been investigated using sodium dodecyl sulphate (SDS) gel electro-phoresis and column chromatography. There is essential agreement that the enzyme is comprised of at least seven subunits, some possibly in multiple copies. This general pattern is found in cytochrome oxidase from all species so far examined (Ref. 8). The three bigger subunits (I-III) are hydrophobic in character and are synthesized on the mitochondrial ribosomes, while the smaller chains are hydrophilic and synthesized on the cytoplasmic ribosomes. The calculation of the overall molecular weight from the molecular weights of the subunits obviously depends on the number of copies of each polypeptide present in the complex. Evidence from *Neurospora* oxidase convincingly indicates that, at least the heavier subunits, are present in a 1:1 ratio. Similar conclusions on bovine cytochrome oxidase have been reached. On this basis, the molecular weight of one functional unit (cyt a a_3) of the bovine enzyme would be approximately 140,000 which could be consistent with a minimum molecular weight of 70,000. This value may be as large as 175,000 if some of the smaller subunits were present in more copies. All the subunits have, at one time or another, been suggested to contain either copper or heme or both. The most convincing evidence, however, comes from amino acid sequence data (Ref. 9). Thus subunit II has strong analogies with the blue copper proteins azurin and

plastocyanin, since the four ligands of copper in plastocyanin (i.e., His 37, Cys 84)
His 87 and Met 92) have been identified in the sequence of subunit II in analogous
positions. Gel electrophoresis experiments in which dissociation of the oxidase
complex was accomplished under relatively nondenaturing conditions, confirmed this
view: under such conditions copper (together with heme) was found to be associated
predominantly with subunit II.

2.5 Functional properties

The activity of cytochrome oxidase is strongly dependent on a number of factors
(cytochrome $\underline{c}$ concentration, ionic strength, ionic composition, pH, lipid content,
etc.) which account for the different values of the activities reported for various
preparations. Under optimum conditions, some oxidase preparations exhibit a
turnover number (based on cyt $\underline{a}_3$) of 400-800 sec^{-1} and the reported rate constants
for the reaction of oxygen with full reduced oxidase (expressed as a biomolecular
reaction between oxygen and cyt $\underline{a}_3$) varies between 4×10^7 and 2×10^8 $M^{-1}s^{-1}$ in
isolated oxidase, mitochondria and whole cells (Ref. 7).

(a) Steady state kinetics. Functional properties of the oxidase are described
by its reactivity with oxygen and cytochrome $\underline{c}$. Two general types of methods have
been developed for this purpose:

(1) Measurements of the oxygen uptake with reduced cytochrome $\underline{c}$ as substrate
    (polarographic or manometric);

(2) Measurements of the rate of oxidation of reduced cytochrome $\underline{c}$ (spectrophoto-
    metric).

The steady-state kinetics of cytochrome oxidase, do not conform to simple
Michaelis-Menten schemes, but show complexities both in the spectrophotometric and
polarographic assay. These have been ascribed, particularly at low ionic strength,
to the inhibitory effect of both reduced and oxidized cytochrome $\underline{c}$ on the reaction,
due to the formation of molecular complexes with the enzyme. A critical analysis
of the steady-state kinetics of cytochrome oxidase in terms of possible reaction
schemes has been recently presented by Errede and Kamen (Ref. 10).

(b) The reaction with cytochrome $\underline{c}$. The second order rate constant for the
reaction between anaerobic oxidized oxidase and reduced cytochrome $\underline{c}$ was determined
by Gibson et al. (Ref. 11) to be 4×10^7 $M^{-1}s^{-1}$ at 21°C in 0.1 M phosphate buffer,
pH 7, a value very close to that for the reaction between reduced oxidase and oxygen.

Yonetani and Ray (Ref. 12) found that the K_m value for reduced cytochrome $\underline{c}$
(8.5 μM) was equal to that of K_I for ferricytochrome $\underline{c}$ (8.3 μM) at pH 6.0 in
0.1 M phosphate buffer. These values diverge at alkaline pH.

The binding between the oxidase and cytochrome $\underline{c}$ is largely electrostatic.
Acetylated and succinylated cytochrome $\underline{c}$ are inactive, whereas guanidylated cytochrome $\underline{c}$ retains full activity. Several authors have stressed the importance of

lysine residues on cytochrome c in the binding process, especially of Lys 13.

(c) Mechanistic problems. From the mechanistic viewpoint, a problem of great
relevance is the identification of the primary electron acceptor, i.e., the "electron
gate" into oxidase. Available evidence (Ref. 8) seems to converge in indicating
that the initial electron enters the oxidase through cytochrome a, and that Cu_A is
a secondary electron acceptor which is reduced internally from cytochrome a. The
structural information concerning a binding site for cytochrome a being on subunit
II, would be consistent with a model postulating that cytochrome a and Cu_A are also
bound to the same subunit.

Experiments on the time course of appearance of photosensitivity have shown
that cytochrome a_3 is reduced slowly when "resting" (i.e., the completely oxidized
form as it is obtained at the end of the isolation procedure) oxidase is mixed
with an excess of cytochrome c (Ref. 11). This reduction, which occurs *via* internal
electron transfer from the electron accepting sites of the complex, is indeed so
slow (k $\sim$ 0.5 s^{-1}) to appear incompatible with steady-state measurements. A possible
explanation of this discrepancy has been provided by showing that in one of the
oxygen intermediates, the "pulsed" oxidase (see below), this rate becomes faster.

Molecular oxygen requires four electrons per molecule in its reduction to water,
whereas the oxidation-reduction components of cytochrome oxidase are nominally one-
electron acceptors. This leads to a difficulty in understanding the mechanism of
the oxygen reaction. Antonini et al. (Ref. 13) proposed that a concerted four-
electron reaction occurred in which both cytochromes and both copper atoms had to
be reduced before oxygen could react. On the basis of potentiometric studies
Lindsay and Wilson (Ref. 14) postulated that carbon monoxide binds to a reduced
cytochrome a_3-reduced copper complex. The competitive relationships between CO
and O_2 suggests that the oxygen binding also occurs only when both are reduced.
If the oxygen forms a bridged compound, this would circumvent the thermodynamically
unfavorable one-electron reduction of O_2 to O_2^- ($E_0 \sim$ 0.32; (Ref. 15)) leading
instead to a two-electron reduction of a bridged peroxide compound. The peroxide
intermediate could then be reduced to water in two one-electron steps or in one
two-electron step (Ref. 7).

2.6 Intermediates in the reaction with oxygen

As with other enzymes involved in complex reactions, understanding of the
catalytic mechanism critically depends on the identification of functional intermediates populated during the catalytic cycle.

(a) Mixed-valence oxidase. A number of methods were used to prepare a species
of mammalian cytochrome oxidase in which only cytochrome a_3 is reduced and in
combination with CO (Ref. 16). The kinetics of CO binding by cytochrome a_3 in
these species is significantly different from that exhibited by the fully reduced

enzyme. The reaction between cytochrome $\underline{a}_3$ and oxygen was followed by flow-flash experiments and reveals a fast, oxygen-dependent rate (k = 8 x 10^7 $M^{-1}s^{-1}$ at low oxygen) followed by a slow process whose rate is independent of oxygen. The authors' (Ref. 16) interpretation of these results was in terms of:
(i) site-site interaction since the ligand binding behavior of cytochrome $\underline{a}_3$ in respect to CO showed a dependence of the redox state of its partners,
(ii) possible single electron steps in the reduction of oxygen.

(b) Oxygenated oxidase. Okunuki (Ref. 17) observed that when oxygen was mixed with a chemically reduced preparation of isolated oxidase, the spectrum of the resulting preparation was not that of the ferric hemoprotein. The new species was characterized by a Soret maximum at near 428 nm and slowly reverted to the spectrum of the ferric compound (Soret maximum at 418 nm). Oril and King (Ref. 18) confirmed, under analogous conditions, the very rapid formation of an "oxygenated compound," but this was a mixture of at least three spectrally different species with different rates of formation and decay. The rate of decay of the species designated compound I was reported to be increased about 20,000 times by ferrocyto-chrome $\underline{c}$, to a rate consistent with its function in mitochondria. Despite extensive efforts, the chemical nature of the "oxygenation compound" remains obscure. Greenwood et al. (Ref. 16) noted that, when cytochrome oxidase is reduced in the presence of CO and all the redox sites are reoxidized by ferricyanide except the one linked in the binding of CO, photodissociation of the CO in the presence of O_2 results in rapid and quantitative formation of the oxygenated compound. Although Greenwood and coworkers (Ref. 16) assumed that the reactive species was $\underline{a}^{3+} Cu_A^{2+} \underline{a}_3^{2+}$, the data of Lindsay and Wilson (Ref. 14) make it probable that the EPR invisible copper was also reduced under their conditions, and that the reactive species was $\underline{a}^{3+} Cu_A^{2+} Cu_B^{1+} \underline{a}_3^{2+}$. The oxygenated compound formed would then be the result of the two-electron reduction of O_2 to a bound peroxide intermediate, or comparable oxidation-reduction species (Ref. 7).

(c) "Pulsed" oxidase. The attribute "pulsed" was assigned to the species obtained upon exposure of reduced oxidase, in the presence of cytochrome $\underline{c}$ and excess ascorbate, to a pulse of O_2 (Ref. 19).

A stoichiometric ratio of 1:1 between oxygen and the functional unit of the oxidase (4 redox sites) could be demonstrated by kinetic titrations in which the reduced enzyme was mixed with different oxygen concentrations (Ref. 20). This result indicates that the pulsed enzyme contains four oxidizing equivalents. The absorption spectrum of the pulsed enzyme, though somewhat similar to the oxidized derivative, shows distinct features, with characteristic differences both in the absorption maximum and in the extinction coefficients. Using a rapid-freezing technique Beinert and coworkers (Ref. 21) reported the identification of a new intermediate trapped after mixing reduced oxidase with oxygen, which has been assimilated to the pulsed oxidase. This intermediate shows an intense and thus an unrecognized EPR signal with g = 5, 1.7 and 1.69 which has been suggested to be due to cytochrome a_3^{3+} in some unknown state, possibly interacting with Cu_B. Spectroscopic differences and similarities between pulsed oxidase and other intermediates in the oxygen reaction have been recently discussed (Ref. 22).

Following the development of the CO binding capacity by cytochrome a_3 as a probe of its reduction, this process was estimated to be 4-5 times faster in the pulsed than in the resting form. Such increase in velocity, which is a consequence of the more efficient intramolecular electron transfer between electron-accepting sites and oxygen-binding sites in the enzyme, may be related to the role of pulsed oxidase in catalysis. This observation has been substantiated by the dynamic characterization of the pulsed form, which qualified it as a catalytically more active form during turnover in all the properly devised experiments of oxygen combination either with the purified enzyme (Ref. 20) or with oxidase molecules embedded in phospholipid vesicles (Ref. 23) and even in mitochondrial fragments (Ref. 24). If the rate-limiting step in the activation process depends on the initial slow reduction of cytochrome a_3, the higher intramolecular electron transfer observed for pulsed-oxidase is consistent with the idea that the pulsed derivative represents a short-cut in reaching the steady-state. If both resting and pulsed oxidase were catalytically competent but with different turnover numbers, the existence of alternative pathways for the electron flux to oxygen may be envisaged and the inter-play between the two forms could provide a smooth and rapid regulation of the catalytic efficiency of the overall system. While the role of protons and other possible effectors on both the activation (R → P) and deactivation (P → R) processes is presently under active investigation, a suceessful numerical simulation of the catalytic properties of Pulsed and Resting oxidase in terms of a minimal kinetic scheme and of a two-state allosteric model has been recently undertaken (Ref. 25).

(d) <u>Low temperature intermediates</u>. Optical and EPR measurements carried out at low temperatures on the reaction between reduced oxidase and oxygen allowed the detection of several intermediates both in the soluble and in the membrane-bound enzyme termed, A, B, and C by Chance and co-workers (Ref. 26). More recently Clore et al. (Ref. 27) studying the O_2 combination after photolysis of the CO derivative of both reduced and mixed valence membrane-bound enzyme, have re-examined the properties of these intermediates. The available data converge in indicating that the first intermediate is an O_2 adduct which is stable at -86°C (k_d ~350 mM). Divergent interpretations, however, exist about the properties of the intermediates observed at higher temperatures, and more than one pathway has been proposed (see Scheme below). Thus, Chance and coworkers (Ref. 26) state that disappearance of the O_2 adduct (compound A in the Scheme) is associated with the formation of the compound B, with a rate which depends on O_2 concentration and tends to a limiting

58

Steps on Oxidation of Cyt Oxidase at low temperature

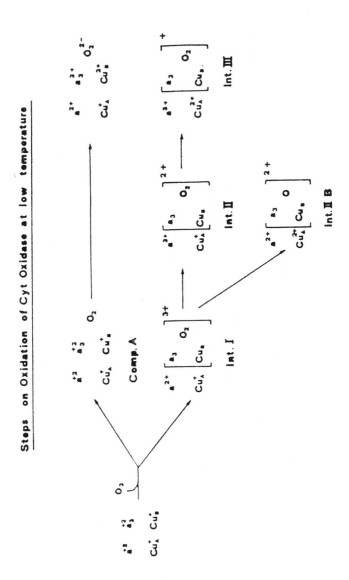

value (1.7 s^{-1} at $-65°C$). The corresponding species in Clore's (Ref. 27) scheme are, respectively, intermediates I and III, while intermediate II is considered a mixture of two species, one of which (IIB) is a dead-end product.

On the basis of their results, Clore et al (Ref. 27) propose a catalytic mechanism for oxidase which specifically takes into account the species identified in the low temperature experiments. However, it should be pointed out that the oxygen intermediates seen at low temperature are not necessarily the relevant ones during turnover, as the flux of electrons within the unit may populate at room temperature other states. This may not apply to the first intermediate (Compound A) which appears, in any model, to be an obligatory structure through which oxygen gains access to the oxidase unit.

3.1 *Pseudomonas* cytochrome oxidase

Pseudomonas cytochrome c oxidase (EC 1.9.3.2) is water soluble and is composed of two identical subunits each containing heme c and heme d (see Fig. 3), as prosthetic group. Whilst the heme c was found to be covalently bound to the protein, the heme d_1 can be removed easily by extraction with acid-acetone.

One of the most recent and reliable isolation procedures, is the one given by Parr et al. (Ref. 28).

3.2 Molecular and spectroscopic properties

Pseudomonas cytochrome oxidase has recently been crystallized and a preliminary X-ray diffraction study at low resolution reported (Refs. 29,30). The two monomers at 65,000 molecular weight each, (Ref. 31) are held together mainly by hydrophobic interactions. This is evidenced by the failure of 3M NaCl, 1M Na_2SO_4 or 6M urea to induce dissociation (Ref. 32). Only when 27 out of the 40 lysines per subunits are succinylated, do the two subunits dissociate by negative charge repulsion.

The absorption spectrum of oxidized *Pseudomonas* cytochrome oxidase (Fig. 4) shows peaks at 411 and 525 nm which together with shoulders at 300 and 560 nm, are typical of an oxidized c type cytochrome. Additionally, there is a peak at 640 nm and a shoulder at 450 nm which may be assigned to the heme d_1 moiety. When reduced, the c heme gives peaks at 417 and 520 nm and a very peculiar twin α band around 550 nm; d_1 heme absorption, however, depend on the reducing agent (Ref. 33). Using ascorbate or acid as reducing agents, absorption peaks at 460 and 655 nm, and a shoulder at 620 nm are observed. Since the purified protein in solution becomes slowly depleted of heme d_1 turning from greenish-brown into brown-red, integrity of the protein can be judged from the ratio of two specific wavelengths where the d_1 and the c hemes absorb in the oxidized form. This ratio is $E_{640}/E_{520} = 1.2$.

EPR and MCD measurements have shown that the two hemes are low spin in the oxidized state (Ref. 34), but heme d_1 becomes high spin when reduced ($S = 2$).

60

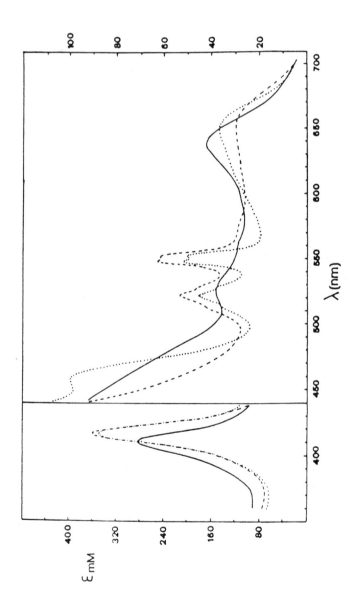

Fig. 4. Absorption spectra in the visible and Soret regions of the oxidized (———), ascorbate-reduced (....), ascorbate-reduced + CO (–·–·–) of *Pseudomonas* cytochrome *c* oxidase in 0.1 M phosphate buffer, pH 7.0 at 25°C. The ordinate gives the absorbance in mM^{-1} cm^{-1} per (*c* *d*)$_2$ heme units.

3.3 Functional properties

(a) Reaction with electron acceptors. The first discovered activity of
Pseudomonas cytochrome oxidase was its ability to reduce molecular oxygen; the
latter finding that it could reduce nitrite to nitric oxide accords much more
favorably, however, with the circumstances under which the enzyme is produced in
bacterial culture (Ref. 35). Both the nitrite reductase and the oxidase activity
are inhibited by cyanide, although only the latter function is inhibited by
carbon monoxide. Such behavior appears contradictory in the light of Kijmoto's
(Ref. 36) conclusion that oxygen and nitrite compete for the same site on the
protein.

The reaction of ascorbate-reduced *Pseudomonas* cytochrome oxidase with O_2 was
studied by using stopped-flow techniques at pH 7.0 and 25°C (Ref. 37). The observed
time courses were complex, the reaction consisting of three phases. Of these, only
the fastest process, with a second order rate constant of 3.3×10^4 M^{-1} s^{-1}, was
dependent on O_2 concentration. The two slower processes were first-order reactions
with rates of 1.0 ± 0.4 s^{-1} and 0.10 ± 0.03 s^{-1}. A kinetic titration experiment
revealed that the enzyme has a relatively low affinity constant for oxygen, approximately 10^4 M^{-1}. Kinetic difference spectra were determined for all three reaction
phases, in order to reveal their different characteristics. The events occurring
during the fast phase of oxidation appear to represent changes at both hemes $\underline{c}$
and $\underline{d}_1$; thus the kinetic results do not allow to say which heme, $\underline{c}$ or $\underline{d}_1$, is the
binding site for oxygen. Ligand-binding evidence, however, suggests that the heme
$\underline{d}_1$ is the most likely site of attack for oxygen. If this assumption is correct,
then the fast oxygen-dependent reaction of the heme $\underline{c}$ implies internal electron-
transfer rates of at least 100 s^{-1}. Rates of this order are greatly in excess
of those that have been observed for the electron transfer from heme $\underline{c}$ to heme $\underline{d}_1$
in the anaerobic reduction of the oxidized enzyme by azurin, i.e., 0.25 s^{-1}.
Although it is clear that the rate of oxygen reduction by the bacterial enzyme is
very much lower than that of the mitochondrial oxidases, this behavior appears to
parallel that of mammalian cytochrome $\underline{c}$ oxidase, in which the presence of the
substrate, oxygen, greatly increases the electron transfer rates within the protein.

(b) Reactions with electron donors. *Pseudomonas* cytochrome is known to oxidize
reduced cytochrome $\underline{c}_{551}$ and reduced azurin. Both substrates react with the enzyme
with a K_m of $\sim 10^{-6}$ M. However, this catalysis is inhibited by the products, oxidized azurin and cytochrome $\underline{c}_{551}$. Studying the reaction between *Pseudomonas* cytochrome oxidase and azurin by more direct methods, Wharton et al. (Ref. 38) have
concluded that direct electron transfer between azurin and the heme $\underline{d}_1$ of the
enzyme does not occur, but that redox changes at this level are brought about
solely by an internal electron transfer mechanism. Analysis of the biomolecular
reaction of the oxidase and azurin showed that direct interaction takes place at

the level of the heme c component. The same authors estimated that electrons may be transferred from heme c to heme d_1 at rates of 0.2-2.0 s^{-1}, but that the reverse reaction rate is 10 s^{-1}. These results parallel those obtained by equilibrium methods, where the reduction potential of the heme d_1 was found to be more negative than that of the heme c.

In addition to the natural electron donors, a number of other reagents are also capable of providing electrons for *Pseudomonas* cytochrome oxidase, like reduced pyocyanine, methylene blue, hydroquinone and ascorbate; both the latter two reductants and NADH in combination with phenazine methosulphate are commonly employed as means of reducing *Pseudomonas* cytochrome oxidase for spectral studies.

(c) Interactions between subunits. Blatt and Pecht (Ref. 39), combining spectrophotometric and potentiometric reductive titrations, measured the redox potentials of the two hemes separately and proposed the existence of allosteric cooperative interactions among the four hemes in the two subunits together with spectroscopic interactions. Heme c was confirmed to have a higher redox potential than heme d_1 and the reduction of the first heme of each type was calculated to contribute about 50% more to the change in absorbance than the second heme of the same type bound to the other subunit.

4.1 Laccase

Laccase (EC 1.10.3.2) was identified in 1883 as the agent responsible for the darkening and hardening of the latex of the lacquer tree. It is present in various plants and microorganisms, notably in fungi. In plants, like the lacquer tree, the physiological function of laccase appears to be that of oxidation of phenolic compounds present in the latex which then form polymers with a protective function. In fungi, laccase is an inducible "extracellular" enzyme present in organisms responsible for wood rotting, and its physiological function may be a "digestive" one.

Laccase is usually purified from the japanese lacquer tree, *Rhus vernicifera* or from the fungus *Polyporus versicolor*. Purification of fungal laccase is an easy procedure since as mentioned, the enzyme appears as inducible extracellular protein in the medium.

4.2 Copper content and molecular properties

The molecular weight of fungal laccase is 64,000; it contains 4 copper atoms per molecule and its carbohydrate content is about 10%.

The molecular weight of tree laccase is less defined ranging from 110,000 to 140,000; consequently the number of copper atoms per molecule varies between 4 and 6. The carbohydrate content is about 45% (Ref. 40).

4.3 The types of copper in Laccase

As other blue oxidases, ascorbic oxidase (and ceruloplasmin), laccase contains copper in different forms (Ref. 41). According to optical and EPR properties the copper atom have been classified as type 1, type 2 and type 3.

Type 1 copper. Type 1 copper is responsible for the intense blue color of laccase due to an intense absorption band with a maximum around 600 nm. The extinction coefficient is 5700 M^{-1} cm^{-1} for the tree enzyme and 4900 M^{-1} cm^{-1} for the fungal enzyme. Type 1 copper has a characteristic EPR spectrum with unusually low values for the hyperfine splitting constant. It has been suggested that sulfur is a ligand of type 1 copper.

Type 2 copper. Type 2 copper gives an EPR spectrum broader than that of type 1 and similar to that generally observed for simple Cu^{2+} complexes. The most characteristic property of type 2 copper is its tendency to interact with anionic ligands such as F^-, N_3^- and CN^-.

Type 3 copper. Type 3 copper is EPR nondetectable. It is now generally accepted that this is due to the presence of two Cu^{2+} atoms with in-pair anti-ferromagnetic coupling. These coppers are believed to be associated with an absorption band at 330 nm.

4.4 Oxidation--reduction and catalytic properties

All the copper atoms present in oxidized laccase can accept electrons since the electron accepting capacity corresponds to the number of copper atoms. The redox potentials of type 1 and type 3 copper in fungal laccase are about 780 mV; in tree laccase they are 394 and 434 mV, respectively (Ref. 42).

Tree and fungal laccases catalyze the oxidation of several diphenols and diamines (Ref. 43). Laccase has a low specificity and also monophenols and ferrocyanide are substrates for the enzyme. It is inhibited by many anions, which bind to type 2 copper. Pre-steady state kinetic studies (Refs. 41,44) have shown that electrons enter the oxidase through type 1 copper. From this site they are transferred to the other coppers, the intramolecular electron transfer being the rate limiting step. The pair of type 3 coppers is probably responsible for oxygen binding.

5.1 Ascorbate oxidase

Ascorbate oxidase (L-ascorbate:O_2 oxidoreductase, EC 1.10.3.3) belongs, together with laccase, to the "blue" copper-containing oxidases (Refs. 41,45,46). It was identified as a distinct enzyme by Szent-Gyorgyi in 1931, and is present in many higher plants. Ascorbate oxidase is not found in animals but ascorbate oxidase activity is present in some microorganisms.

5.2 Isolation and molecular properties

The enzyme is generally purified from squashes (*Cucurbita pepo condensa, Cucurbita pepo medullosa*) and cucumber (*Cucumis sativus*) (Ref. 47). The yield is about 1 mg/kg of fresh squash. The best preparations of the enzyme have a copper content near 0.35% corresponding to the presence of 8 copper atoms per mole of enzyme (Ref. 48). However, copper contents corresponding from 6 to 12 copper atoms have also been reported.

The molecular weight of ascorbate oxidase at neutral or alkaline pH is 140,000. The acid pH polymerization may occur. The $s_{20,w}$ value is 6.55 at pH ≥ 7 and increases to about 10 at pH near 5. After treatment with sodium dodecyl sulfate (SDS) subunits of molecular weight about half that of the native enzyme ($\sim 70,000$) are obtained. Treatment with SDS and mercaptoethanol give smaller fragments with molecular weight from 38,000 to 28,000. The enzyme contains carbohydrate (2-10%), and has an acid isoelectric point.

5.3 Catalytic properties

Ascorbate oxidase catalyzes the oxidation of ascorbic acid (Vitamin C) by molecular oxygen according to the reaction:

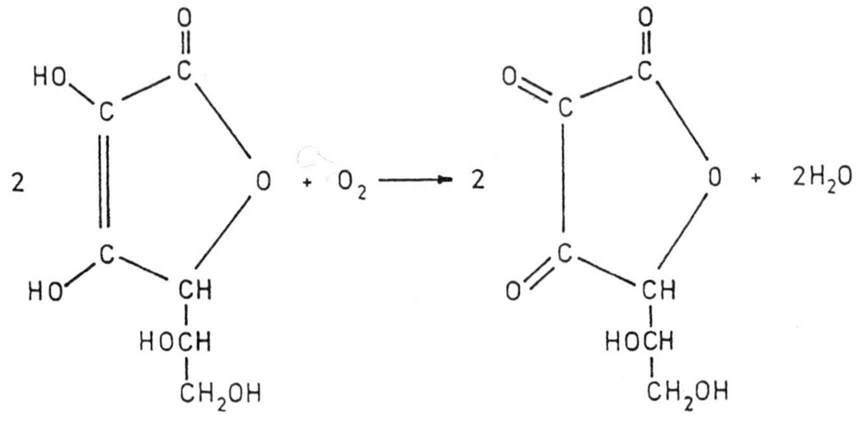

However, many other compounds are oxidized by O_2 in the presence of ascorbate oxidase. The enzyme acts on compounds which contain a lactone ring with a vicinal enediol adjacent to a carbonyl group. Other cyclic compounds are also oxidized: 2,5-dichlorohydroquinone, 2,6-dichlorohydroquinone and 2,6-dichloroindophenol.

It has been suggested that the physiological substrates of ascorbate oxidase may be o-diphenolic compounds, oxidation of which being responsible for the darkening processes in vegetables. Ascorbate oxidase can also oxidize ferrocyanide.

The activity of the enzyme is expressed in Dawson units: one Dawson unit corresponds to 1.5×10^{-8}M of ascorbate oxidized per second in air and at saturation with ascorbate. The best enzyme preparations have an activity corresponding to 3800-4000 Dawson units/mg protein.

5.4 Steady-state kinetics

With ascorbate as a substrate the turnover number is 500,000 min^{-1} at 25° and K_m 2×10^{-4}M independently of pH between 4.5 and 7.4 (Ref. 49). With ferrocyanide, the turnover number is 1,500 M^{-1} and K_m 3×10^{-3}M but depends largely on pH, k_{cat} at pH 7.4 being three orders of magnitude lower than at pH 4.5.

K_m for oxygen is different with ascorbate ($K_m \sim 2 \times 10^{-4}$M) and ferrocyanide ($K_m \sim 10^{-5}$M). The different steady-state parameters for ascorbate and ferrocyanide may imply different catalytic pathways for the two substrates.

The activity of ascorbate oxidase is inhibited by anions such as F^- and N_3^-.

5.5 Catalytic mechanism

As other "blue" oxidases, ascorbate oxidase contains the three types of copper classified as type 1, type 2 and type 3 (Ref. 50); type 1 being paramagnetic and with a very high extinction coefficient around 600 nm, type 2 being also paramagnetic but uncolored, and type 3 consisting of a pair of copper atoms undetectable by EPR due to antiferromagnetic coupling. Present experimental evidence indicates that in ascorbate oxidase about 50% of the copper atoms are EPR detectable comprising three type 1 and one type 2 copper atoms per molecule. Thus if ascorbate oxidase contains 8 copper atoms per molecule these are three type 1, one type 2 and two pairs of type 3. The involvement of the various types of copper atoms in catalysis can be inferred by redox measurements and pre-steady state kinetic experiments (Refs. 51,52).

Redox titrations with ascorbate give a mid-point potential for type 1 copper of 334 mV, but titrations with ferrocyanide show heterogeneity in the redox properties of the type 1 coppers. Pre-steady state kinetic studies were performed using reductic acid (cyclopentane-1,2,3-trione) and ferrocyanide, since with ascorbate the reduction of type 1 copper was too rapid. Both with reductic acid and ferrocyanide, in the absence of oxygen, a rapid bleaching of the blue color (at 610 nm) is observed. Reoxidation of reduced type 1 copper on reaction with oxygen is also very rapid. In analogy with laccase, present evidence suggests that electrons enter the enzyme through type 1 copper and oxygen reacts with type 3 copper. However, the situation with ascorbate oxidase is not yet clear.

REFERENCES

1. Malmstron, B.G. (1974) Quant. Revs. Biophys., 6, 389-431.
2. Lemberg, M.R. (1969) Physiol. Revs., 49, 48-121.
3. Keilin, D. (1966) The History of Cell Respiration and Cytochromes (prepared by J. Keilin) Cambridge University Press, Cambridge, England.
4. Lemberg, M.R. and Barret, J.V. (1973) Cytochromes, New York: Academic Press.
5. Van Gelden, B.F., Orme Johnson, W.H., Hansen, R.E., and Beinert, H. (1967) Proc. Natl. Acad. Sci. USA, 58, 1073-1079.
6. Beinert, H. (1966) in The Biochemistry of Copper (Peisach, J., Aisen, P., and Blumberg, W., eds.) New York: Academic Press, pp. 213-234.
7. Wilson, D.F. and Erecinska, P. (1979) in The Porphyrins, Vol. VII, New York: Academic Press.
8. Brunori, M., Antonini, E. and Wilson, M.T. (1981) in Metal Ions in Biological Systems, Vol. 13 (Sigel, H., ed.) New York: Marcel Dekker.
9. Sacher, R., Steffens, G.J., and Buse, G. (1979) Hoppe-Seylers Z. Physiol. Chem., 360, 1385-1392.
10. Errede, B. and Kamen, M.D. (1978) Biochemistry, 17, 1015-1031.
11. Gibson, Q., Greenwood, C., Wharton, D.C., and Palmer, G. (1965) J. Biol. Chem., 240, 888-894.
12. Yonetani, T. and Ray, G.S. (1965) J. Biol. Chem., 240, 3392-3398.
13. Antonini, E., Brunori, M., Greenwood, C., and Malmstrom, B. (1970), Nature 228, 936-937.
14. Lindsay, J.G. and Wilson, D.F. (1974) FEBS Letts., 48, 45-49.
15. George, P. (1965) in Oxidases and Related Redox Systems (King, T.E., Mason, H.S., and Morrison, M., eds.) University Park Press.
16. Greenwood, C., Wilson, M.T., and Brunori, M. (1974) Biochem. J., 137, 205-215.
·17. Okunuki, K. (1966) Comp. Biochem. Physiol., 14, 232-240.
18. Orii, Y. and King, T.E. (1976) J. Biol. Chem., 251, 7847-7493.
19. Antonini, E., Brunori, M., Colosimo, A., Greenwood, C., and Wilson, M.T. (1976) in Oxygen and Physiological Function (Jobsis, F.F., ed.) Professional Information Library, Dallas, pp. 53-61.
20. Brunori, M., Colossimo, A., Rainoni, G., Wilson, M.T., and Antonini, E. (1979) J. Biol. Chem., 254, 10769-10775.
21. Beinert, H., Shaw, R.W., and Hansen, R.E. (1978) J. Biol. Chem., 253, 6637-6640.
22. Colosimo, A., Brunori, M., Sarti, P., Antonini, E. and Wilson, M.T. (1981) Is. J. Chem., 21, 30.
23. Brunori, M., Colosimo, A., Sarti, P., Antonini, E., Lalla, M.W., and Wilson, M.T. (1982) in Oxidases and Related Redox Systems (King, T.E., Mason, H.S. and Morrison, M., eds.) Pergamon Press.
24. Bonaventura, C., Bonaventura, J., Brunori, M., and Wilson, M.T. (1978) FEBS Letts., 85, 30-34.
25. Wilson, M.T., Peterson, J., Antonini, E., Brunori, M., Colosimo, A., and Wyman, J. (1981) Proc. Natl. Acad. Sci. USA, 78, 7115-7118.
26. Chance, B., Saronio, C., Waring, A., and Leigh, J.S. (1978) Biochim. Biophys. Acta, 502, 37-55.
27. Clore, M.G., Andreasson, L.E., Karlsson, B., Aasa, R., and Malmstron, B.G. (1980) Biochem. J., 185, 139-154.
28. Parr, S.R., Barber, D., Greenwood, C., Phillips, B.W., and Melling, J. (1976) Biochem. J., 157, 432-430.
29. Takano, T., Dickerson, R.E., Schichman, S.A., and Meyer, T.E. (1979) J. Mol. Biol., 133, 185-187.
30. Akey, C.W., Moffat, K., Wharton, D.C., and Edelstein, S.T. (1980) J. Mol. Biol., 136, 19-43.
31. Silvestrini, M.C., Colosimo, A., Brunori, M., Walsh, T.A., Barber, D., and Greenwood, C. (1979) Biochem. J., 183, 701-709.
32. Kuronen, T. and Ellfolk, N. (1972) Biochim. Biophys. Acta, 275, 308-318.

33. Barber, D. (1978) Ph.D. Thesis, University of East Anlgia, Norwich, England.
34. Walsh, T.A., Johnson, M.K., Greenwood, C., Barber, D., Springale, J.P., and Thompson, A.J. (1979) Biochem. J., 177, 29-35.
35. Yananaka, T. (1964) Nature, 204, 253-255.
36. Kijmoto, S. (1968) Ann. Rep. Works Osaka Univ., 16, 19.
37. Greenwood, C., Barber, B., Parr, S.F., Antonini, E., Brunori, M., and Colosimo, A. (1978) Biochem. J., 173, 11-17.
38. Wharton, D.C., Gudat, J.C., and Gibson, Q.H. (1973) Biochim. Biophys. Acta, 292, 611-620.
39. Blatt, Y. and Pecht, I. (1981) Biochemistry, 21, 364-372.
40. Reinhammar, B. (1970) Biochim. Biophys. Acta, 205, 35-47.
41. Reinhammar, B. (1979) in Advances in Inorganic Chemistry (Eichorn, E. and Marzilli, F., eds.) New York: Elsevier-North Holland, pp. 91-118.
42. Reinhammar, B. (1972) Biochim. Biophys. Acta, 275, 245-259.
43. Levine, W.G. (1966) in The Biochemistry of Copper (Peisach, J., Aisen, P. and Blumberg, W.E., eds.) New York: Academic Press, pp. 371-387.
44. Malmstrom, B., Finazzi-Agro, A. and Antonini, E. (1969) Eur. J. Biochem., 9, 383-391.
45. Mondovi, B. and Avigliano, L. (1983) in Copper Proteins (Lontie, R., ed.) CRC Press, Inc., in press.
46. Malmstrom, B.G., Andreasson, L.E. and Reinhammer, B. (1975) in The Enzymes, Vol. XIIB (Boyer, P.D., ed.), New York: Academic Press, pp. 507-579.
47. Marchesini, A. and Kroneck, P.M.H. (1979) Eur. J. Biochem., 101, 65-76.
48. Petersen, L.C. and Degn, H. (1978) Biochim. Biophys. Acta, 526, 85-92.
49. Krul, K.G. and Dawson, C.R. (1977) Bioinorg. Chem., 1, 71-77.
50. Malkin, R. and Malmstrom, B.G. (1970) Adv. Enzymol., 33, 177-244.
51. Avigliano, L., Rotilio, G., Urbanelli, S., Mondovi, B. and Finazzi-Agro, A. (1978) Arch. Biochem. Biophys., 185, 419-422.
52. Andreasson, L.E. and Reinhammar, B. (1976) Biochim. Biophys. Acta, 445, 579-597.

CHAPTER 4   DIOXYGENASES AND MONOOXYGENASES

MITSUHIRO NOZAKI[*] AND OSAMU HAYAISHI[+]
[*]Department of Biochemistry, Shiga University of Medical Science, Seta, Ohtsu,
Shiga 520-21, Japan; [+]Department of Medical Chemistry, Kyoto University Faculty
of Medicine, Yoshida, Sakyo-ku, Kyoto 606, Japan

INTRODUCTION

Oxygen is one of the most important elements in life and plays a central role in
the metabolism and the generation of energy in all aerobic organisms. One function
of oxygen is to act as an ultimate hydrogen acceptor in the process of biological oxidation of nutrients. During this process, oxygen undergoes four-electron reduction to
generate two molecules of water and energy is conserved in the form of ATP. Numerous
enzymes known as dehydrogenases or oxidases are involved in this process. Oxygen is
also involved in the transformation of biologically essential substances and foreign
compounds. In this process, molecular oxygen is directly incorporated into various
compounds. The enzymes involved in such reactions are referred to as oxygenases
(Refs. 1,2).

In 1955, two groups of investigators independently demonstrated that oxygen atoms
in the atmosphere were enzymatically incorporated into the substrates by the use of
^{18}O as a tracer. Mason and collaborators found that during the oxidation of
3,4-dimethylphenol to dimethylcatechol by phenolase, the oxygen atom incorporated
into the substrate was derived exclusively from molecular oxygen (Eq. (1)) (Ref. 3).
Hayaishi and associates found that the two atoms of oxygen incorporated into *cis, cis*
muconic acid produced from catechol by the action of pyrocatechase were both derived
from molecular oxygen (Eq. (2)) (Ref. 4).

Since the demonstration of isotopically labelled oxygen insertion, a large number
of oxygenases have been found in all types of living organisms. Their importance was

established in the biogenesis of cellular constituents as well as important regulatory effectors, transformation of foreign compounds such as drugs and carcinogens,
and for the degradation of hydrocarbons, therapeutic chemicals and end moieties
of plant and animal metabolism.

Cofactors involved in oxygenase reactions are flavin, heme, nonheme iron, copper,
pteridine and so forth, and the nature of these cofactors has recently been elucidated by application of new physical, chemical and biological probes for assessment
of the structure and function. Thus, oxygenase systems play a major role in
elucidating the chemical mechanisms of "oxygen activation" in biological systems.

In this section, discussion will mainly be focused on flavin, heme and nonheme
iron-containing oxygenases, and on the interaction of oxygen with the cofactors
involved in these oxygenase-catalyzed reactions. For the physiological significance
and general properties and function of oxygenases, the readers are referred to
monographs (Refs. 5-10) or other review articles (Refs. 11-21).

CLASSIFICATION

As in the cases of phenolase and pyrocatechase, respectively, oxygenases are classified into two major groups, monooxygenases and dioxygenases, depending on whether
one or two atoms of oxygen are inserted per molecule of substrate (Ref. 22).

(A) Monooxygenase. In monooxygenase reactions, molecular oxygen (dioxygen)
reacts with the substrate and one atom of oxygen is incorporated into the substrate,
whereas the other atom of oxygen is reduced to water by a reductant essential for
the reaction, is shown in Eq. (3), where H_2X and S denote the reducing agent and
substrate, respectively.

$$S + O_2 + H_2X \longrightarrow SO + H_2O + X \tag{3}$$

Since both oxygenation and oxidation reactions are involved in the reaction, monooxygenases are sometimes referred to as "mixed function oxidases." The term
"hydroxylase" is also used for some monooxygenases which catalyze the formation
of a hydroxyl group as a result of monooxygenation. In some monooxygenase
reactions, the substrate itself serves as an electron donor as well as oxygen
acceptor (Eq. (4)), where SH_2 denotes the substrate.

$$SH_2 + O_2 \longrightarrow SO + H_2O \tag{4}$$

This type of enzymes may be referred to as "internal monooxygenases." Most other
monooxygenases, however, require various kinds of external hydrogen (or electron)
donors as in Eq. (3); they are, therefore, referred to as "external monooxygenase."

(b) <u>Dioxygenases</u>. Dioxygenases catalyzing the incorporation of two atoms of molecular oxygen into the substrate are also classified into two groups. In most cases, one substrate acts as an oxygen acceptor and a single molecule of the substrate receives 2 atoms of oxygen as shown in Eq. (5),

$$S + O_2 \longrightarrow SO_2 \tag{5}$$

where S donates substrate.

In some dioxygenase reactions, however, one atom each of the oxygen molecule is incorporated into two different molecules of one substrate (Eq. (6)) or into two different substrate molecules (Eq. (7)).

$$2S + O_2 \longrightarrow 2SO \tag{6}$$

$$S + S' + O_2 \longrightarrow SO + S'O \tag{7}$$

The term "intramolecular dioxygenases" may be used for the dioxygenases catalyzing the reaction shown in Eq. (5) and "intermolecular dioxygenases" for those catalyzing the reaction shown either in Eq. (6) or Eq. (7), respectively.

In the reaction represented in Eq. (7), one of the two substrates is invariably α-ketoglutarate, which is converted to succinate by the incorporation of one atom of oxygen with concomitant decarboxylation. Therefore, the overall reaction may be schematically shown as in Eq. (8) and the enzymes catalyzing this type of reaction are sometimes referred to as "α-ketoglutarate requiring dioxygenases."

$$
S + \begin{array}{c} COOH \\ | \\ CH_2 \\ | \\ CH_2 \\ | \\ C{=}O \\ | \\ COOH \end{array} + O_2 \longrightarrow SO + \begin{array}{c} COOH \\ | \\ CH_2 \\ | \\ CH_2 \\ | \\ COOH \end{array} + CO_2 \tag{8}
$$

(C) <u>Cofactors involved in oxygenases (Ref. 21)</u>. Cofactors involved in monooxygenases and dioxygenases are summarized in Tables 1 and 2, respectively. All the internal monooxygenases that have to date been purified and characterized contain flavin coenzymes, and the substrate itself serves as the hydrogen donor. The externa hydrogen donors required for the external monooxygenases include reduced NAD(P), ascorbic acid and sulfhydryl compounds. Cofactors involved in the external monooxygenases are flavin, pteridine, heme, nonheme iron and copper. In some monooxygenase reactions, enzymes and/or electron carrier systems other than monooxygenase itself are involved in the transfer of electrons or hydrogens to the cofactor involve

TABLE 1

Monooxygenases and their cofactors[a]

Type of Reaction	Cofactors	Electron donors	Electron transport system[b]	EC No.[c]
(1) Internal monooxygenases oxidative decarboxylation	FAD or FMN	substrate		1:13:12
(2) External monooxygenases				
(i) hydroxylation	FAD	NAD(P)H	–	1:14:13
	P450	NADPH	NADPH-Cyt. P450 reductase (fp)	1:14:14
	P450	NAD(P)H	NADPH-Fe-S reductase(fp), Fe-S	1:14:15
	Biopterine, NHI	NADPH	dehydrobiopterine reductase	1:14:16
	NHI	NADH	NADH-rubredoxin reductase(fp), rubredoxin (NHI)	
	Cu	Ascorbic acid	–	1:14:17
(ii) desaturation	NHI	NADH	NADH-Cyt.b_5 reductase(fp), Cyt.b_5(Hp)	1:14:99:5
(iii) demethylation	NHI	NADH	NHI-FAD	1:14:99:15
(iv) N-or S-oxide formation	FAD	NADPH	?	1:14:13:8
(v) epoxide formation	NHI-FAD	NADPH	?	1:14:99:7

[a] The following abbreviations are used: fp: flavoprotein; NHI: nonheme iron protein; Hp: hemoprotein; Fe-S: iron-sulfur protein.
[b] A dash means that electron carriers other than monooxygenases are not involved in the reaction and electron donors directly reduce cofactors involved in the monooxygenase.
[c] Enzyme Commission number (EC No.) refers to the new numbering system recommended in 1978 by the Nomenclature Committee of the Internal Union of Biochemistry. A question mark means that an involvement of an electron transport system is not known yet.

A major function of dioxygenases is the cleavage of the aromatic ring with the insertion of two atoms of molecular oxygen. The indole ring cleaving enzymes, tryptophan 2,3-dioxygenase and indoleamine 2,3-dioxygenase, contain heme as a sole cofactor. A flavonol-cleaving enzyme, quercetinase, contains copper, and a pyridine ring-cleaving enzyme 2-methyl-3-hydroxypyridine-5-carboxylate dioxygenase, contains flavin as a cofactor. With the exception of these enzymes, most, if not all, of the other ring cleaving dioxygenases contain nonheme iron as the sole cofactor. Among these, some enzymes contain the ferrous form of iron and some the ferric form. In the so-called double hydroxylation reactions, a hydrogen donor, NAD(P)H, and an electron transport system are required, and the terminal dioxygenases appear to be nonheme iron proteins. All the α-ketoglutarate requiring dioxygenases that have been charac-

TABLE 2

Dioxygenases and their cofactors[a]

Type of reactions	Cofactors	EC No.
(1) Intramolecular dioxygenases		
(i) ring cleavage reaction	Fe(II)	1:13:11
	Fe(III)	1:13:11
	Heme	1:13:11
	Cu	1:13:11
	FAD, NAD(P)H	1:14:12
(ii) double-hydroxylation reaction	NHI, NADH, NHI-FAD	1:14:12
(iii) oxygenation reactions of sulfur and sulfur compounds	Fe(III)	1:13:11:1
	NAD(P)H, Fe(II)	1:13:11:20
(iv) lipid peroxidation	Fe(II)	1:13:11:12
	Heme	
(v) miscellaneous	Heme, tryptophan, GSH	1:14:99:1
(2) Intermolecular dioxygenases (i) α-ketoglutarate-requiring reactions	Fe(II), ascorbic acid	1:14:11
(ii) denitration	FAD, NHI	

[a] See the legend to Table 1 for details.

terized require ferrous iron and ascorbic acid. Another intermolecular dioxygenases catalyzing the reaction schematically shown in Eq. (6), 2-nitropropane dioxygenase, reportedly contains FAD and nonheme iron. The role of these cofactors in the oxygenative reactions will be discussed in detail in a later section.

FLAVIN-CONTAINING OXYGENASES

Flavins are common cofactors to oxidoreductases and oxygenases. In the former reactions, flavins are reduced by a specific substrate and then either react with O_2 to form H_2O_2, or transfer one or two electrons (or hydrogen atoms) to an electron (or hydrogen) acceptor. In contrast to these enzymes, in the latter reactions, flavins are also involved in the activation of oxygen and its incorporation into the substra[...] In many monooxygenase-catalyzed reactions, one atom of the oxygen molecule is incorporated into the substrate to form an oxygenated product and the other atom is reduced to H_2O.

(A) Internal monooxygenases. Internal monooxygenases catalyze oxygenative decarboxylation of lactate and amino acids including lysine, arginine and tryptophan with insertion of one atom of oxygen into the substrate. All of these enzymes contain flavin as a sole cofactor; lactate monooxygenase contains FMN and others FAD. The general reaction catalyzed by the monooxygenases is shown in Eq. (9).

$$\underset{\overset{|}{XH}}{\overset{\overset{H}{|}}{R-C-COOH}} + O_2 \longrightarrow R-C\overset{\overset{O}{\diagup}}{\underset{XH}{\diagdown}} + CO_2 + H_2O \qquad (9)$$

Accordingly, lactate gives acetate and amino acids give corresponding acid amides as products with concomitant formation of CO_2 and H_2O. The dehydrogenated substrate bound to the enzyme is considered to be an intermediate of the reaction.

Lysine monooxygenase catalyzes the reaction shown in Eq. (10) under aerobic conditions (Ref. 23).

$$\begin{array}{c} CH_2NH_2 \\ | \\ (CH_2)_3 \\ | \\ CHNH_2 \\ | \\ COOH \end{array} + O_2 \longrightarrow \begin{array}{c} CH_2NH_2 \\ | \\ (CH_2)_3 \\ | \\ CONH_2 \end{array} + CO_2 + H_2O \qquad (10)$$

The enzyme exhibits a typical flavoprotein absorption spectrum with maxima at 274, 385 and 400 nm (Ref. 23). Careful analyses of this enzyme ruled out the presence of a metal cofactor and it proved to be a simple flavoprotein with FAD as the sole prosthetic group. This finding suggested that flavin is not merely an electron carrier but that it could serve as the site of oxygen activation (Ref. 24).

Under anaerobic conditions, the enzyme-bound FAD is fully reduced by lysine. Introduction of oxygen after complete reduction of the enzyme-bound FAD results in the formation of an equimolar amount of α-ketoaminocaproic acid which is nonenzymatically cyclized to form piperidine-2-carboxylic acid (Eq. (11)) (Ref. 25).

$$\begin{array}{c} CH_2NH_2 \\ | \\ (CH_2)_3 \\ | \\ CHNH_2 \\ | \\ COOH \end{array} \xrightarrow[\text{EFADH}_2]{\text{EFAD}} \begin{array}{c} CH_2NH_2 \\ | \\ (CH_2)_3 \\ | \\ C=NH \\ | \\ COOH \end{array} \xrightarrow[\text{NH}_3]{\text{H}_2\text{O}} \begin{array}{c} CH_2NH_2 \\ | \\ (CH_2)_3 \\ | \\ C=O \\ | \\ COOH \end{array} \underset{\longleftarrow}{\overset{-H_2O}{\longrightarrow}} \qquad (11)$$

This reaction is analogous to that catalyzed by L-amino acid oxidase and the dehydrogenated lysine, an imino acid, appears to be an intermediate of this reaction. The anaerobic reduction of the enzyme-bound FAD by an equimolar concentration of lysine is an extremely slow process. This can be explained by the findings that lysine acts as an effector as well as a substrate. The enzyme appears to have both a regulatory site and a catalytic site and the regulatory site has to be occupied by lysine or nonsubstrate effectors such as ε-aminocaproate to be in a catalytically active state (Ref. 26).

When the enzyme is pretreated with various sulfhydryl blocking reagents, then oxygenation of lysine is greatly reduced. Instead, the modified enzyme catalyzes the oxidative deamination of lysine producing α-ketoaminocaproic acid, NH_3 and H_2O_2, in

almost stoichiometric amounts. When the sulfhydryl blocking reagents are removed
from the modified enzyme, monooxygenase activity is restored (Ref. 27). Thus in
addition to the monooxygenase reaction, lysine monooxygenase catalyzes the oxidase
reaction under certain conditions. This thesis was further strengthened by the
finding that the monooxygenase catalyzes a typical oxidase reaction aerobically
with ornithine as a substrate and forms α-keto-δ-amino-n-valerate with simultaneous
formation of ammonia and H_2O_2 in stoichiometric amounts (Eq. (12)) (Ref. 28).

$$
\begin{array}{c}
CH_2NH_2 \\
| \\
(CH_2)_2 \\
| \\
CHNH_2 \\
| \\
COOH
\end{array}
+ O_2 \longrightarrow
\begin{array}{c}
CH_2NH_2 \\
| \\
(CH_2)_2 \\
| \\
C=O \\
| \\
COOH
\end{array}
+ NH_3 + H_2O_2
\qquad (12)
$$

These results are compatible with the interpretation that the primary reaction of
lysine monooxygenase may be the reduction of the enzyme-bound FAD with the formation
of an α-imino acid as an intermediate. Under anerobic conditions, the α-imino acid
analogue of lysine is released from the enzyme and hydrolyzed to form an α-keto acid.
Under aerobic conditions, the imino acid and $FADH_2$ complex reacts with oxygen to form
a ternary complex on the enzyme surface and an oxygenated product, CO_2 and H_2O, may
be formed in a concerted manner. In fact, during the steady state of the aerobic
reaction of lysine monooxygenase, the characteristic spectrum observed may be attributable to a ternary complex of enzyme, lysine and oxygen (Ref. 29).

Lactate monooxygenase, another internal monooxygenase, contains FMN and catalyzes
the reaction shown in Eq. (13) (Refs. 30,31).

$$
\begin{array}{c}
CH_3 \\
| \\
H-C-OH \\
| \\
COOH
\end{array}
+ O_2 \longrightarrow
\begin{array}{c}
CH_3 \\
| \\
COOH
\end{array}
+ CO_2 + H_2O
\qquad (13)
$$

Like lysine monooxygenase, enzyme-bound FMN of lactate monooxygenase is reduced by
lactate under anaerobic conditions with stoichiometric formation of the dehydrogenated
product, pyruvate, with concomitant formation of H_2O_2 (Ref. 32). However, pyruvate
failed to serve as the substrate for the enzyme. On the other hand, when the free
reduced enzyme is complexed with 2-^{14}C-labelled pyruvate, and O_2 is introduced into
the complex, little H_2O_2 is detected and a stoichiometric amount of [14]CH_3COOH is
formed (Ref. 33). From these findings, Lockridge et al. (Ref. 33) suggested that the
form of the enzyme reacting with O_2 is a complex of the reduced enzyme and keto acid,
and that locally produced high concentrations of H_2O_2 react with the dehydrogenated
substrate to form an oxygenated product with concomitant decarboxylation. The non-
enzymic decarboxylation of keto acid by H_2O_2 which leaves behind one oxygen in the
product has long been known (Ref. 34). In this case, primary reaction of the mono-

oxygenase would be a typical flavoprotein oxidase and the oxidase products would mutually react to form an oxygenated and decarboxylated product.

(B) <u>External monooxygenase</u>. Most of the flavin containing external monooxygenases so far studied are of bacterial origin and catalyze the hydroxylation reaction of aromatic substrates. These enzymes are simple flavoproteins in the sense that no other detectable organic coenzymes or transition metal elements are present in these enzymes, nor are they required for the catalase (Ref. 24).

Salicylate hydroxylase is a typical example of this type of enzyme and catalyzes the reaction shown in Eq. (14) (Ref. 35).

$$
\text{(benzene ring with COOH and OH)} + NADH + H^+ + O_2 \longrightarrow \text{(benzene ring with OH and OH)} + NAD^+ + CO_2 + H_2O \tag{14}
$$

The enzyme purified from *Pseudomonas putida* has a molecular weight of 51,000 and contains one mole of FAD per mole of the enzyme. Accordingly, the enzyme exhibits a typical flavoprotein absorption spectrum with maxima at 375 and 450 nm (Ref. 35). When the substrate, salicylate is added to the enzyme in the absence of NADH, the absorption maxima shift to 385 and 455 nm, respectively, with a shoulder at around 480 nm, suggesting the formation of an enzyme-substrate complex. The enzyme-bound FAD is fully reduced by an anaerobic addition of an equimolar amount of NADH. When salicylate is added to the reduced enzyme thus obtained, followed by the addition of oxygen, the stoichiometric formation of catechol occurs (Ref. 36). Similar results are obtained when the chemically reduced enzyme is used (Ref. 37). All these observations suggest that reduction of the enzyme-bound FAD by NADH is a partial reaction in the overall reaction. On the other hand, the enzyme catalyzes the oxidation reaction of NADH in the absence of the substrate (Ref. 38). However, the Km value of NADH is 1.1 mM in the absence of the substrate and is about 400 times greater than that in the presence of the substrate (2.6 μM). Moreover, the reduction rate of the enzyme-bound FAD by NADH is greatly enhanced in the presence of the substrate. Thus, the following reaction scheme (Fig. 1) is proposed (Ref. 39).

The rate-limiting step of the overall reaction appears to be in the reoxidation of the reduced enzyme-salicylate complex with O_2, which is found to reach a limiting value of 21 sec^{-1} as the O_2 concentration is increased. This value is all but identical with the molecular activity of the catalytic reaction, suggesting the presence of an intermediate X_2, which may well be a complex of reduced flavin, substrate and O_2. Likewise, an intermediate, X_1, is proposed in the reduction of the oxidized enzyme-salicylate complex by NADH. Besides the substrate, NADH oxidation is enhanced by other substrate analogues, including benzoate or dihydroxybenzoate. However, these substrate analogues are not hydroxylated and merely serve as nonsubstrate effectors, producing H_2O_2 (Ref. 40).

A similar reaction mechanism has been proposed for p-hydroxybenzoate hydroxylase,

76

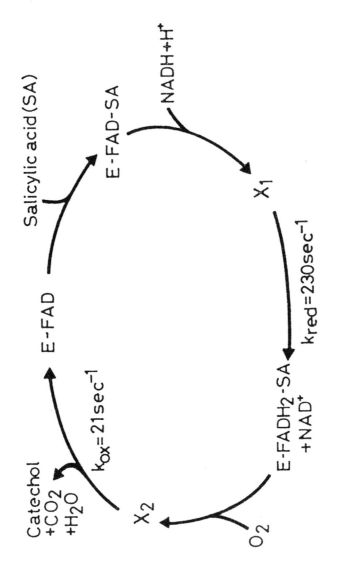

Fig. 1. Proposed reaction mechanism for salicylate hydroxylase (Ref. 39).

which catalyzes the following reaction (Eq. (15)) (Ref. 18,41).

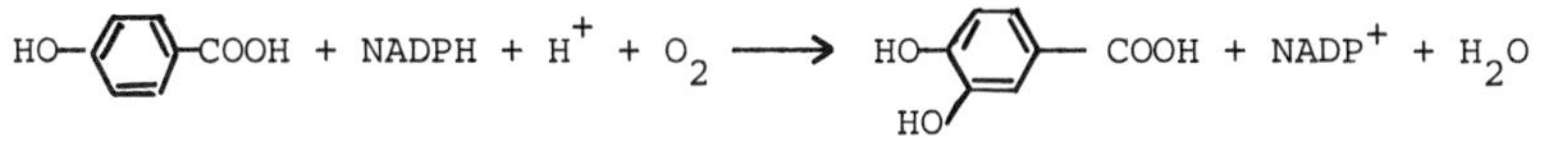

$$HO-\langle\bigcirc\rangle-COOH + NADPH + H^+ + O_2 \longrightarrow HO-\langle\bigcirc\rangle-COOH + NADP^+ + H_2O \qquad (15)$$

The reduction of enzyme-bound FAD by NADPH is also enchanced in the presence of substrate or nonsubstrate effectors with this enzyme (Refs. 42,43). The effectors
activate only the oxidase activity with the hydroxylation reaction being uncoupled and
producing H_2O_2. Such uncoupling of flavin reduction from substrate hydroxylation
appears to be a common phenomenon for this type of external monooxygenases (Ref. 18).
Thus, it is reasonable to speculate that a common reduced flavin species is involved
in both oxidase and hydroxylase reactions. In the absence of hydroxylatable substrate
this reduced flavin is reoxidized by O_2 to form oxidized flavin and H_2O_2. In the
presence of a hydroxylatable substrate, rapid kinetic studies have enabled the
spectral characterization of oxygenated intermediates when the reduced enzyme-
substrate complex is reacted with O_2. Oxygenated intermediates were detected with
p-hydroxybenzoate (Ref. 44) and 2,4-dihydroxybenzoate (Ref. 45) as substrates. No
such oxygenated intermediates have been detected with the free reduced enzyme or with
the enzyme complex with nonsubstrate effectors. With 2,4-dihydroxybenzoate as a
substrate, three different intermediates were detected (Fig. 2) (Ref. 46). The first
intermediate with an absorption maximum at 385 nm was postulated to be the 4a-
hydroperoxyflavin by comparing with spectral properties of the model compounds.

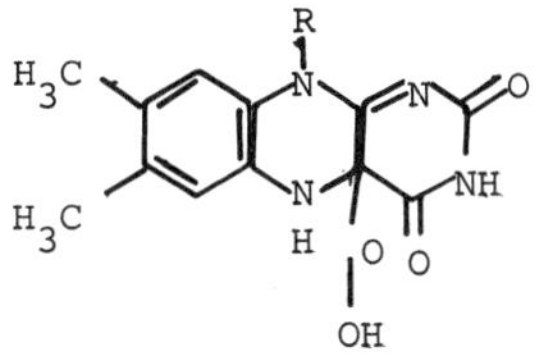

The rapid-quench experiments indicate that oxygen atom transfer from the first intermediate to the protein-bound substrate occurs coincidentally with the formation of
intermediate II. As only one atom of molecular oxygen is transferred in the hydroxylation reaction, it is postulated that intermediate II represents a complex of
hydroxydihyroflavin and a precursor of the product. The deprotonation may occur
during the enzyme-bound state, thereby resulting in the formation of intermediate III,
a complex of the product and enzyme with the flavin in the form of a hydroxydihydro-
flavin. By elimination of H_2O and the release of product, reversion would then be
made to the oxidized enzyme (Ref. 46). A similar oxygenated flavin intermediate has
been found with other external flavin monooxygenases, melilotate hydroxylase and
phenol hydroxylase (Ref. 18).

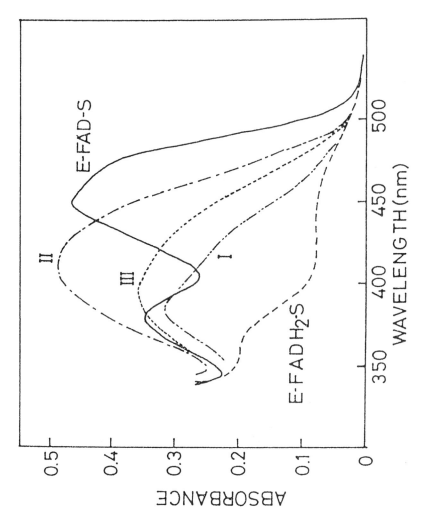

Fig. 2. Intermediates in the reaction of oxygen with reduced p-hydroxybenzoate hydroxylase complex with 2,4-dihydroxybenzoate. Data of Entsch, Massey and Ballou (Ref. 46).

(C) Dioxygenases. FAD-dependent dioxygenase, 2-methyl-3-hydroxypyridine-5-carboxylic acid oxygenase, purified from *Pseudomonas* MA1, catalyzes the following reaction (Eq. (16)).

$$HO \diagup COOH + NADH + H^+ + O_2 \rightarrow HO - C \diagup COOH + NAD^+ \qquad (16)$$

The crystalline oxygenase is homogenous and contains 2 moles of FAD per mole of enzyme, based on the molecular weight of 166,000 (Ref. 47). Under anaerobic conditions, the FAD in the enzyme is reduced by NADH; admission of oxygen reoxidizes the enzyme slowly, whereas on addition of oxygen and compound I, rapid reoxidation of the enzyme occurs with formation of the open chain product (compound II). When free FAD, FMN or riboflavin is added to the reaction mixture, oxidation of NADH remains dependent on the presence of the oxygenase and compound I, but is partially uncoupled from the oxygenation of compound I. Under these conditions, free reduced flavine appear. Such uncoupling may lead to appearance of artifactual species of activated oxygen or flavin that play no intermediate role in the oxygenase reaction (Ref. 48).

2-Nitropropane dioxygenase, catalyzing the reaction shown in Eq. (17) is another flavin-containing dioxygenase.

$$2 \; H-\overset{CH_3}{\underset{CH_3}{C}}-NO_2 + O_2 \longrightarrow 2 \; \overset{CH_3}{\underset{CH_3}{C}}=O + 2 \; HNO_2 \qquad (17)$$

The enzyme purified to homogeneity from *Hansenula mrakii* (IFO 0895) contains 1 mole of FAD and 1 g atom of nonheme iron per mole of enzyme, based on the molecular weight of 62,000 (Ref. 49). Stoichiometrical studies together with the results of ^{18}O experiments show that two atoms of molecular oxygen are incorporated into two molecules of the product formed from 2-nitropropane. Accordingly, the enzyme may be classified as an intermolecular dioxygenase. The enzyme-bound FAD is reduced by the substrate, 2-nitropropane, under anaerobic conditions, but the enzyme-bound Fe(III) is not affected. The role of these cofactors in the catalysis is not clear at present. However, the addition of superoxide dismutase to the reaction system resulted in a significant decrease in nitrate formation from 2-nitropropane. A O_2^- trapper, cytochrome c, is also a potent inhibitor of the reaction with concomitant reduction of the cytochrome. The enzyme is also inhibited by epinephrine and the absorbance at 480 nm is increased during the inhibition. Further, the enzyme catalyzes the oxidation of 2-nitropropane by KO_2 under anaerobic conditions. These findings indicate that the enzyme reaction is mediated by O_2^- formed through the enzymic univalent reduction of molecular oxygen with 2-nitropropane (Ref. 50).

HEME-CONTAINING OXYGENASES

Proteins containing heme prosthetic groups play diverse roles in all living organisms. They are involved in oxygen carriage as in hemoglobin and myoglobin, electron transfer as in cytochromes, reduction of oxygen as in cytochrome oxidase, reduction of peroxides as in catalases and peroxidases, and in oxygen transfer as in oxygenases. Included among oxygenases are cytochrome P450s which act as terminal components in multienzyme systems involved in monooxygenation of a wide variety of organic compounds, and the indole ring-cleaving enzymes, tryptophan 2,3-dioxygenase, and indoleamine-2,3-dioxygenase which are hemoproteins. Differing from oxygen carrying proteins, these hemoprotein oxygenases function to activate molecular oxygen enabling the incorporation of oxygen into an organic compound, although the oxygen carrying proteins also catalyze monooxygenation reactions under certain conditions (Ref. 51).

(A) Monooxygenase. Cytochrome P450s are carbon monoxide-binding pigments origi- nally found in liver microsomes by Klingenberg (Ref. 52) and Garfinkel (Ref. 53), and were identified as a protohemoprotein by Omura and Sato (Ref. 54). The cytochromes are widely distributed in nature and are involved in detoxification of foreign chemicals, conversion of precarcinogenic chemicals to carcinogens, and metabolic conversion of steroid compounds (Ref. 55). Thus, studies on the cytochrome P450 have produced important and fruitful knowledge in the fields of biochemistry, pharmacology and endocrinology. Recent developments in this field have been reviewed in a large number of original papers, review articles and symposia (Refs. 7-10,19,20).

Cytochrome P450 is the terminal component in the multienzyme systems which consist of electron transfer systems funnelling electrons initially from NAD(P)H, to the terminal monooxygenase. The electron transport from the pyridine nucleotide to the hemoprotein is mediated by two different mechanisms. In one group, the electron trans- port system consists of a flavoprotein and an iron-sulfur protein for the reduction of the cytochrome as in mitochondrial and bacterial systems. In another group, a flavoprotein directly transfers electrons to the cytochrome from pyridine nucleotide, as in the case of microsomal systems.

The mammalian cytochrome P450 systems are membrane bound and cannot be purified without the use of detergents or other solubilizing agents (Refs. 56,57). However, the bacterial P450 system functioning in methylene hydroxylation of D-camphor from *Pseudomonas putida* (Eq. (18)) are soluble proteins, and all three components of the mutienzyme complex, cytochrome P450 cam, putidaredoxin reductase (a flavoprotein) and putidaredoxin (an iron-sulfur protein) have been obtained in crystalline forms (Ref. 20). Thus, extensive studies on the mechanism of action of this cytochrome system have been carried out using these preparations.

$$\text{(camphor structure)} + \text{NADH} + \text{H}^+ + O_2 \rightarrow \text{(hydroxylated camphor structure)} + \text{NAD}^+ + H_2O \qquad (18)$$

Fig. 3 illustrates the reaction cycle of the cytochrome P450 cam (Refs. 58,59). The resting state of the enzyme having a Soret peak at 417 nm is a low-spin Fe(III) form, which interacts with the substrate, D-camphor, resulting in the formation of an enzyme-substrate complex (ES complex). The ES complex has a Soret peak at 391 nm and is a high-spin Fe(III) form. The complex undergoes reduction by electrons originating from NADH and transferred by a flavoprotein, NADH-putidaredoxin reductase, and an iron-sulfur protein, putidaredoxin. The reduced ES complex having a Soret peak at 408 nm, then reacts with dioxygen to form an oxycytochrome P450, which shows absorption maxima at 418, 555, and 580 nm. Carbon monoxide can bind to the reduced ES complex in a competitive manner with oxygen and gives a Soret peak at 446, thus accounting for the name of this class of enzyme. The introduction of the second electron to the oxy form results in the formation of the hydroxylated product and water in a concerted process, and the enzyme back in its original Fe(III) low-spin form.

The oxy-complex of the cytochrome P450 is formed only in the presence of the substrate and its absorption spectrum is similar to those of oxyhemoglobin and oxy-myoglobin, known to bind oxygen directly to the heme iron and to that of an oxygenated form of tryptophan 2,3-dioxygenase as will be discussed later (Refs. 60,61)(Table 3). Thus, the oxygenated complex is believed to be in an equilibrium between $Fe(II)O_2$ and $Fe(III)O_2^-$ forms, the heme iron being the binding and activation site of oxygen.

A similar reaction cycle has been proposed for mammalian cytochrome P450 systems by Estabrook et al. (Ref. 62) and an oxycytochrome P450 intermediate was demonstrated (Ref. 63) using the microsomal drug-metabolizing system. In the microsomal system, NADPH serves as the electron donor and a synergetic effect of NADH is observed for the cytochrome P450 catalyzed reactions. Based on such findings, it was proposed that the second electron for the reaction cycle is provided by NADH *via* cytochrome b_5 (Ref. 64).

In addition to the NADPH and oxygen-dependent monooxygenation reactions, cytochrome P450 has been demonstrated to catalyze peroxide-dependent reactions of various compounds (Ref. 65,66). When liver microsomes are incubated with ethylmorphine and hydrogen peroxide, in the absence of NADPH and in the presence of sodium azide to inhibit microsomal catalase, formaldehyde, a product of N-demethylation of ethylmorphine is formed concomitant with a stoichiometric utilization of hydrogen peroxide (Ref. 67). This reaction is not dependent on the presence of oxygen and is not inhibited by carbon monoxide, but the reaction product is analogous to that obtained

82

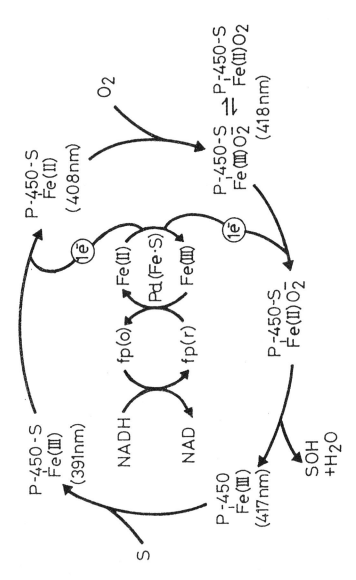

Fig. 3. Oxidation-reduction cycle of cytochrome P-450 cam. The symbols fp(o) and fp(r) represent oxidized and reduced forms of a flavoprotein, NADH-putidaredoxin reductase, respectively; and Pd. denotes putidaredoxin, an iron-sulfur protein (Fe-S).

TABLE 3

Absorption maxima of oxygenated hemoproteins[a]

Hemoprotein	Absorption maxima (nm)		
	γ	β	α
Oxyhemoglobin	415	542	576
Oxymyoglobin	418	544	582
Peroxidase compound III	418	546	581
ESO$_2$ complex of TPO	418	545	576
ESO$_2^-$ complex of P-450	418	555	580
EO$_2$ complex of IDO	415	542	576

[a]The following abbreviations are used: ESO$_2$: a ternary complex of enzyme, sub-strate and oxygen; EO$_2$: enzyme oxygen complex; TPO: tryptophan 2,3-dioxygenase; IDO: indoleamine 2,3-dioxygenase.

by the NADPH-dependent cytochrome P450 system. On the other hand, the formation of hydrogen peroxide during the aerobic oxidation of NADPH has also been demonstrated by liver microsomes. The hydrogen peroxide formation is inhibited by inhibitors of the cytochrome P450 system, carbon monoxide and metyrapone, indicating that the reaction can be attributed to cytochrome P450 (Ref. 67). However, since there is no significant synergetic effect of NADH for the formation of hydrogen peroxide, Estabrook et al. proposed that the hydrogen peroxide is formed by dismutation of superoxide anion dissociated from the oxycytochrome P450 in which Fe(II)O$_2$ and Fe(III)O$_2^-$ are in equilibrium (Ref. 67).

The formation of hydrogen peroxide from NADPH is markedly attenuated by the presence of substrates such as ethylmorphine, which undergoes N-dimethylation by cytochrome P450. In contrast, other substrates enhance the rate of hydrogen peroxide formation without an increase in the rate of substrate monooxygenation (Refs. 68,69). This "uncoupling" phenomenon may be analogous to that observed with the flavin con-taining monooxygenases discussed above.

As catalase associated with the microsomal fraction degrades hydrogen peroxide as rapidly as it is formed, the hydrogen peroxide formation from NADPH, and the peroxi-datic reaction of cytochrome P450 may have nothing to do with the NADPH- and oxygen-dependent reaction of cytochrome P450; nevertheless, these observations may provide a clue to the understanding of the active form of oxygen in the system.

(B) Dioxygenases. Dioxygenases that catalyze the cleavage of the indole ring of tryptophan derivatives are hemoproteins. Recent review articles concerning these enzymes are available (Refs. 16,17,21,71). Recently, lipoxygenase from fungus was also found to be a hemoprotein (Refs. 71,72). In this section, discussion is focused on the indole-ring cleaving enzymes.

Tryptophan 2,3-dioxygenase catalyzes the cleavage of the pyrrole ring of tryptophan to form formylkynureine (Eq. (19)).

$$
\text{(indole structure)} - CH_2 - \underset{\underset{NH_2}{|}}{CH}COOH + O_2 \rightarrow \text{(benzene structure)} \quad (19)
$$

The enzyme has been purified either from cells of *Pseudomonas*, grown in the presence of tryptophan (Refs. 73,74) or from the livers of glucocorticoid- and L-Tryptophan-treated rats (Ref. 75). The enzymes from both sources are hemoproteins and show absorption spectra characteristic of ferriheme protein (Refs. 73-76). Feigelson and associates reported that not only heme but also copper is an essential cofactor in both bacterial and hepatic enzymes (Refs. 77,78). On the other hand, Ishimura and Hayaishi found only minute quantities of copper in their preparation and regarded these amounts as being adventitious (Ref. 79). These controversies have been resolved by recent joint experiments. The obtained results show that copper is not essential for the catalytic activity, and that heme is the sole cofactor of the enzyme (Ref. 8).

The purified Pseudomonad enzyme exhibits a typical spectrum of a high-spin proto-hemoprotein, both in its ferric and ferrous states. The heme in the enzyme is autox-idizable in the absence of the substrate, tryptophan, and the enzyme is usually isolated in the ferric form (Ref. 73). The ferric enzyme is catalytically inactive unless reducing agents such as H_2O_2 or ascorbic acid, are added, suggesting that the ferrous form of the enzyme is catalytically active (Ref. 73). When the substrate tryptophan is added to the ferrous state of the enzyme under anaerobic conditions, slight shifts of the Soret band to a longer wavelength with some hypochromicity are observed indicating the formation of an enzyme-substrate complex. This enzyme-substrate complex binds with oxygen to form a new spectral species with peaks at 418 545, and 576 nm. This new spectral species can also be observed during the steady state of the reaction (Fig. 4)(Ref. 81) and is established to be a ternary complex o oxygen, tryptophan and the enzyme, an obligatory intermediate of the reaction by mean of rapid reaction spectrophotometry and kinetic analysis (Ref. 73).

The absorption maxima of the new spectral species are almost identical to those o oxygenated hemoproteins such as oxyhemoglobin, oxymyoglobin, peroxidase compound III and oxycytochrome P450 (Table 3). As in the case of cytochrome P450, the oxygenated form of tryptophan 2,3-dioxygenase is observed only in the presence of the substrate tryptophan. Thus, a sequential order of substrate binding is suggested in which tryptophan combines with the enzyme first and then reacts with oxygen to form the oxygenated intermediate (Ref. 73). Steady state kinetic analyses of the reaction are also consistent with an ordered Bi-Uni mechanism in which tryptophan binds before oxygen (Ref. 82).

The binding of the substrate to the enzyme enhances the reactivity of the enzyme-heme, thereby increasing the affinity of the heme toward ligands such as molecular oxygen, carbon monoxide and cyanide. Thus, L-tryptophan is not a mere substrate but

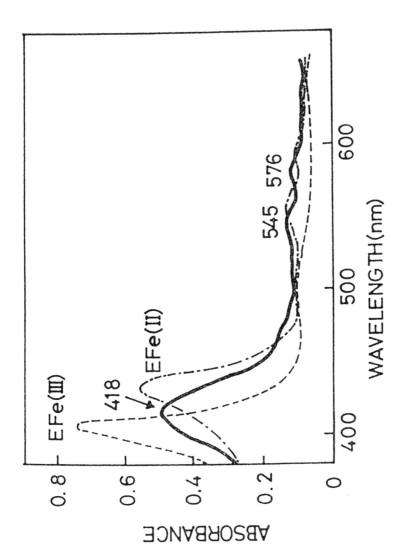

Fig. 4. Absorption spectra of tryptophan 2,3-dioxygenase. E Fe(III) and E Fe(II) represent the ferric and ferrous form of the enzyme, respectively, in the presence of L-tryptophan. Thick solid line represents the spectrum during the steady state of the reaction (Ref. 81).

also functions as an activator of the enzyme-heme in either the ferric or ferrous
state (Refs. 81-83). Furthermore, the activity of the enzyme is shown to be a sigmoidal function of L-tryptophan concentration, but the addition of a nonmetabolizable
tryptophan analogue, α-methyltryptophan, normalizes the signoidal curve to a hyperbolic one (Ref. 70). These findings, suggest the presence of two types of tryptophan
binding sites on the enzyme, catalytic and allosteric, and there appears to be a
positive cooperativity between two sites.

Indoleamine 2,3-dioxygenase (IDO) is another heme-containing dioxygenase that
catalyzes the cleavage of the indole ring of tryptophan derivatives (Eq. (19)). However, it is distinctly different from tryptophan 2,3-dioxygenase (TPO). TPO has been
found only in the liver and is specific only to the L-form of tryptophan, although
recent experiments indicate that the D-isomer is also oxygenated to varying degrees
(Ref. 84). IDO is ubiquitously distributed in various organs and tissues and
exhibits broad specificity toward indole derivatives including D- and L-isomers of
tryptophan, 5-hydroxytryptophan, serotonin, tryptamine and so forth (Ref. 85). Moreover, TPO utilizes molecular oxygen while IDO utilizes superoxide anion as well as
molecular oxygen for activity, as will be discussed below.

IDO requires methylene blue and ascorbic acid as cofactors (Ref. 86). Xanthine
oxidase with hypoxanthine, which is known to generate superoxide anion, can replace
ascorbic acid while hydrogen peroxide or its generating system can not (Ref. 86). A
highly purified preparation of IDO from rabbit intestine is inhibited by the presence
of a highly purified preparation of superoxide dismutase (Ref. 87). When the superoxide anion produced by electrolytic reduction of molecular oxygen or by potassium
superoxide (KO_2) is added to the reaction mixture in the absence of ascorbic acid,
the enzyme catalyzes the conversion of tryptophan to formylkynurenine (Ref. 88).
Moreover, experiments with ^{18}O-labelled potassium superoxide ($K^{18}O_2$) and molecular
oxygen ($^{18}O_2$) reveal that O_2^- is utilized and incorporated into the product of the
reaction and that molecular oxygen is also incorporated into the product, albeit to
a lesser extent (Ref. 89).

When potassium superoxide dissolved in dimethylsulfoxide is slowly infused into a
solution containing the native ferric form of enzyme, a new spectral species having
absorption maxima at 415, 542, and 576 nm is observed (Ref. 90). An identical spectral
species is also observed when molecular oxygen is introduced into a cuvette containing
the ferrous form of enzyme. Absorption maxima of the spectral species are almost
identical to those observed with other oxygenated hemoproteins (Table 3), indicating
that the new spectral species is a resonance form between heme-superoxide complex
$[Fe(III)O_2^-]$ and heme-dioxygen complex $[Fe(II)O_2]$. Thus, the oxygenated complex of
the enzyme is formed in the absence of the organic substrate, tryptophan. This
situation is quite different from the case of TPO or cytochrome P450, in which the
oxygenated complex is formed only in the presence of the substrate. However, this
binary complex of IDO is relatively stable, and the half life is approximately 20

minutes at pH 7.0 and 24° and it decomposes instantaneously upon addition of the substrate, tryptophan (Ref. 90). Moreover, steady state kinetic analyses reveal that the anzyme follows an ordered sequential Bi-Uni mechanism in which the organic substrate is bound to the enzyme before oxygen (Ref. 88). This sequence is analogous to that reported in the case of TPO and nonheme iron-containing dioxygenases as discussed below.

All these results taken together with the kinetic evidence (Ref. 91), Hayaishi and associates proposed that reaction mechanism of this enzyme, as shown in Fig. 5 (Refs. 51,91). First, the enzyme binds rapidly with the substrate, then the ES complex reacts with superoxide to form a ternary complex which is in equilibrium with the ferrous oxygen substrate complex. This complex is also produced by the binding of molecular oxygen with the ferrous form of enzyme and substrate complex. Once the ternary complex is produced, it decomposes to yield the reaction product, generating the ferrous form of enzyme. The first order rate constant for the decomposition is estimated to be 2.0 s^{-1} and is in good agreement with the turnover number of the enzyme, indicating that the decomposition of the ternary complex is the rate limiting step of the overall reaction. However, the ferrous form of the enzyme is slowly oxidized to the ferric form during catalysis: the latter form remains inactive in the absence of the superoxide anion. Thus, the enzyme utilizes both molecular oxygen and the superoxide anion.

Recently Hayaishi's group found that IDO and TPO catalyze NADPH-dependent hydroxylation reaction of aniline, analogous to that catalyzed by cytochrome P450 (Ref. 51). A similar reaction was also described with hemoglobin by Mieyal and coworkers (Refs. 92,93). This reaction may be comparable to the peroxidatic reaction catalyzed by the microsomal cytochrome P450 system, since it is inhibited by catalase. Nevertheless, this observation suggests that the metal dioxygen adduct is one of the so-called active forms of oxygen in hemoprotein catalyzed oxygenation and is a common step in both dioxygenase and monooxygenase catalyzed reactions.

NONHEME IRON-CONTAINING DIOXYGENASES

Cleavage of the benzene rings is a function that appears to depend almost entirely on nonheme iron-containing dioxygenases. When a benzene ring is cleaved by a dioxygenase, hydroxylation of the benzene ring usually proceeds to form catechol derivatives. Catechol derivatives are cleaved by one of two different modes by individual dioxygenases. Some enzymes rupture the bond between two hydroxylated carbon atoms to form muconic acid derivatives, a reaction referred to as intradiol cleavage. Other enzymes cleave between a hydroxylated carbon atom and an adjacent carbon carrying hydrogen, and this reaction is referred to as extradiol cleavage (Ref. 94).

Pyrocatechase catalyzing the reaction shown in Eq. (2) is a typical example of the intradiol dioxygenase. Protocatechuate 3,4-dioxygenase is another example of the intradiol type and catalyzes the conversion of protocatechic acid to β-carboxymuconic

88

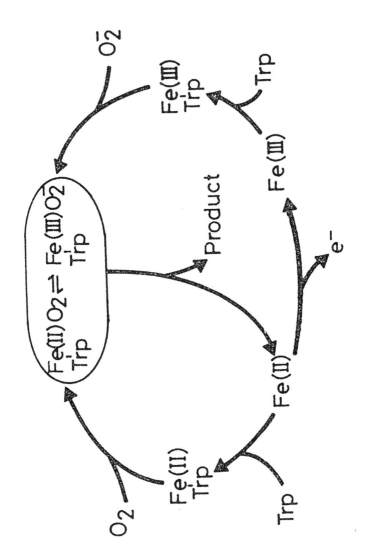

Fig. 5. Possible reaction sequence of indoleamine 2,3-dioxygenase (Refs. 90,91).

acid with the insertion of two atoms of molecular oxygen (Eq. (20)). Metapyrocatechase is a typical example of the extradiol type enzyme and catalyzes the oxygenative
cleavage of catechol to form α-hydroxymuconic semialdehyde (Eq. 21). These dioxygenases purified from *Pseudomonas* have been obtained in crystalline forms and are the
subjects of extensive studies regarding chemical structures and reaction mechanisms
(Refs. 21,95,96).

$$\tag{20}$$

$$\tag{21}$$

Both intradiol and extradiol types of enzymes contain nonheme iron as the sole
cofactor. However, dioxygenases catalyzing the intradiol cleavage are distinctly red
and contain the ferric form of iron, while those catalyzing the extradiol cleavage
are colorless and contain the ferrous form of iron.

Steady state kinetic analyses and binding studies of these two types of dioxygenase
reactions are consistent with the sequential ordered Bi-Uni mechanism shown in Eq.
(22) in which an organic substrate first combines with the enzyme to form an ES
complex and then, reacts with oxygen to form a ternary complex of enzyme, substrate
and oxygen, regardless of the valence state of the iron bound to the enzyme (Ref. 97).

$$\tag{22}$$

Since protocatechuate 3,4-dioxygenase is one of the most extensively studied nonheme iron-containing dioxygenases, discussion will mainly be focused on the structure
and function of this enzyme. For details of other nonheme iron-containing oxygenases
readers are referred to monographs (Refs. 5-7) or other review articles (Refs. 16,17,
21,95,96).

(A) Protein chemical structure. Photocatechuate 3,4-dioxygenase obtained in a
crystalline form from p-hydroxybenzoate-induced cells of *Pseudomonas aeruginosa* (Ref.
98) has a molecular weight of approximately 700,000 and contains 8 g atoms of ferric
iron and eight substrate binding sites per mole of enzyme. The enzyme is dissociated
into homogenous protomers of approximately 90,000 daltons by an alkaline treatment and
the protomers are dissociated further into four smaller subunits of two nonidentical
types $(\alpha_2\beta_2)$. The molecular weights of the α and β subunits are estimated to be
22,500 and 25,000 and their isoelectric points to be 5.2 and 9.5, respectively (Ref.
99).

There are distinct differences between amino acid compositions of each subunit. The amino acid composition of the native enzyme obtained by direct analysis agrees quite well with that calculated from the compositions of the α and β subunits based on the assumed subunit structure of $(\alpha_2\beta_2)_8$, indicating that the native enzyme consists of 8 protomers, each of which is composed of a pair of two nonidentical subunits $(\alpha_2\beta_2)$. This protomer appears to contain one atom of ferric iron, forming one active site of the enzyme (Refs. 99,100).

The β-subunit contains 238 amino acid residues, 4 of which are methionines. Therefore, cyanogen bromide cleavage of the S-carboxymethylated β-subunit gives 5 peptides. The sequences of these cyanogen bromide peptides are determined by analyses of the peptides obtained by tryptic, staphylococcal proteolytic and thermolytic digestions. The alignment of the cyanogen bromide peptides is established by examining the overlapping of sequences of the 3 methionine containing tryptic peptides, one of which contains 2 methionine residues. Thus, the total sequence of the β-subunit has been established as shown in Fig. 6 (Refs. 101,102). Likewise, the total amino acid sequence of the α-subunit which consists of 200 residues was determined by Kohlmiller and Howard (Fig. 6)(Ref. 103). The complete amino acid sequence of protocatechuate 3,4-dioxygenase was thus established by two different groups. This is the first oxygenase whose complete amino acid sequence is determine

Figure 7 shows the comparison of sequences of α and β subunits. There is no apparent homology between the two sequences, but the COOH-terminal half consists of several identical sequences, enclosed in frames in the figure, rather than in the NH_2-terminal half. It is of interest to note that pyrocatechase, another intradiol dioxygenase, also consists of two nonidentical subunits, α and β, and that both subunits shows evident homology in their NH_2-terminal sequence up to residue 21 (Ref. 104). On the other hand, an extradiol type of enzyme, metapyrocatechase, appears to consist of 4 identical subunits (Ref. 105).

A summary of subunit structures of these catechol dioxygenases is shown in Table 4. A preliminary X-ray analyses of protocatechuate 3,4-dioxygenase has recently appeared (Ref. 106).

(B) Spectral analyses. As described above, steady state kinetic analyses of catechol dioxygenases confirmed an ordered Bi-Uni mechanism where the organic substrate first combines with the enzyme to form an enzyme-substrate complex, and then reacts with oxygen to form a ternary complex of oxygen, substrate and enzyme, an oxygenated intermediate (Ref. 97). In order to confirm the involvement of such intermediates in the dioxygenase-catalyzed reactions, spectral and kinetic studies were carried ou using protocatechuate 3,4-dioxygenase.

The enzyme shows a broad absorption between 400 and 650 nm. The visible absorpti spectrum of the enzyme exhibits an increase in absorbance with a slight red shift of the peak by the addition of the substrate, protocatechuic acid, under anaerobic conditions, indicating the formation of an enzyme-substrate complex (Ref. 107). Whe

α-Subunit

```
                                    10                                         20
Pro-Ile-Glu-Leu-Leu-Pro-Glu-Thr-Pro-Ser-Gln-Thr-Ala-Gly-Pro-Tyr-Val-His-Ile-Gly-
                                    30                                         40
Leu-Ala-Leu-Glu-Ala-Ala-Gly-Asn-Pro-Thr-Arg-Asp-Gln-Glu-Ile-Trp-Asn-Arg-Leu-Ala-
                                    50                                         60
Lys-Pro-Asp-Ala-Pro-Gly-Glu-His-Ile-Leu-Leu-Leu-Gly-Gln-Val-Tyr-Asp-Gly-Asp-Gly-
                                    70                                         80
His-Leu-Val-Arg-Asp-Ser-Phe-Leu-Glu-Val-Trp-Gln-Ala-Asp-Ala-Asp-Gly-Glu-Tyr-Gln-
                                    90                                        100
Asp-Ala-Tyr-Asn-Leu-Glu-Asn-Ala-Phe-Asn-Ser-Phe-Gly-Arg-Thr-Ala-Thr-Thr-Phe-Asp-
                                   110                                        120
Ala-Gly-Glu-Trp-Thr-Leu-His-Thr-Val-Lys-Pro-Gly-Val-Val-Asn-Asn-Ala-Ala-Gly-Val-
                                   130                                        140
Pro-Met-Ala-Pro-His-Ile-Asn-Ile-Ser-Leu-Phe-Ala-Arg-Gly-Ile-Asn-Ile-His-Leu-His-
                                   150                                        160
Thr-Arg-Leu-Tyr-Phe-Asp-Asp-Glu-Ala-Gln-Ala-Asn-Ala-Lys-Cys-Pro-Val-Leu-Asn-Leu-
                                   170                                        180
Ile-Glu-Gln-Pro-Gln-Arg-Arg-Glu-Thr-Leu-Ile-Ala-Lys-Arg-Cys-Glu-Val-Asp-Gly-Lys-
                                   190                                        200
Thr-Ala-Tyr-Arg-Phe-Asp-Ile-Arg-Ile-Gln-Gly-Glu-Gly-Glu-Thr-Val-Phe-Phe-Asp-Phe
```

β-Subunit

```
                                    10                                         20
Pro-Ala-Gln-Asp-Asn-Ser-Arg-Phe-Val-Ile-Arg-Asp-Arg-Asn-Trp-His-Pro-Lys-Ala-Leu-
                                    30                                         40
Thr-Pro-Asp-Tyr-Lys-Thr-Ser-Ile-Ala-Arg-Ser-Pro-Arg-Gln-Ala-Leu-Val-Ser-Ile-Pro-
                                    50                                         60
Gln-Ser-Ile-Ser-Glu-Thr-Thr-Gly-Pro-Asn-Phe-Ser-His-Leu-Gly-Phe-Gly-Ala-His-Asp-
                                    70                                         80
His-Asp-Leu-Leu-Leu-Asn-Phe-Asn-Asn-Gly-Gly-Leu-Pro-Ile-Gly-Glu-Arg-Ile-Ile-Val-
                                    90                                        100
Ala-Gly-Arg-Val-Val-Asp-Gln-Tyr-Gly-Lys-Pro-Val-Pro-Asn-Thr-Leu-Val-Glu-Met-Trp-
                                   110                                        120
Gln-Ala-Asn-Ala-Gly-Gly-Arg-Tyr-Arg-His-Lys-Asn-Asp-Arg-Tyr-Leu-Ala-Pro-Leu-Asp-
                                   130                                        140
Pro-Asn-Phe-Gly-Gly-Val-Gly-Arg-Cys-Leu-Thr-Asp-Ser-Asp-Gly-Tyr-Tyr-Ser-Phe-Arg-
                                   150                                        160
Thr-Ile-Lys-Pro-Gly-Pro-Tyr-Pro-Trp-Arg-Asn-Gly-Pro-Asn-Asp-Trp-Arg-Pro-Ala-His-
                                   170                                        180
Ile-His-Phe-Gly-Ile-Ser-Gly-Pro-Ser-Ile-Ala-Thr-Lys-Leu-Ile-Thr-Gln-Leu-Tyr-Phe-
                                   190                                        200
Glu-Gly-Asp-Pro-Leu-Ile-Pro-Met-Cys-Pro-Ile-Val-Lys-Ser-Ile-Ala-Asn-Pro-Glu-Ala-
                                   210                                        220
Val-Gln-Gln-Leu-Ile-Ala-Lys-Leu-Asp-Met-Asn-Asn-Ala-Asn-Pro-Met-Asn-Cys-Leu-Ala-
                                   230
Tyr-Arg-Phe-Asp-Ile-Val-Leu-Arg-Gly-Gln-Arg-Lys-Thr-His-Phe-Glu-Asn-Cys
```

Fig. 6. Complete amino acid sequence of protocatechuate 3,4-dioxygenase (Refs. 101-103).

```
                                                                                  6
α                                                          P I E L L P
β  P A Q D N S R F V I R D R N W H P K A L T P D Y K T S I A R S P R Q A L V S I P
                                                                                 40

   E T P S Q T A G P Y V H I G L A L E A A G N P T R D Q E I W N R L A K P D A P G   46
   Q S I S E T T G P N F S H L G F G A H D H D L L L N F N N G G L P I G E R I I     79

   E H I L L G Q V Y D G C D G H L V R D S F L E V W Q A D A D G E Y Q D A Y N L      85
   V A G R V V D D Q Y G K P V P N T L V E M W Q A N A G G R Y R H K N D R Y L A P L L 119

   E N A F N S F G R T A T T F D A G E W T L H T V K P G V V N N A A G V P M A       123
   D P N F G G V G R C L T D S D G Y Y S F R H I K P G P Y P W R N G P N D W R P     158

   P H I N I S L F A R G I N I H L H T R L Y F D D E A Q A N A K C P V L N L T I E Q 163
   A H I H F G I S G P S I A T K L L I H T Q L Y F Q G D P L I P H C P I V K S I A N 197

   P Q R R E T L I A K R C E V D G K T A Y R F D I R I Q G E G E T V F P D           199
   P E A V Q L I A K L D M N N A N P M N C L A Y R F D I V L R G Q R K T H F E N     237

   F  200
   C  238
```

Fig. 7. Comparison of sequences of α and β subunits of protocatechuate 3,4-dioxygenase. Some gaps are introduced to achieve maximum homology, and identical residues are enclosed in frames (Ref. 102).

TABLE 4

Properties of catechol dioxygenases

	Pyrocatechase	Protocatechuate 3,4-dioxygenase	Metapyrocatechase
Ec No.	1:13:11:1	1:13:11:13	1:13:11:2
Source material	*Pseudomonas arvilla* C-1	*Pseudomonas aeruginosa*	*Pseudomonas arvilla*
Type of cleavage	Intradiol	Intradiol	Extradiol
Valence of Fe	Fe(III)	Fe(III)	Fe(II)
Molecular weight	60,000	700,000	140,000
Subunit structure	$\alpha\beta$	$(\alpha_2\beta_2)_8$	α_4
	$\alpha = 30,000$	$\alpha = 22,500$	$\alpha = 35,000$
	$\beta = 32,000$	$\beta = 25,000$	
Active site	$\alpha\beta$-Fe(III)	$\alpha_2\beta_2$-Fe(III)	α-Fe(II)

the ES complex is mixed with a buffer solution containing oxygen, a short-lived new spectral species characterized by a broad absorption band with a maximum between 500 and 520 nm appears after 3 msec, and the original spectrum of the ES complex is restored upon the exhaustion of oxygen (Ref. 108). A spectrum similar to the new spectral species is also observed with slow reacting substrates such as 3,4-dihydro-xyphenylacetic acid and 3,4-dihydroxyphenylpropionic acid during the steady state (Ref. 109). These spectra are distinct from those of the enzyme, enzyme-substrate complex or a mixture of both and appear only in the presence of both organic substrate and oxygen. Detailed kinetic analyses of the enzyme with the slow reacting substrate reveal that the new spectral species is indeed an obligatory intermediate and is a ternary complex of oxygen, substrate and enzyme, i.e., an oxygenated intermediate (Ref. 109). In order to form the oxygenated intermediate, an organic substrate must be present. This situation is the same as those observed with heme-containing oxygenases mentioned above, and is consistent with the reaction sequence shown in Eq. (22). The decomposition of the oxygenated intermediate appears to be the rate-limiting step for the overall reaction since the rate constant agrees quite well with the turnover number based on the active site of the enzyme.

(C) <u>Iron site structure</u>. The iron in the intradiol enzyme is reported to be high-spin ferric in a rhombic environment (Ref. 107,110). However, there had been controversial reports as to the ligands of the iron bound to the enzyme; Blumberg and Peisach suggested on the basis of ESR spectroscopy, a tetrahedral arrangement of 4 cysteinyl sulfur atoms (Ref. 111), while Que et al. suggested coordination of nitrogen or oxygen atom, but not sulfur, to the ferric iron, based on their Mössbauer studies (Ref. 112). In order to clarify this discrepancy, resonance Raman spectral studies of the enzyme were carried out (Ref. 113). When the enzyme is excited at the 488 nm line of an argon ion laser, four prominent Raman lines are observed at 1177, 1265, 1505 and 1605 cm^{-1}, but none of these lines are detectable for the apo and colorless ferrous enzymes. Thus, the appearance of these Raman lines apparently requires the presence of ferric iron. These Raman lines are attributable to the ring vibration of ferric iron coordinated by tyrosine ligands by comparison with spectra of model iron phenolate complexes (Ref. 113). Since these Raman lines are not disturbed by the addition of substrate under anaerobic conditions, the tyrosine ligation is not altered in the enzyme-substrate complex (Ref. 113), in which the iron remains in a high-spin ferric form (Ref. 112). The substrate may coordinate to the iron via the orthodihydroxy grouping (Ref. 114). Raman spectra of the ESO_2 complex with various substrate analogues reveal that the visible spectrum is still dominated by the tyrosine-iron charge transfer interactions (Refs. 114,115). In this complex iron still remains high-spin ferric (Ref. 112).

Raman spectra similar to those obtained with protocatechuate 3,4-dioxygenase have been observed with another intradiol dioxygenase, pyrocatechase (Ref. 96), which contains high-spin ferric iron, thus, the iron site structure of this enzyme is probably identical to that of protocatechuate 3,4-dioxygenase.

On the other hand, an extradiol dioxygenase, metapyrocatechase, is colorless, shows no significant signal in ESR spectra, and is extremely unstable to oxidants such as O_2 or H_2O_2, unless 10% acetone is present (Ref. 116). Thus, the iron in the active enzyme is likely to be in the ferrous form (Ref. 117). However, another extradiol enzyme, protocatechuate 4,5-dioxygenase reportedly contains either low spin Fe(II) or antiferromagnetically coupled high spin Fe(III), as determined in Mössbauer studies (Ref. 118). Recent Mössbauer studies on the native metapyrocatechase (Ref. 119) revealed that the relatively high isomeric shift, $\delta = 1.31$ mm/s and the large quadrupole splitting, $E_Q = 3.28$ mm/s clearly verify the presence of high-spin Fe(II) in this enzyme. The observed values of isomeric shift and quadrupole splitting of metapyrocatechase are very close to those of the reduced form of protocatechuate 3,4-dioxygenase (Ref. 112) and to reduced hemerythrin (Ref. 120), but not to that of rubredoxin (Ref. 121)(Table 5). Thus, it seems probable that the iron in metapyrocatechase resides in an environment similar to those of proto-catechuate 3,4-dioxygenase and hemerythrin, in which a tyrosine residue coordinates to the iron as a phenolate anion. The ES complex of metapyrocatechase shows a Mössbauer spectrum essentially identical to that of the native enzyme and with no ESR signals, thereby implying that the substrate does not alter either the coordination environment around the Fe(II) or the valence state of the iron upon its binding to the protein (Ref. 119).

The Mössbauer data of protocatechuate 4,5-dioxygenase (Ref. 118) are quite different from those of metapyrocatechase, although both enzymes are colorless, ESR silent and catalyze the extradiol cleavage of the catechol ring. Whether the difference in spectroscopic observations in these two extradiol dioxygenases are due

TABLE 5

Mössbauer data of various iron-containing proteins

Iron-containing proteins	$T_{(K)}$	$\delta_{(mm/s)}$	$\Delta E_{0\,(mm/s)}$	Reference
Metapyrocatechase	4	1.31	3.28	(119)
Protocatechuate 3,4-dioxygenase (reduced form)	4	1.21	3.13	(112)
Hemerythrin (reduced form)	4	1.20	2.89	(120)
Rubredoxin (reduced form)	4	0.70	3.25	(121)
Protocatechuate 4,5-dioxygenase	100	0.42 0.60 or 0.49 0.52	0.64 0.63 0.80 0.45	(118)

to the purity of enzyme, i.e., iron contamination, or to different characteristics of the individual enzymes, needs further experimentation. However, Lipscomb and Wood (Ref. 122) recently reported that Mössbauer spectra of several preparations with different specific activities show a direct correlation between the ferrous iron concentration and activity and suggested that the enzyme has an active site ferrous iron.

(D) Extradiol cleavage of catechols by intradiol dioxygenases. It has been believed that the site of cleavage of an aromatic ring is strictly specific for each enzyme; the ferric iron-containing dioxygenases exclusively cleave the catechol ring in the intradiol manner, whereas the ferrous iron-containing dioxygenases cleave it in the extradiol manner. However, a ferric iron-containing dioxygenase, pyrocatechase, from Pseudomonas arvilla C-1 catalyzes both intradiol and extradiol cleavage when 3-substituted catechols are used as the substrate (Ref. 123). The enzyme catalyzes exclusively intradiol cleavage with catechol or 4-substituted catechols as substrates, but it catalyzes both intradiol and proximal extradiol cleavage (C_2 - C_3 cleavage) on 3-substituted catechol derivatives with the intradiol to extradiol cleavage ratio of 17 for 3-methylcatechol and 5 for 3-methoxycatechol. In any case, no distal extradiol cleavage (C_1 - C_6 cleavage) is observed.

The extradiol cleavage of 3-methylcatechol by the intradiol enzymes was confirmed by Hou et al. (Ref. 124) with pyrocatechase from various microorganisms. Que also reported that when o-aminophenol is added to pyrocatechase from Pseudomonas arvilla, ring cleavage between C_1 and C_6 yields an intermediate which cyclizes rapidly to picolinic acid (Ref. 125). Thus, pyrocatechase from Pseudomonad catalyzes the following cleavage reactions on various catechol derivatives:

OH   OH   OH   OH   OH   OH   NH$_2$ OH

R   R

Both intradiol and extradiol cleavage reactions on pyrogallol, 3-hydroxycatechol,
are expected to produce the same reaction product, α-hydroxymuconic acid. However,
an extradiol enzyme, metapyrocatechase, gives a product having an absorption
maximum at 290 nm at pH 7.5. This initial product is gradually converted to a more
stable compound having an absorption peak at 239 nm. At an alkaline pH, the absorption peak shifts to 350 nm. On the other hand, an intradiol enzyme, protocatechuate
3,4-dioxygenase, gives a product having an absorption peak at 300 nm at pH 7.5.
However, upon the addition of alkali (pH 12.0), a new spectral species having a peak
at 350 nm appears which is found to be the same as the species noted in the case
of metapyrocatechase. Therefore, primary reaction products of pyrogallol resulting f
the action of metapyrocatechase and protocatechuate 3,4-dioxygenase are not identical, but in an alkaline medium, both primary reaction products are converted to the
same compound, having an absorption maximum at 350 nm. These results taken together
with the identification of the primary products by optical, infrared and NMR spectro-
scopies, and by thin layer chromatographies, in comparison with the authentic samples
suggest that the primary product obtained by the action of metapyrocatechase is
α-hydroxymuconic acid and that obtained by protocatechuate 3,4-dioxygenase is
2-pyrone-6-carboxylic acid, respectively (Ref. 126). Pyrocatechase from *Pseudomonas
arvilla* gives a mixture of nearly equimolar amounts of these two compounds, suggestin
that the enzyme also catalyzes both intradiol and extradiol cleavage with pyrogallol
as substrate (Fig. 8).

(E) Formation of 2-pyrone-6-carboxylic acid from pyrogallol. To elucidate the
reaction mechanism for the formation of 2-pyrone-6-carboxylic acid from pyrogallol by
the action of protocatechuate 3,4-dioxygenase, tracer experiments were carried out
using oxygen-18 gas. The results indicated that 1 atom of ^{18}O is incorporated into
2-pyrone-6-carboxylic acid which is isolated as its methyl ester. Mass and infrared
spectroscopy clearly showed that the isotopic oxygen is distributed in both oxygens
of the ester moiety, but neither of the oxygens of the lactone moiety contains an
isotopic oxygen, indicating that the free dicarboxylic acid is not involved in the
formation of the lactone (Ref. 126). The present experimental results may be
explained by the reaction mechanism shown in Fig. 9. In this scheme, the presence
of an enol group is important and tautomerization of the enol to the keto form in
the fifth step may make it possible to form the lactone. When the tautomerization
of the enol group is hampered in some way by the specificity of the enzyme, the
seven-numbered lactone would be cleaved to form the muconic acid derivatives. This
may be the first experimental evidence for the participation of the seven-membered
lactone, as proposed by Hamilton (Ref. 127) in the case of dioxygenase reaction.

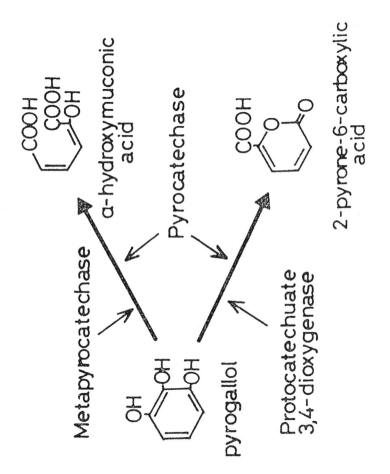

Fig. 8. Cleavage of pyrogallol by extradiol and intradiol dioxygenases.

98

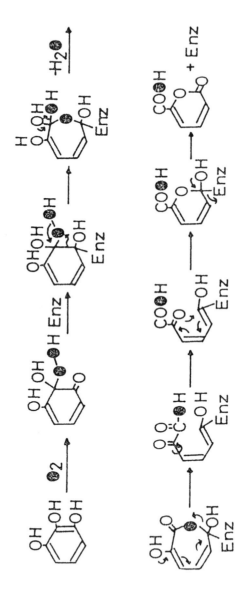

Fig. 9. Proposed mechanism for the formations of 2-pyrone-6-carboxylic acid from pyrogallol by the action of protocatechuate 3,4-dioxygenase.

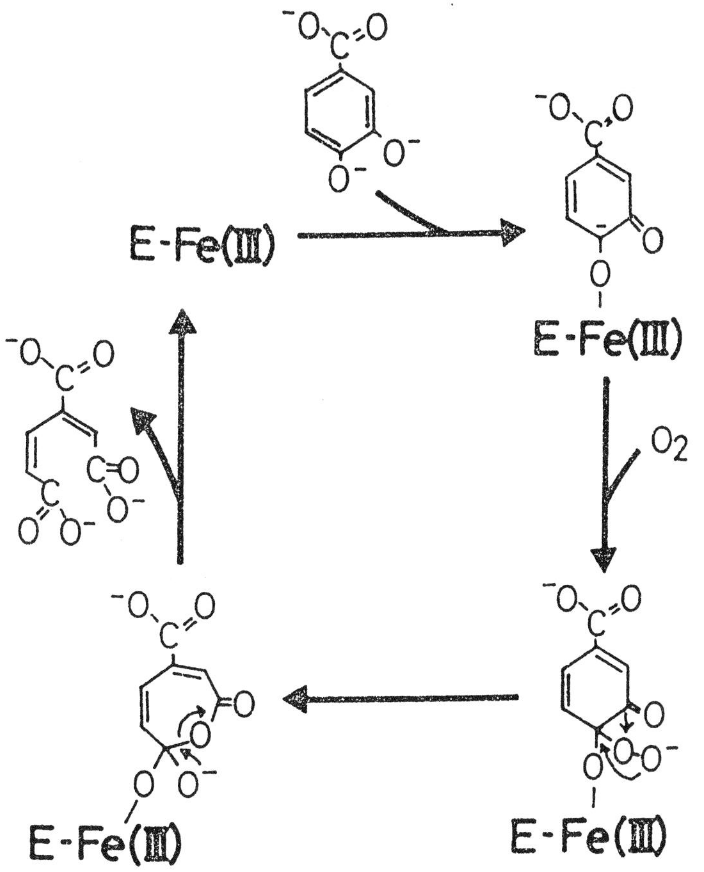

Fig. 10. Proposed reaction mechanism of protocatechuate 3,4-dioxygenase.

(F) <u>Proposed mechanism</u>. In light of all the aforementioned data, we propose the
reaction mechanism of protocatechuate 3,4-dioxygenase as shown in Fig. 10. The
enzyme contains high-spin ferric iron in the active site and the enzyme reacts with
organic substrate first to form an ES complex. The iron appears to be involved in
the formation of the ES complex as the binding site for the substrate. The ES
complex then reacts with oxygen to form a ternary complex (ESO_2). Since the iron
appears to remain in the ferric form in the ES and ESO_2 complexes, and there is no
precedent for the formation of a ferric iron-oxygen complex, oxygen might react
with the activated substrate rather than with the ferric iron to form a peroxide.
This peroxide intermediate undergoes a rearrangement to form a seven-membered lactone
as originally proposed by Hamilton (Ref. 127), and which then breaks down to form
the ring fission product.

Whether or not this same reaction mechanism is applicable to other dioxygenase
reactions needs further experiments.

CONCLUDING REMARKS

In the foregoing sections, we discussed recent findings regarding the structure
and reaction mechanism of three different classes of oxygenases, flavin-, heme- and
nonheme iron-containing oxygenases. Regardless of the cofactor involved in these
oxygenase reactions, oxygenated forms of enzyme have been demonstrated to be an
obligatory intermediate. In all cases, the enzyme binds oxygen only in the presence
of substrate to form a ternary complex of ESO_2, thereby suggesting that the binding
of the substrate to the enzyme leads to a conformational change, facilitating the
oxygen binding. Either substrate or oxygen or both are probably activated in the
ternary complex and react together to form the oxygenated end product.

There have been numerous arguments as to the nature of the so-called "active form
of oxygen"; whether it is singlet oxygen, superoxide anion, oxene, or other species
of oxygen, but no definite evidence has so far been available. Evidence has been
presented to indicate that superoxide anion, O_2^-, may be involved in some oxygenase
reactions. However, whether or not the free superoxide anion is an active form
of oxygen in these oxygenases-catalyzed reactions remains to be elucidated. Nevertheless, demonstration of the enzymatically active species of the oxygenated intermediate may open the way to clarification of the activation mechanism of oxygen:
Dioxygen adduct to the cofactor involved in the reaction may be the so-called
activated oxygen and may be a common form of active oxygen in both dioxygenase-
and monooxygenase-catalyzed reactions.

ACKNOWLEDGMENT

The authors are grateful to M. Ohara for critical reading of the manuscript.

REFERENCES

1. Hayaishi, O., Rothberg, S., and Methler, A.H. (1956) Abstr. 130th Meeting Am. Chem. Soc., 53C.
2. Hayaishi, O. (1962) in Oxygenases, Hayaishi, O., ed., New York: Academic Press, pp. 1-29.
3. Mason, H.S., Fowlks, W.L., and Peterson, L. (1955) J. Am. Chem. Soc., 77, 2914-2915.
4. Hayaishi, O., Katagiri, M., and Rothberg, S. (1955) J. Am. Chem. Soc., 77, 5450 -5451.
5. Hayaishi, O., ed. (1962) Oxygenases, New York: Academic Press.
6. Block, K. and Hayaishi, O., eds. (1966) Biological and Chemical Aspects of Oxygenases, Tokyo: Maruzen.
7. Hayaishi, O., ed. (1974) Molecular Mechanisms of Oxygen Activation, New York: Academic Press.
8. Boyd, G.S. and Smellie, R.M.S., eds. (1972) Biological Hydroxylation Mechanisms, New York: Academic Press.
9. Ullrich, V., Roots, I., Hildebrandt, A., Estabrook, R.W., and Conney, A.W., eds. (1976) Microsomes and Drug Oxidations, New York: Pergamon Press.
10. Sato, R. and Omura, T., eds. (1978) Cytochrome P-450, Tokyo: Kodansha.
11. Mason, H.S. (1957) Adv. Enzymol., 19, 79,233.
12. Hayaishi, O. (1962) Ann. Rev. Biochem., 31, 25-46.
13. Mason, H.S. (1965) Ann. Rev. Biochem., 34, 595-634.
14. Hayaishi, O. (1966) Pharmacol. Rev., 18, 71-75.
15. Hayaishi, O. and Nozaki, M. (1969) Science, 164, 389-396.
16. Nozaki, M. and Ishimura, Y. (1975) in Microbial Iron Metabolism, Nielands, J.B., ed., New York: Academic Press, pp. 417-444.
17. Hayaishi, O., Nozaki, M., and Abbott, M.T. (1975) in The Enzymes, Vol. XII, Boyer, P., ed., New York: Academic Press, pp. 119-189.
18. Massey, V. and Hemmerich, P. (1975) in The Enzymes, Vol. XII, Boyer, P., ed., New York: Academic Press, pp. 191-252.
20. Gunsalus, I.C. and Slgar, S.G. (1978) Adv. Enzymol., 47, 1-44.
21. Nozaki, M. (1979) Top. Curr. Chem., 78, 145-186.
22. Hayaishi, O. (1964) Proc. Plenary Sessions, 6th Intern. Congr. Biochem., N.Y. Vol. 33, pp. 31-43.
23. Takeda, H., Yamamoto, S., Kojima, Y. and Hayaishi, O. (1969) J. Biol. Chem., 244, 2935-2941.
24. Yamamoto, S., Takeda, H., Maki, Y., and Hayaishi, O. (1969) J. Biol. Chem., 244, 2951-2955.
25. Yamamoto, S., Nakazawa, T., and Hayaishi, O. (1972) J. Biol. Chem., 247, 3434-3438.
26. Flashner, M.I.S. and Massey, V. (1974) J. Biol. Chem., 249, 2587-2592.
27. Yamauchi, T., Yamamoto, S., and Hayaishi, O. (1973) J. Biol. Chem., 248, 3750-3752.
28. Nakazawa, T., Hori, K., and Hayaishi, O. (1972) J. Biol. Chem., 247, 3439-3444.
29. Yamamoto, S., Hirata, H., Yamauchi, T., Nozaki, M., Hiromi, K., and Hayaishi, O. (1971) J. Biol. Chem., 246, 5540-5542.
30. Sutton, W.B. (1955) J. Biol. Chem., 216, 749-761.
31. Hayaishi, O. and Sutton, W.B. (1957) J. Am. Chem. Soc., 79, 4809-4810.
32. Sutton, W.B. (1957) J. Biol. Chem., 226, 395-405.
33. Lockridge, O., Massey, V., and Sullivan, P.A. (1972) J. Biol. Chem., 247, 8097-8106.
34. Hamilton, G. (1971) in Progress in Bioorganic Chemistry, Vol. 1, Kaiser, T. and Kezdy, F., eds., New York: Wiley, pp. 83-157.
35. Yamamoto, S., Katagiri, M., Maeno, H., and Hayaishi, O. (1965) J. Biol. Chem., 240, 3408-3413.
36. Takemori, S., Yasuda, H., Mihara, K., Suzuki, M., and Katagiri, M. (1969) Biochim. Biophys. Acta, 191, 58-68.
37. Takemori, S., Yasuda, H., Mihara, K., Suzuki, M., and Katagiri, M. (1969) Biochim. Biophys. Acta, 191, 69-76.

38. Katagiri, M., Maeno, H., Yamamoto, S., Hayaishi, O., Kitao, T., and Oae, S. (1965) J. Biol. Chem., 240, 3414-3417.
39. Takemori, S., Nakamura, M., Suzuki, K., Katagiri, M., and Nakamura, T. (1972) Biochim. Biophys. Acta, 284, 382-393.
40. White-Stevens, R.H. and Kamin, H. (1972) J. Biol. Chem., 247, 2538-2570
41. Hosokawa, K. and Stanier, R.Y. (1966) J. Biol. Chem., 241, 2453-2460.
42. Howell, L.G. and Massey, V. (1970) Biochem. Biophys. Res. Commun., 40, 887-893.
43. Spector, T. and Massey, V. (1972) J. Biol. Chem., 247, 4679-4687.
44. Spector, T. and Massey, V. (1972) J. Biol. Chem., 247, 7123-7127.
45. Spector, T. and Massey, V. (1972) J. Biol. Chem., 247, 5632-5636.
46. Entsch, B., Massey, V., and Ballou, D.P. (1974) Biochem. Biophys. Res. Commun., 57, 1018-1025.
47. Sparrow, L.G., Ho, P.P.K., Sundaran, T.K., Zach, D., Nyns, E.J., and Snell, E. E. (1969) J. Biol. Chem., 244, 2590-2600.
48. Kishore, G.M. and Snell, E.E. (1979) Biochem. Biophys. Res. Commun., 87, 518-523.
49. Kido, T., Soda, K., Suzuki, T., and Asada, K. (1976) J. Biol. Chem., 251, 6994-7000.
50. Soda, K., Kido, T., and Asada, K. (1977) in Biochemical and Medical Aspects of Active Oxygen, Hayaishi, O. and Asada, K., eds., Toky1: University of Tokyo Press, pp. 119-133.
51. Hayaishi, O., Takikawa, O., Sono, M., and Yoshida, R. (1980) in Microsomes, Drug Oxidations and Chemical Carcinogenesis, Coon, M.J., Conney, A.H., Estabrook R.W., Gelboin, H.V., Gillette, J.R., and O'Brien, P.J., eds., New York: Academic Press, pp. 1-13.
52. Klingenberg, M. (1958) Arch. Biochem. Biophys., 75, 376-386.
53. Garfinkel, D. (1958) Arch. Biochem. Biophys., 77, 493-509.
54. Omura, T. and Sato, R. (1963) Biochim. Biophys. Acta, 71, 224-226.
55. Estabrook, R.W., Cooper, D.Y., and Rosenthal, O. (1963) Biochem. Z., 338, 741-755.
56. Imai, Y. and Sato, R. (1974) Biochem. Biophys. Res. Commun., 60, 8-14.
57. Haugen, D.A. and Coon, M.J. (1976) J. Biol. Chem., 251, 7929-7939.
58. Gunsalus, I.C., Meeks, J.R., Lipscomb, J.D., Debrunner, P., and Münck, E. (1974) in Molecular Mechanisms of Oxygen Activation, Hayaishi, O., ed., New York: Academic Press, pp. 559-613.
59. Peterson, J.A. (1979) in Biochemical and Clinical Aspects of Oxygen, Caughey, W.S., ed., New York: Academic Press, pp. 227-273.
60. Ishimura, Y., Ullrich, V., and Peterson, J.A. (1971) Biochem. Biophys. Res. Commun., 42, 140-146.
61. Peterson, J.A., Ishimura, Y., and Griffin, B.W. (1972) Arch. Biochem. Biophys., 149, 197-208.
62. Estabrook, R.W., Schenkman, J.B., Cammer, W., Remmer, H., Cooper, D.Y., Narasimhulu, S., and Rosenthal, O. (1966) in Biological and Chemical Aspects of Oxygenases, Bloch, K., and Hayaishi, O., eds., Tokyo: Maruzen, pp. 153-170.
63. Estabrook, R.W., Baron, J., Peterson, J.A., and Ishimura, Y. (1972) in Biological Hydroxylation Mechanisms, Boyd, G.S. and Smellie, R.M.S., eds., New York: Academic Press, pp. 159-185.
64. Hildebrandt, A. and Estabrook, R.W. (1971) Arch. Biochem. Biophys., 143, 66-79.
65. Estabrook, R.W. and Werringloer, J. (1977) in Drug Metabolism Concepts, Jerina, D.M., ed., American Chemical Society, pp. 1-26.
66. Blake, R.C., II and Coon, M.J. (1979) in Biochemical and Clinical Aspects of Oxygen, Caughey, W.S., ed., New York: Academic Press, pp. 263-273.
67. Estabrook, R.W. and Werringloer, J. (1977) in Microsomes and Drug Oxidations, Ullrich, V., Roots, I., Hildebrandt, A.G., Estabrook, R.W., and Conney, A., eds., Oxford: Pergamon Press, pp. 748-757.
68. Ullrich, V. and Diehl, H. (1971) Eur. J. Biochem., 20, 509-512.
69. Hildebrandt, A.G., Speck, M., and Roots, I. (1973) Biochem. Biophys. Res. Commun., 54, 968-975.
70. Feigelson, P. and Brady, F.O. (1974) in Molecular Mechanism of Oxygen Activation Hayaishi, O., ed., New York: Academic Press, pp. 87-133.

71. Satoh, T., Matsuda, Y., Takashio, M., Satoh, K., Beppu, T., and Arima, K. (1976) Agr. Biol. Chem., 40, 953-961.
72. Matsuda, Y., Satoh, T., Beppu, T., and Arima, K. (1976) Agr. Biol. Chem., 40, 963-976.
73. Ishimura, Y., Nozaki, M., Hayaishi, O., Nakamura, T., Tamura, M., and Yamazaki, I. (1970) J. Biol. Chem., 245, 3593-3602.
74. Poillon, W.N., Maeno, H., Koike, K., and Feigelson, P. (1969) J. Biol. Chem., 244, 3447-3456.
75. Schutz, G. and Feigelson, P. (1972) J. Biol. Chem., 247, 5327-5332.
76. Tanaka, T. and Knox, W.E. (1959) J. Biol. Chem., 234, 1162-1170.
77. Brady, F.O., Monaco, M.E., Forman, H.J., Schutz, G., and Feigelson, P. (1972) J. Biol. Chem., 247, 7915-7922.
78. Maeno, H. and Feigelson, P. (1965) Biochem. Biophys. Res. Commun., 21, 297-302.
79. Ishimura, Y. and Hayaishi, O. (1973) J. Biol. Chem., 248, 8610-8612.
80. Ishimura, Y., Makino, R., Ueno, R., Sakaguchi, K., Brady, F.O., Feigelson, P., Aisen, P., and Hayaishi, O. (1980) J. Biol. Chem., 255, 3835-3837.
81. Ishimura, Y., Nozaki, M., Hayaishi, O., Tamura, M., and Yamazaki, I. (1967) J. Biol. Chem., 242, 2574-2576.
82. Forman, H.J. and Feigelson, P. (1971) Biochemistry, 10, 760-763.
83. Ishimura, Y., Nozaki, M., Hayaishi, O., Tamura, M., and Yamazaki, I. (1968) Advan. Chem., 77, 235-241.
84. Watanabe, Y., Fujiwara, M., Yoshida, R., and Hayaishi, O. (1980) Biochem. J., 189, 393-405.
85. Hirata, F. and Hayaishi, O. (1972) Biochem. Biophys. Res. Commun., 47, 1112-1119.
86. Yamamoto, S. and Hayaishi, O. (1967) J. Biol. Chem., 242, 5260-5266.
87. Hirata, F. and Hayaishi, O. (1971) J. Biol. Chem., 246, 7825-7826.
88. Ohnishi, T., Hirata, F., and Hayaishi, O. (1977) J. Biol. Chem., 252, 4643-4647.
89. Hayaishi, O., Hirata, F., Ohnishi, T., Henry, J.P., Rosenthal, I., and Katoh, A. (1977) J. Biol. Chem., 252, 3548-3550.
90. Hirata, F., Ohnishi, T., and Hayaishi, O. (1977) J. Biol. Chem., 252, 4637-4642.
91. Taniguchi, T., Sono, M., Hirata, F., Hayaishi, O., Tamura, M., Hayaishi, K., Iizuka, T., and Ishimura, Y. (1979) J. Biol. Chen., 254, 3288-3294.
92. Mieyal, J.J., Ackerman, R.S., Blumer, J.L., and Freeman, L.S. (1976) J. Biol. Chem., 251, 3436-3441.
93. Mieyal, I.J. and Blumer, J.L. (1976) J. Biol. Chem., 251, 3442-3446.
94. Nozaki, M., Kotani, S., Ono, K., and Senoh, S. (1970) Biochim. Biophys. Acta 220, 213-223.
95. Nozaki, M. (1974) in Molecular Mechanisms of Oxygen Activation, Hayaishi, O., ed., New York: Academic Press, pp. 135-165.
96. Que, L., Jr. (1980) Structure and Bonding, 40, 39-72.
97. Hori, K., Hashimoto, T., and Nozaki, M. (1973) J. Biochem., 74, 375-384.
98. Fujisawa, H. and Hayaishi, O. (1968) J. Biol. Chem., 243, 2673-2681.
99. Yoshida, R., Hori, K., Fujiwara, M., Saeki, Y., Kagamiyama, H., and Nozaki, M. (1976) Biochemistry, 15, 4048-4053.
100. Nozaki, M., Yoshida, R., Nakai, C., Iwaki, M., Saeki, Y., and Kagamiyama, H. (1976) in Iron and Copper Proteins, Yasunobu, K.T., Mower, H.F., and Hayaishi, O., eds., New York: Plenum Press, pp. 127-136.
101. Iwaki, M., Kagamiyama, H., and Nozaki, M. (1979) J. Biochem., 86, 1159-1162.
102. Iwaki, M., Kagamiyama, H., and Nozaki, M. (1981) Arch. Biochem. Biophys., in press.
103. Kohlmiller, N.A. and Howard, J.B. (1979) J. Biol. Chen., 254, 7309-7315.
104. Nakai, C., Kagamiyama, H., Saeki, Y., and Nozaki, M. (1979) Arch. Biochem. Biophys., 195, 12-22.
105. Nakai, C., Kagamiyama, H., and Nozaki, M., unpublished data.
106. Satyshur, K.A., Rao, S.T., Lipscomb, J.D., and Wood, J.M. (1980) J. Biol. Chem., 255, 10015-10016.
107. Fujisawa, H., Uyeda, M., Kojima, Y., Nozaki, M., and Hayaishi, O. (1972) J. Biol. Chem., 247, 4414-4421.

108. Fujisawa, H., Hiromi, K., Uyeda, M., Nozaki, M., and Hayaishi, O. (1971) J. Biol. Chem., 246, 2320-2321.
109. Fujisawa, H., Hiromi, K., Uyeda, M., Okuno, S., Nozaki, M., and Hayaishi, O. (1972) J. Biol. Chem., 247, 4422-4428.
110. Nakazawa, T., Nozaki, M., Hayaishi, O., and Yamano, T. (1969) J. Biol. Chem., 244, 119-125.
111. Blumberg, W.E. and Peisach, J. (1973) Ann. N.Y. Acad. Sci., 222, 539-560.
112. Que, L., Jr., Lipscomb, J.D., Zimmerman, R., Münck, E., Orme-Johnson, N.R., and Orme-Johnson, W.H. (1976) Biochim. Biophys. Acta, 452, 320-334.
113. Tatsuno, Y., Saeki, Y., Iwaki, M., Yagi, T., Nozaki, M., Kitagawa, T., and Otsuka, S. (1978) J. Am. Chem. Soc., 100, 4614-4615.
114. Felton, R.H., Cheung, L.D., Phillips, R.S., and May, S.W. (1978) Biochem. Biophys. Res. Commun., 85, 844-850.
115. Que, L., Jr., and Heistand, R.H., II (1979) J. Am. Chem. Soc., 101, 2219-2221.
116. Nozaki, M., Kagamiyama, H., and Hayaishi, O. (1963) Biochem. Z., 338, 582-590.
117. Nozaki, M., Ono, K., Nakazawa, T., Kotani, S., and Hayaishi, O. (1968) J. Biol. Chem., 243, 2682-2690.
118. Zabinski, R., Münck, E., Champion, P.M., and Wood, J.M. (1972) Biochemistry, 3212-3219.
119. Tatsuno, Y., Saeki, Y., Nozaki, M., Otsuka, S., and Maeda, Y. (1980) FEBS Lett., 112, 83-85.
120. Okamura, M.Y., Klotz, I.M., Johnson, C.E., Winter, M.R.C., and Williams, R.J.P. (1969) Biochemistry, 8, 1951-1958.
121. Debrunner, P.G., Münck, E., Que, L., Jr., and Schulz, C.E. (1976) in Iron-Sulfur Proteins, Vol. 3, Lovenberg, W., ed., New York: Academic Press, pp. 381-417.
122. Lipscomb, J.D. and Wood, J.M. (1979) in 3rd International Symposium on Oxidases and Related Oxidation-Reduction Systems, Albany, New York, in Pergamon Press, Oxford.
123. Fujiwara, M., Golovleva, L.A., Saeki, Y., Nozaki, M., and Hayaishi, O. (1979) J. Biol. Chem., 250, 4848-4855.
124. Hou, L.T., Patel, R., and Lillard, M.O. (1977) Appl. Environ. Microbiol., 33, 725-727.
125. Que, L., Jr. (1978) Biochem. Biophys. Res. Commun., 84, 123-129.
126. Saeki, Y., Nozaki, M., and Senoh, S. (1980) J. Biol. Chem., 255, 8465-8471.
127. Hamilton, G.A. (1974) in Molecular Mechanisms of Oxygen Activation, Hayaishi, O., ed., New York: Academic Press, pp. 405-451.

CHAPTER 5   THE BIOCHEMISTRY AND PHARMACOLOGY OF OXYGEN RADICAL
             INVOLVEMENT IN EICOSANOID PRODUCTION

K. D. RAINSFORD AND B. P. SWANN
Lilly Research Centre Limited, Windlesham, Surrey GU20 6PH, U.K.

Inflammatory reactions to tissue injury or infection comprise a wide variety
of cellular responses and biochemical reactions. Among these the generation of "active
oxygen" species (including oxygen-derived free radicals) and their subsequent
enzymically-controlled and/or spontaneous reaction with long-chain unsaturated fatty
acids appears to be one of the main events in inflammation. The enzyme-controlled
reactions involve participation of the cyclo-oxygenase pathway, peroxidases, lipo-
oxygenases and other systems involved in the production and catabolism of eicosanoids
including prostaglandins (see Fig. 1). Active oxygen species are also produced
from the action of peroxidases on hydroperoxy fatty acids initially formed from
peroxidation of unsaturated fatty acids. Thus a cycle of initial fatty acid
oxidation by active oxygen species followed by their regeneration and later
rearrangement would appear theoretically to offer potential for amplification of
the inflammatory response (Fig. 1).

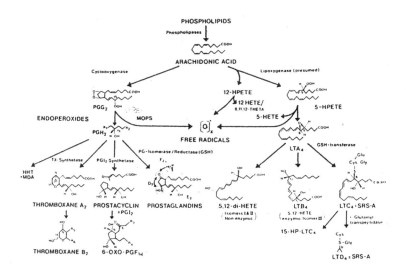

Fig. 1. Molecular events involved in the production of prostaglandins, thromboxanes
and leukotrienes showing sites of free radical production. R_1-R_6 denotes the
respective carbon chain segments derived from the precursors. HPETE = hydroperoxy-
eicosatetraenoic acid; HETE = hydroxyeicosatetraenoic acid; MOPS = Multisubstrate
oxidizing peroxidases (of Egan et al. (Ref. 186); HHT = 12-L-hydroxy 5,8,10-heptade-
catrienoic acid; MDA = malondialdehyde; GSH = glutathione.

The object of this review is to (1) focus attention on these reactions involving the participation of active oxygen species in arachidonic acid oxidation; (2) suggest what active oxygen species may be involved and discuss their actual or probable formation; and (3) indicate likely ways whereby pharmacological intervention could be employed to modulate or regulate the response to achieve a desirable therapeutic end. We do not propose to discuss the functions of the prostanoids except in relation to regulation of the formation of active oxygen species *via* hydroperoxy fatty acids. Excellent reviews have been published on the wider aspects of prostanoid production and the reader is referred to these (Refs. 1-3). Aspects of the chemistry, metabolism and biological functions of superoxide anion and related species appear elsewhere in this book and are also featured in a recent symposium (Refs. 4,5).

EICOSANOID METABOLISM AND ITS REGULATION

(a) Arachidonic acid release. Arachidonic acid (20:4) is the principal fatty acid precursor of all the dienoic prostanoids, thromboxanes, hydro(per)oxy fatty acids and leukotrienes which are produced by the cyclo-oxygenase and lipoxygenase pathways (Fig. 1) in inflammatory cells. These include polymorpho-nuclear (neutrophil) leucocytes, macrophages/monocytes, platelets (Refs. 6-14), synovial fluid (Ref. 15) and synovial fibroblasts (Ref. 16). Furthermore, the main products of these pathways, prostaglandins E_2, F_2, I_2 (prostacyclin) and thromboxane B_2 are present in high concentrations in joint effusions of patients with rheumatoid and other arthritic conditions (Refs. 17-19), or following experimentally induced inflammation or nerve stimulation (Refs. 1,8).

Arachidonic acid itself is derived from the essential fatty acid, linoleic acid (18:2) by chain elongation and desaturation (Ref. 1). The stereospecificity of this precursor is illustrated by the fact that high dietary levels of 9-*trans*, 12-*trans*-linoleate will inhibit production of both the *cis*, *cis*-isomer and arachidonic acid (Ref. 20). Arachidonic acid is released from esterified precursors (phospholipids, triglycerides or cholesterol esters) by the action of a phospholipase A_2 or possibly cholesterol esterases (Ref. 1). The release of arachidonic acid is blocked by anti-inflammatory glucocorticoids (Refs. 21-23). This effect is due to (1) direct inhibition of phospholipase A_2 activity (Ref. 24) and (2) the glucocorticoid-induced synthesis *de novo* of a polypeptide, macrocortin, which specifically inhibits the activity of phospholipase A_2 (Ref. 25). Phospho-lipase activity is also inhibited by cholesterol (Ref. 26). Tissue lipases involved in arachidonic acid release from triglycerides are inhibited by nicotinic acid (Ref. 27). Indomethacin and its analogues also directly inhibit phospholipase A_2 activity in polymorphs (Refs. 28,29).

(b) Cyclo-oxygenase activity. The pathway for the synthesis of prostanoids and thromboxanes proceeds through the combined cyclo-oxygenase/peroxidase reactions of prostaglandin (PG) endoperoxide synthetase (EC 1.14.99.1) (Refs. 2,30). This enzyme catalyzes the addition (in two steps) of two molecules of dioxygen at the 11- and 15-positions of arachidonic acid with rearrangement of the double bond at the 11-12 position. The product formed its prostaglandin G_2 (PGG_2) in which oxygen is linked as an endoperoxide bridge across the 9-11 position of arachidonic acid with a peroxy group at the 15-position (Ref. 1). Subsequent peroxidase activity, inherent at the same active site of the synthetase enzyme, converts the 15-hydroperoxy group of PGG_2 to the 15-hydroxy group in PGH_2 and liberates an oxygen radical species, which is a central component in the continuing formation of prostanoids (Fig. 1).

The purified PG endoperoxide synthetase requires an iron porphyrin center for cyclo-oxygenase activity (Refs. 30,31). It has been postulated that this cofactor is responsible for the binding and positioning of the arachidonic acid substrate to the enzyme (Ref. 32). The metal center may well function in this role as perferryl iron $(FeO)^{2+}$ (see later section on this topic). Among other metallo-porphyrins (Mn, Co, Zn) only the manganese protoporphyrin is capable of replacing the iron requirement for enzyme activity (Ref. 2). This species, however, does not exhibit the peroxidase activity inherent in the iron-porphyrin system.

(c) Peroxidase activity and reactions of $(O)_x$. The peroxidase-like conversion of PGG_2 to PGH_2 (Refs. 2,30,31), results in release of an oxidizing radical species $(O)_x$ which is thought to irreversibly self-deactivate the cyclo-oxygenase enzyme. The exact identity of $(O)_x$ has yet to be determined but the first suggestion for the nature of $(O)_x$ was a hydroxyl radical (Ref. 33). More recent studies have shown that PG endoperoxide synthetase exhibits a broad spectrum requirement for hydroperoxide activation before biosynthesis of PGs can occur. Even hydrogen peroxide can act as a substrate (Ref. 34). The iron species must aid the removal of the 13L-hydrogen from arachidonic acid to give a dienyl radical (Ref. 35). The dienyl radical acts as a site for addition of molecular oxygen and may be intercepted by suitable trapping systems (Ref. 36). Details of the mechanism whereby arachidonic acid is transformed to PGG_2 and the role of hydroperoxide activation are still not clear. The most recent overall view is provided by Hemler and Lands (Ref. 37). The consequence of the peroxidase activity of the heme iron in the cyclo-oxygenase system is the probable formation of a perferryl iron species (Refs. 38,39). This species is known to participate in many reactions involving peroxides. Two intermediates, commonly known as Compounds I and II have been identified, which are two and one oxidation levels respectively above that in the starting iron (III) center (Ref. 40).

The stereochemical features of the active site of cytochrome c peroxidase have recently been elucidated in detail (Ref. 41). Important roles are assigned to

certain histidine residues in the protein and a critical requirement is for an
arginine residue to aid cleavage of the RO-OH bond (see Fig. 2). The product is
a perferryl iron system which can be formally written as $Fe^{IV}-O^-$. The second
oxidation equivalent can either be transferred to an adjacent tryptophan residue,
as in cytochrome c peroxidase, or incorporated into the porphyrin ring itself
via oxidation to a π-cation radical as in the case of horseradish peroxidase
(Refs. 42,43). Alternative formulations based on cleavage of one iron-pyrrole
bond with oxygen atom insertion have been proposed (Ref. 44).

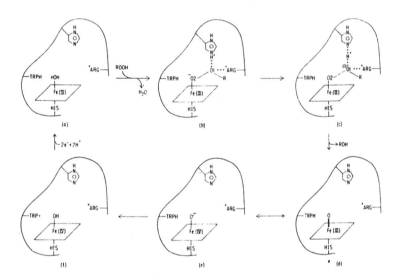

Fig. 2. Postulated mechanism of peroxidase activity involving the heme moiety,
based on the studies of the analogous reactions in cytochrome c peroxidase devised
by Poulos and Kraut (Ref. 41). This diagram is adapted from the original and is
reproduced in part with their permission. Addition of PGG$_2$ (= R-OOH) occurs between
the histidine and arginine residues and the Fe(III) porphyrin as in (b). The
subsequent cleavage of the fatty acid peroxide oxygen bond (c) and release of PGH$_2$
(= R-OH) is accompanied by formation of the perferryl iron, Fe(IV)-O$^-$, species
(d) → (e). This can either transfer one electron to an adjacent tryptophan as
in (f) or oxidize the porphyrin ring to a π-cation radical. Either species is of
sufficient high oxidation potential to abstract two hydrogen atoms from the
β-CH$_2$ unit of two independent 1,4-penta diene systems to generate the initial
carbon radical precursors of the prostaglandins. This process returns the heme
to its initial oxidation level for a further catalytic cycle. The structure of
the peptide chain to which the heme is prosthetically bound may aid the selectivity
of the oxidative hydrogen abstraction step. The formation of (d), (e) *via* (c)
explains the requirement for hydroperoxide activation of the cyclo-oxygenase
enzyme prior to PG synthesis initiation.

Recently model systems containing perferryl iron species have been prepared
(Ref. 45) and a study begun of their oxidizing properties (Ref. 46). It should be
noted that similar perferryl iron systems have been proposed as intermediates in
Fenton-type reactions and this area continues to be one of considerable controversy.

Again the nature of the ligands around the iron seem to influence which oxygen
species are produced and their relative reativity (Refs. 47-49). These species
are also related to the catalytic centers of cytochrome P-450 (Ref. 49) and
catalase (Ref. 44).

As well as PGG_2 several other hydroperoxides serve as precursors for the
perferryl iron in PG synthetase including 15-HPETE, 12-HPETE, and even hydrogen
peroxide (Ref. 34). If $(O)_x$ is ultimately shown to be a major factor in the
inflammatory response then the HPETE to HETE reaction may be of particular interest
in view of the increasing importance attached to lipoxygenase products in
inflammation. Whilst formation of HPETEs is not affected by most nonsteroidal
anti-inflammatory (NSAI) drugs there is evidence to show that the subsequent
peroxidase transformation of HPETEs to HETEs may be inhibited (Refs. 50,51).

Further elucidation of the possible contribution of HPETEs to the generation of
$(O)_x$ must await more definitive data on the nature of the iron centers involved in
their formation, their conversion to HETEs and on the relative contributions of
the lipoxygenase to cyclooxygenase pathways of arachidonic acid metabolism in any
particular pathological situation. In view of the importance of the leukotrienes
this area should receive intense investigation during the 1980s. It should also
be pointed out that other iron species are capable of converting hydroperoxides of
unsaturated fatty acids to the corresponding hydroxy derivatives.

(d) Reactions of $(O)_x$ generated from PG synthetase. The $(O)_x$ species has been
detected by electron paramagnetic resonance (EPR) spectroscopy in microsomal
preparations quenched by freezing to -196°C. The spectra gave no discernible
structure and as accurate "g" measurements could not be made it was impossible to
establish its identity (Ref. 39). A variety of molecules which are known to
scavenge hydroxyl (OH•) or related radicals, e.g., phenol, methional, paracetamol,
tryptophan and 2-methylamino-4-𝑡-butyl-6-iodophenol (MK-447) accelerate the
conversion of PGG_2 to PGH_2 (Refs. 30,33,52-54). Furthermore these phenols, as
well as some related compounds with anti-oxidant activity, prolong the lifetime
of the enzyme by protecting it from self-destruction and so enhancing overall
production of prostaglandins (Refs. 2,37).

Another approach has been to study the stoichiometry of the peroxidase reaction
in the presence of the sulphide form of the pro-drug, sulindac (Ref. 39). Sulindac
itself is only weakly effective as an inhibitor of PG synthesis but is converted
metabolically from the sulphoxide to sulindac sulphide, 𝑐𝑖𝑠-5-fluoro-2-methyl-1-
[4-(methylthio)benzilidene]indene-3-acetic acid (Refs. 55,56). The sulphide is
in turn re-oxidized in vivo and effectively acts as a scavenger of active oxygen
species in the peroxidase reaction in the PG endoperoxide synthetase pathway. The
quantitative oxidation of sulindac sulphide proceeds with the reduction of the
hydroperoxy fatty acid and occurs in the absence of molecular oxygen (Ref. 34).
Scission of the hydroperoxy group occurs to yield an oxygen atom in the sulindac

molecule, with retention of the other in the hydroxy fatty acid. This was confirmed in studies of the distribution of ^{18}O-hydroperoxy PGE_2 (labelled at the C-15 position). The most recent suggestion from this group is that the oxidation of sulindac sulphide is more readily explained by the formation of an oxygen-iron complex such as perferryl iron (FeO)$^{2+}$ (Ref. 39).

It should be made clear that (O)$_x$ produced *via* the PG synthetase/peroxidase pathway is a potent oxidizing agent. Many compounds have been shown to act as co-substrates during the PG synthetase reaction. The exact mechanism operating in any particular case may, however, vary. For example it has been shown that the co-oxidation of diphenylisobenzofuran proceeds *via* a radical chain pathway (Ref. 57) the oxidation of sulindac suophide to sulindac involves oxygen transfer (see above) whereas that of *trans*-7,8-dihydroxy-7,8-dihydrobenzo(a)pyrene does not (Ref. 58). The conclusion is that one cannot assume a particular mechanism operates based solely on precedents established in unrelated systems.

An important feature of (O)$_x$ is its reaction with the enzyme systems involved in PG biosynthesis with possible consequences in regulation of the overall biosynthetic pathway. It is known that the PG synthetase enzyme itself is irreversibly inactivated during the biosynthetic process if sufficient (O)$_x$ is produced. A claim has been made that on average about 5,000 arachidonic acid molecules are oxygenated per enzyme molecule prior to destruction (Ref. 33). A differential effect on the isomerase enzymes involved in the transformation of PGH_2 has been reported as prostacyclin synthetase is irreversibly inhibited whereas thromboxane A_2 synthetase is unaffected (Refs. 59,60). Likewise there is data suggesting the co-formation of "hydroxyl" radicals during PG biosynthesis as determined by various techniques (Refs. 61-63). It is important to rationalize whether the techniques used to measure "hydroxyl" radical production could discriminate between this species and the oxygen in the preferryl iron centre of the cyclo-oxygenase enzyme.

(e)   Inhibition of endoperoxide conversion. The cyclo-oxygenase activity of PG endoperoxide synthetase is markedly inhibited by many acid NSAI drugs (Table 1) (Ref. 64), anti-inflammatory steroids (Ref. 65), the arachidonic acid analogue eicosa-5,8,11,14-tetraynoic acid (ETYA), and related fatty acids (Refs. 66-68); various cannabinoids (Ref. 69); gold salts (Ref. 70); psychotropic drugs (Ref. 72; tartrazines (in food coloring agents (Ref. 72); o-hydroxyethylated rutosides (Ref. 73); flavanoids (Ref. 74) and phenolic compounds (Ref. 75).

At first sight it would seem that no common structural basis could exist for the inhibition of the cyclo-oxygenase enzyme system by such a variety of compounds. Some authors have, however, suggested that there are certain structural requirements (e.g., presence of specifically-oriented aromatic, phenolic and carboxylic acid groups) for inhibitory action of compounds at putative cyclo-oxygenase active sites (Ref. 76-80).

The structural tolerance of the cyclo-oxygenase enzyme for fatty acids has been delineated by Berthuis et al. (Ref. 81) and Van Dorp and Christ (Ref. 82) and forms an important basis for understanding the structural requirements for inhibiting this enzyme. An acid group was essential as methyl arachidonate and arachidonyl alcohol were not substrates. Only the C_{19} and C_{21} analogs of arachidonic acid could substitute for the C_{20} compound. $CH_3(CH_2)_n(CH=CHCH_2)_4(CH_2)_2CO_2H$ where n is 3-5 are substrates for the enzyme but lower (C_{18}) and higher (C_{22}) homologs are not.

TABLE 1

Inhibition by Nonsteroid Anti-inflammatory Drugs of Prostaglandin Production in Microsomes In Vitro and Macrophages in Culture[a]

Drug	IC$_{50}$ (μM)	
	Macrophages	Sheep seminal vesicle Microsomes
Acetylsalicylic acid	6.6	83.2
Azapropazone	11.2	3.0
Benoxaprofen	9.8	N.A.
BW-755c	0.3	N.A.
Diclofenac	0.0096	0.30
Diflunisal	1.4	7.9
Fenclofenac	1.6	N.A.
Flufenamic acid	0.016	2.4
Flurbiprofen	0.0033	0.71
Ibuprofen	0.56	1.5
Indomethacin	0.0017	0.40
Ketoprofen	0.022	0.12
Naproxen	0.28	6.2
Phenylbutazone	5.5	12.9
Piroxicam	0.10	N.A.
Sulindac	3.7	N.A.
Sulindac sulphide	0.006	2.19
Tolmetin	1.0	N.A.

[a]Data from Ref. 185, IC$_{50}$ denotes the concentration (in μM) required to produce inhibition of the production of prostaglandins in macrophages in culture (i.e., an intact cell system) contrasted with concentrations required to inhibit microsomal prostaglandin production in vitro. N.A. = not available.

The effect of chain branching was studied by utilization of appropriately substituted methyl analogs and similar derivatives. Substitutions by a methyl group at C-2, C-3 and C-19 was possible but no cyclization was observed with the C-4 and C-18 compounds. Interestingly cis-8,11,14-eicosatriene-5-ynoic acid was a substrate also. This may reflect tolerance to substitution in the plane of the 5,6-double bond but not with substitution away from this plane as would result by methyl replacement at an sp^3 hybridized carbon center in the chain. Since many NSAI drugs have aromatic rings attached to a propionic acid side chain they may still be capable of binding to the cyclo-oxygenase enzyme with their acid group competing for the C-1 carboxylic acid binding site on the enzyme. Studies with arachidonic acid analogs with methyl substitution on the 5,6-double bond would help clarify this hypothesis.

Other pertinent data is provided by the structural requirements for cyclo-oxygenase inhibition by triynoic acids (Ref. 68). No C_{18} acid with a single acetylene bond was an inhibitor and of a series of diynoic acids only octadeca-9, 12-diynoic acid was effective. Of the four isomeric octadeca-9,12-enynoic acids three were active. The inactive isomer, octadeca-9-*cis*-12-ynoic acid, can easily be seen to occupy a very different spatial configuration as a consequence of its 9-*cis* double bond.

The inhibition of cyclo-oxygenase activity by an extensive series of phenolic compounds was studied by Dewhirst (Ref. 75). It was considered from these results that inhibition was decreased by ring substituents which were electron-donating and also enhanced the hydrophobicity of the molecule. The inhibitory activity could be prevented by masking the phenolic hydroxyl group. Enhancement of inhibitory activity could be achieved by adding a short bridge to a second aromatic group. In this respect the presence of a second aromatic nucleus for enhanced inhibitory activity is in agreement with the postulated interaction of NSAI drugs with the cyclo-oxygenase receptor site by Gund and Shen (Ref. 77).

However, there is definitely a paradoxical situation with the phenolic compounds. On the basis of studies with MK-447 (Refs. 53,54) phenolic compounds would be expected to enhance the conversion of PGG_2 to PGH_2 and thus *stimulate* the production of prostaglandins/thromboxanes. In early studies on PG production in microsomal preparations it was found necessary to add either adrenaline, tryptophan, indole, hydroquinone, serotonin or some such phenolic or anti-oxidant-like substance in order to stimulate or "optimize" prostaglandin production and prevent the irreversible degradation of the cyclo-oxygenase enzyme from PGG_2 generated "radicals" (Ref. 33). Phenolic compounds such as those studied by Dewhirst (Ref. 75) could prevent the enzyme destruction and thus enhance prostaglandin production as well as directly inhibiting enzyme activity. Some clues as to the inhibitory/stimulatory actions of MK-447 have been provided recently by the work of Harada et al. (Ref. 83) At low concentrations there would appear to be a radical scavenging effect (i.e., stimulation of PG production) whereas at high concentrations there is a direct inhibitory effect of the drug on the cyclo-oxygenase activity. It would appear that the effects of phenolic compounds on cyclo-oxygenase activity could depend on (1) their activity as free radical scavengers, and (2) the interaction of these compounds with the active or other effector/modulator sites of the cyclo-oxygenase enzyme to prevent substrate interaction. A second specific action of a drug on the cyclo-oxygenase enzyme is seen with aspirin. This drug (but not its metabolite, salicylate) inhibits the cyclo-oxygenase by an irreversible acetylation of the enzyme protein (Ref. 84). The acetylation of the enzyme by aspirin occurs at the same concentrations as required to inhibit the cyclo-oxygenase activity and acetylation is also blocked by the potent cyclo-oxygenase inhibitor, indomethacin. This suggests that the inhibitory site of NSAI drugs is common with that of the site of acetylation by aspirin.

Fatty acids (e.g., linolenic, linoleic, oleic and decanoic acids) are, as with some NSAI drugs, reversible cyclo-oxygenase inhibitors (Refs. 85,86). The highest inhibitory activity is seen with 5-cis, 8-cis, 12-trans, 14-ciseicosatetraenoic acid. This is the closest structure to the product of the initial peroxidation at the 11-position in arachidonic acid but cannot itself undergo attack (Ref. 87). Thus an anionic receptor has been postulated as one of the groups present at the binding site of both inhibitor and substrate (Ref. 77). Methyl esters of acidic NSAI drugs do not interfere with the binding of the fatty acid substrate to the enzyme (Ref. 88). This would indicate a requirement for an anionic group at the putative fatty acid binding site on this enzyme. However, the methyl esters of the NSAI drugs do not cause the time-dependent destruction of cyclo-oxygenase activity shown with certain parent NSAI acids (Ref. 88). Thus, it appears there are two components of the inhibition of this enzyme activity. One is related to inhibition of fatty acid binding at the active site either by structurally analogous fatty acids or lipophilic drugs (i.e., not necessarily acids). The other is the irreversible destruction of the enzyme by acidic drugs. The most recent studies on the interaction of NSAI drugs with the cyclo-oxygenase system suggest that they interact at sites which is supplementary to the binding of these drugs to the catalytic site and this is obligatory for efficacy as cyclo-oxygenase inhibition. This may also explain the selectivity of many such drugs in inhibiting the cyclo-oxygenase but not the lipoxygenase pathway (Refs. 79,80).

(f) Catabolism of prostaglandins and thromboxanes. The rate of catabolism of the prostaglandins and thromboxanes will influence not only their formation but also the proportion of radicals generated as products of the cyclo-oxygenase/peroxidase pathways involved in their synthesis. Inhibitory effects of drugs on the degradation of prostanoids would be expected to decrease the production of free radicals by simple mass action effects in slowing down prostaglandin and thromboxane production. The principal features of the degradation of prostaglandins E and F have been summarized by Oates et al. (Ref. 89).

The principal enzyme in PGE/F catabolism is the 15-hydroxy dehydrogenase (PGDH). Many NSAI drugs inhibit this enzyme, but often at concentrations above that required to inhibit cyclo-oxygenase in vitro (Refs. 90,91). Total PGF_2 metabolism is also inhibited in vitro by NSAI drugs at high concentrations, and at low concentrations by sulphasalazine (IC_{50} = 50 μM) and diphloretin phosphate (20 μM) (Ref. 92). Sulphasalazine (but not its principal metabolites sulphapyridine and 5-aminosalicylic acid) specifically inhibits PGDH instead of the other enzymes in prostaglandin catabolism (Ref. 92). While sulphasalazine does have some, albeit weak, effects on the cyclo-oxygenase enzyme systems, it does seem to be the most specific inhibitor of PGDH of the compounds so far studied. This may account for the therapeutic actions of this drug in reducing the elevated prostaglandin levels in ulcerative colitis and Crohn's disease (Refs. 92,93). The elevated levels of prostaglandins observed in the colonic mucosa in this disease may be a reflection of radical production. Hence the beneficial effects of sulphasalazine may be due to indirect impairment of radical generation.

(g) Leukotriene synthesis--the lipoxygenase pathway. In addition to arachidonic acid being susceptible to attack by oxygen at the 11- and 15-positions (as in the cyclo-oxygenase pathway), there are other positions where unsaturated carbon atoms exist in positions which are favorable for activation for oxygenation. Principally, these include the 5- and 12-positions and the resultant monohydroperoxyeicosaetraenoic acids (HPETEs) are the first steps in the lipoxygenase pathways; these being quite separate from the cyclo-oxygenase pathway as previously discussed (Fig. 1). The products of the lipoxygenase pathways can yield extremely biologically active compounds which have a different spectrum of activity compared with those from the cyclo-oxygenase pathway.

The enzyme lipoxygenase (EC 1.13.1.13) catalyzes the oxidation of unsaturated fatty acids (or esters thereof) having a 1,4-cis, cispentadiene system (Ref. 94). It can be seen that three such groupings are present in arachidonic acid (Fig. 1). A lipoxygenase has been isolated and characterized from platelets (Ref. 95) where 12-H(P)ETE is the principal product. Also, lipoxygenase activity is observed in the purified prostaglandin cyclo-oxygenase from sheep vesicular glands with substrates incapable of endoperoxide formation (Ref. 96). These studies suggest that the mammalian lipoxygenase reactions are quite different to the reactions of plant lipoxygenases, which possess non-heme iron-containing enzymes (Refs. 97,98). They also suggest that endoperoxide formation and PG biosynthesis may be a specialized case of more general lipoxygenase reaction sequences. Evidence implicating lipo-oxygenase activity has been derived from biosynthetic studies in isolated cells with radiolabelled arachidonic acid and/or by GC/MS identification of the products (Refs. 12,95,99-105). There have not been any reports to date of isolation of the 5-lipoxygenase enzyme or other enzymes involved in the pathways of leukotriene biosynthesis (Ref. 105). Studies are needed on the purified enzymes in this lipoxygenase pathway before definite pronouncements can be made about the nature of the enzymes involved in the biosynthesis of the leukotrienes and related hydro(per)oxy fatty acids. This is also important in relation to free radical $(O)_x$ production, and we can only speculate on the origins of a hydroxyl or some such equivalent radical being generated from the conversion of the various HPETEs to HETEs as shown in Fig. 1. Inhibitors of this conversion will clearly influence the production of the $(O)_x$ species in this pathway and hence control the cellular reactions elicited by $(O)_x$ as well as the other responses induced by the individual HETEs. The reactivities of the $(O)_x$ species could vary depending on the nature of ligands attached to the iron centre and the tertiary structure of the surrounding protein for each particular lipoxygenase.

(h) Inhibition of hydro(per)oxy fatty acid and leukotriene biosynthesis. Several authors have reported that certain compounds inhibit the formation of one or more of the products of the lipoxygenase pathway and have described these compounds as "lipoxygenase inhibitors." As the enzyme systems have not been isolated or the complete conditions for optimal assay of lipoxygenase activity and kinetic properties determined, some authors have resorted to studying the effects of drugs or compounds on soybean lipoxygenase activity. Baumann and co-workers (Ref. 74) showed that the inhibitory effects of 3',4'-dihydroxyflavone and 1,5-dihydroxynaphthalene were identical in soybean lipoxygenases with that on the lipoxygenase activity present in homogenates of rat lung and spleen. This is of interest since the specificity of the lipoxygenase from these sources with respect to site of actions on arachidonic acid is quite different (Ref. 106). It suggests that there may be some general properties of lipoxygenase inhibitors.

Principal effects of the Eicosanoids with respect to Inflammation

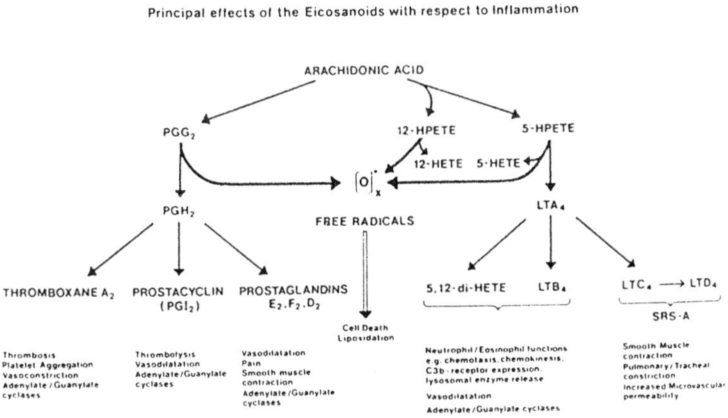

Fig. 3. Sites of inhibitory actions of drugs on the biosynthesis of eicosanoids and free radical scavenging by phenolic compounds. Abbreviations for hydroxy fatty acids as in Fig. 1. BW755c = 3-amino-1-(m-(trifluoromethyl)-phenyl)2-pyrazalor; MK-447 = 2-aminomethyl-4-t-butyl-6-idophenol; ETYA = 5,8,11,14-Eicosatetraynoic acid (this also inhibits the cyclo-oxygenase enzyme); NDGA = nordihydroguaiaretic acid; NSAIDs = nonsteroidal anti-inflammatory drugs.

Given the above-mentioned reservations concerning the lack of information on mammalian lipoxygenases it is possible to identify some presumptive lipoxygenase inhibitors (Fig. 3; Table 2). A variety of phenolic and flavanoid compounds appear to be selective inhibitors of lipoxygenase activity compared with their effects on the prostaglandin cyclo-oxygenase enzyme system (Table 2; Ref. 74). Compound MK-447 which enhances the conversion of PGG_2-PGH_2 is, by comparison with its potent effects on lipoxygenase activity, a relatively weak inhibitor of cyclo-oxygenase activity (Table 2). Also phenidone and compound BW 755c (which Higgs and co-workers (Ref. 107 consider is a selective inhibitor of the lipoxygenase pathway) are both potent inhibitors of cyclo-oxygenase activity.

TABLE 2

Inhibition of Lipoxygenase Activity, Compared With That on Prostaglandin Cyclo-oxygenase, By Some Anti-Inflammatory/Analgesic, Flavanoid and Anti-Oxidant Compounds[a]

Drug/Compound	IC_{50} lipoxygenase (µM)	IC_{50} PG-synthetase (µM)
I. Anti-Inflammatory/Analgesic Drugs		
Acetylsalicylic acid	1000	330
BW 755c	7.4	3.1
Diclofenac	1000	0.8-1.0
Indomethacin	1000	5.6
Mefenamic acid	300	0.8-1.0
MK 447 (2-aminomethyl-4-t-butyl-6-iodophenol)	130	1000
Naproxen	1000	0.8-1.0
Paracetamol	1000	560
Phenylbutazone	1000	15
II. Flavanoids		
(+)-Catechin (cyanidanol) (= 3,3',4',5,7-flavanpentol)	1000	130
3',4',-Dihydroxyflavone	33	100
Epicatechin	330	120
Galangin (= 3,5,7-trihydroxyflavone)	150	120
Luteolin (= 3',4',5,7-tetrahydroxyflavone)	30	100
7-Monohydroxyethylquercetin	200	1000
7-Monohydroxyethylrutin	300	1000
Morin (2',3',4',5,7-pentahydroxyflavone)	250	120
Rutin	200	1000
Silybin	150	1000
3',4',5,7-Tetrahydroxyethylquercetin	80	1000
3',4,7-Trihydroxyethylquercetin	300	1000
III. Miscellaneous		
1,5-Dihydroxynaphthalene	20	130
2,3-Dihydroxynaphthalene	60	130
1,3-Dihydroxynaphthalene	500	130
Diphenylthiocarbazone	400	1000
Phenidone	200	63

[a]Data from Ref. 74. IC_{50} denotes the concentration required for 50% inhibition.

Perhaps one of the most interesting groups of lipoxygenase inhibitors are the flavanoid compounds, though not all of these are specific inhibitors compared with their effects on the cyclo-oxygenase system (Ref. 74). These results suggest that certain arrangements of phenolic moieties may be basic to the inhibitory actions of both flavanoid and nonflavanoid compounds. Also, by analogy with the effects of phenolic compounds on the peroxidase reaction in PG synthetase, it is possible that some of the phenolic or flavanoid compounds may have dual actions in both inhibiting lipoxygenases and scavenging the free radicals generated in the con- version of HPETEs to HETEs.

Some, but not all, NSAI drugs that inhibit cyclo-oxygenase activity also inhibit soybean lipoxygenase activity (Table 2) and these may inhibit lipoxygenase activity in mammalian cells (Ref. 108). Although several authors have evaluated the soybean lipoxygenase enzyme, which specifically converts arachidonic acid to 15-HPETE, the relevance of these studies to either mode of action or design of lipoxygenase inhibitors for mammalian systems is very dubious (Ref. 109). Some acetylenic fatty acids and 15-hydroxy-5,8,11,13-eicosatetraenoic acid have been shown to be potent and selective inhibitors of platelet lipoxygenase-like activity (Refs. 110-112). Recent results also suggest that in some systems ETYA inhibits the enzyme that converts 5-HPETE to LTA_4 rather than the 5-lipoxygenase (Ref. 114).

Endogenous inhibitors of lipoxygenase activity have been identified in plasma and serum from various sources (Ref. 114) though the effects of some of the proteins implicated with this activity may be attributed to binding of the arachidonic acid substrate.

BIOLOGICAL AND PHARMACOLOGICAL IMPORTANCE OF FREE RADICAL PRODUCTION

(a) Pathophysiological consequences of eicosanoid-generated free radicals. Elevated production of prostaglandins, HETEs and/or leukotrienes occur in a wide variety of pathological conditions. The immense variety of reaction initiated by the products of eicosanoid metabolism in respect to inflammatory reactions can only be briefly summarized here (see Fig. 4). Some recent studies have shown the existence of specific receptors for the prostanoids. Differential stimulation of receptors on adenylate and guanylate cyclases has been demonstrated by individual prostaglandins and the di-HETEs (Fig. 4). Some of these actions of prostaglandins on cyclic nucleotide production are mutually antagonistic. For example, elevation of prostaglandin E_2 levels causes stimulation of adenylate cyclase activity so causing enhanced production of cAMP (Refs. 115,116). In contrast, prostaglandin $F_{2\alpha}$ causes stimulation of cGMP production (Refs. 115,117).

In addition to the biological effects caused by the enhanced production of various eicosanoids during inflammation, it can be seen from Fig. 4 that there is potential for stimulating production of the oxygen radical $(O)_x$ species accompanying this increased eicosanoid synthesis. The concept that this $(O)_x$ species had an

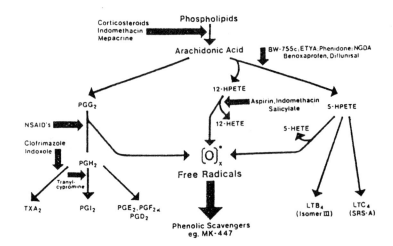

Fig. 4. General aspects of the actions of the products formed from the oxidation of arachidonic acid. Abbreviations as in Fig. 1. It should be noted that interaction between the individual prostanoids and leukotrienes can account for enhancement or antagonism of some of the actions of these products (e.g., see Ford-Hutchinson et al. (Ref. 187).

important role in inflammation was first suggested by Kuehl and co-workers (Refs. 53-54) and was discussed earlier in this review. A recent review article gives an excellent overview of the data in this area (Ref. 110).

(b) Generation and measurement of $OH^\cdot/(O)_x$ production. The mechanisms involved in the generation of $OH^\cdot/(O)_x$ species in biological systems are still speculative. However, a role for their participation and amplification of an inflammatory process may be anticipated by O_2^-, $OH^\cdot$ and $(O)_x$ being involved in the following reactions:

(1) Depolymerization of hyaluronic acid and synovial fluid by hyaluronidases activated by free radicals (Ref. 119). It is known that the viscosity of synovial fluid decreases in rheumatoid arthritis (Ref. 120) and that hyaluronidase is normally not active in synovial fluid at physiological pH values (Ref. 121).

(2) Labilization of lysosomal membranes (Ref. 122).

(3) Lipid peroxidation and subsequent generation of chemotactic factors (Refs. 123-125). This has been shown to occur in synovial fluid of rheumatoid arthritis patients (Ref. 15).

(4) Impairment of leukocyte function (Ref. 126).

(5) Impairment of lymphocyte function (Ref. 127).

(6) Destruction of lysosomal enzyme inhibitor proteins and damage to nucleic acids (Refs. 128-130).

The individual radicals are produced in different cellular compartments so that the above-mentioned biochemical effects are presumably specific to the sites at which the radicals are generated. For instance extracellular superoxide and hydroxyl radical production is evident during polymorph and monocyte-macrophage activation. We presume from the in vitro studies performed on microsomal prostaglandin synthesis that the major site of generation of $(O)_x$ species is in the endoplasmic reticulum with the added possibility that this radical may be released into the cytoplasm. Thus damage elicited by this species may be an intracellular event and it is quite probable that attack on intracellular organelles (e.g., lysosomes) or lipid components (causing their peroxidation) could be major factors in the development of cellular damage.

Amongst the pathways in the body capable of producing $OH^\bullet$ or related species are the following:

(1) A myeloperoxidase dependent system that utilizes H_2O_2 and a halide ion – thought is is uncertain whether the ultimate species produced is $OH^\bullet$ or $HOC\ell$ or utilizes iodide (Refs. 131,132). Myeloperoxidase is unusual as a peroxidase in that it has two heme centers (Refs. 133,134).

(2) The reaction between Fe^{2+} salts and H_2O_2. Iron complexes can catalyze this process, perhaps the most physiologically significant are transferrin and lactoferrin (Refs. 135-137). It has been claimed that ascorbate could be the physiological agent in vivo that reduces the Fe^{3+} to Fe^{2+} (Ref. 138).

(3) The use of hydroperoxides in a similar manner to that in (2) above (Ref. 139).

(4) The formation of perferryl iron compounds in prostaglandin cyclo-oxygenase reactions and possibly in lipoxygenase reactions as mentioned previously.

(5) Porphyrin ligands are known to function like the dismutase enzymes capable of converting O_2^- to H_2O_2 (Refs. 140,141). Reaction of many porphyrins with H_2O_2 can lead to a powerful oxidizing species and irreversible opening of the porphyrin ring (Refs. 141-143).

(6) Xanthine oxidase mediated systems (Ref. 144).

It is clear that there is a significant overlap between these processes and especially in respect of the $(O)_x$ species generated in eicosanoid metabolism. Ultimately it is the specificity of the analytical methods utilized that can distinguish these possibilities. Unfortunately there are few critical reviews of this aspect in the literature (Refs. 139,145). All of these methods can only be employed in analysis of subcellular fractions and isolated cell systems. Perhaps the most useful of these are the use of spin traps (Refs. 146,147) and the production of ethylene or methane from 2-keto-4-thiomethylbutyrate or dimethyl sulphoxide respectively (Refs. 131,148,149).

(c) Rationale for pharmacological intervention. From the point of view of inflammation, blockade of prostaglandin cyclo-oxygenase activity may not be a desirable factor in inflammation (or other conditions) since this may lead to an imbalance in other pathways so enhancing the possibility of leukotriene, H(P)ETE or $(O)_x$ production. For these purposes a drug that has a balanced effect on the production of all the eicosanoids metabolism would seem to have more desirable properties as an anti-inflammatory agent. This could be combined with an oxygen $(O)_x$ scavenging entity to prevent the potentially cyclical responses (lipid peroxidation, loss of cellular integrity and eventual cell death) resulting from the release of this species in eicosanoid metabolism. Some of the newer NSAI drugs and flavanoids may combine these properties. To achieve specific non-involvement or inhibition of some of the inflammatory cell reactions it appears necessary to have drugs which inhibit the production and effects of leukotrienes and the HETEs (compare Fig. 2). In other pathological states, it may be desirable to have these functions enhanced, for example, in stimulating the cell-mediated cytoxicity against tumor cells or helminth parasites.

We could envisage a range of drugs developed in order to specifically control the production of one or more of these products in certain cellular locations. Alternatively, it may be difficult to achieve control of the production of particular combinations of the products of the eicosanoid pathway in the required sites without appropriate delivery of the drug to that site in the body (e.g., with target-directed liposomes). Hence, it may be more appropriate to combine certain drugs in order to achieve therapeutic aims.

To achieve these aims it is important to establish: (1) the identity and localization of production of the $(O)_x$ radical species; (2) the importance of its production especially in relation to effects of other mediators of inflammation; and (3) the structure-activity relationships underlying the control of $(O)_x$ radical production.

Apart from the inflammatory conditions (e.g., arthritis), enhanced prostaglandin production occurs in (1) metastatic tumors (Ref. 150); (2) Bartter's syndrome--a familial condition where glomerular hyperplasia develops from over-production of renal prostaglandins which stimulates production of renin, angiotensin II and aldosterone leading to decreased plasma potassium (Refs. 151-154); (3) renal hypertension (Refs. 155-158); (4) ulcerative colitis and Crohn's disease (Refs. 159,160); (5) radiation and endotoxin-induced diarrhea (Refs. 161,162); and (6) dysmenorrhea (Ref. 163). The treatment of these conditions with anti-inflammatory drugs results in some alleviation of the symptoms of these conditions, depending on the relative importance of the prostaglandin pathways and presumably other products of eicosanoid metabolism generated in the pathogenesis of these diseases (Refs. 92,150,165-168). The indirect effects of the NSAI drugs in these conditions may, in part, be due to blockade of free radical production.

Elevation of leukotrienes C_4 and D_4 and prostaglandins occurs in asthmatic conditions, anaphylaxis and other immediate-type hypersensitivity reactions

(Refs. 168-171). Purified LTC_4 and LTD_4 (both components of slow reacting sub-stance of anaphylaxis, SRS-A) have both been shown to elicit allergic responses characteristic of immediate-type hypersensitivity reactions, including the potent bronchoconstriction (see Fig. 4, Refs. 172,173). Prostacyclin and other prosta-glandins appear to modulate the release of SRS-A (Ref. 174) so that there appears to be some interrelationship in the biological effects of the various products of eicosanoid metabolism. Disodium cromoglycate, isamoxole and some other drugs appear capable of depressing SRS-A production and more important, its biological effects (Refs. 175-180). It is clear that blocking production, of effects, of leukotrienes (SRS-A) is one way towards blunting the responses in immediate-type hypersensitivity reactions. Examination of Fig. 2 shows that the free oxygen radical $(O)_x$ could also be formed as a result of the accelerated lipoxygenase and cyclo-oxygenase activities in the production of SRS-A and prostaglandins. The actions of SRS-A antagonists/inhibitors on such free radical production has yet to be determined but could clearly be of importance.

The gastric ulcerogenic effects of anti-inflammatory drugs have some parallels with inflammatory reactions induced in other compartments in the body. Inhibition of prostaglandin production has been considered as one mechanism of the ulcerogenic actions of these drugs (for review see Ref. 181). Many acidic NSAI drugs are potent irritants and in addition to their inhibitory effects on prostaglandin production may "prime" the eicosanoid synthesizing system by acting as irritant-inducing arachidonate generators. If selective effects of NSAI drugs occur on the cyclo-oxygenase pathway then a diversion of arachidonate may occur to other parts of the eicosanoid pathway (e.g., to form hydro(per)oxy fatty acids) so enhancing the formation of free radicals on the conversion of HPETEs to HETEs.

Compound MK-447 and other phenolic scavengers have been shown to decrease the gastric ulcerogenicity of indomethacin and other irritant NSAI drugs (Ref. 181). Since this compound inhibits lipoxygenase activity as well as scavenging free radicals it appears that MK-447 could correct the disproportionate effects of ulcerogenic NSAI drugs on arachidonate metabolism (resulting from inhibition of prostaglandin production alone) accompanying enhanced production of the free $(O)_x$ radicals. Hence the generation of this species may be an important factor in ulcerogenesis produced by these drugs (Ref. 181).

CONCLUSIONS

It is apparent from the above discussion that possible avenues are open for modulating the actions of the biological mediators of the products of accelerated cicosanoid metabolism, namely:

(1) Block the actions of the products of the pathway of eicosanoid metabolism, e.g., prostaglandins, SRS-A, etc.

(2) Selectively inhibit one or more of the pathways of cicosanoid metabolism.

(3) Scavenge the free radical $(O)_x$ species which are generated in the peroxidase reactions.

(4) Design drugs to remove reative fragmentation products of fatty acid metabolism (e.g., malondialdehyde, 4-hydroxynonenal). While these metabolites have not been discussed in this review, they have considerable cytoxic activity (Refs. 182-184).

Clearly, there are requirements for selectivity in order to achieve the inhibitory effects on particular components of eicosanoid metabolism. Also, there is the problem of delivering compounds to specific organs and sub-cellular sites in order to achieve the selectivity required to regulate these reactions. Certainly compounds which influence oxygen species production in vitro and in vivo from the various potential precursors, including that from eicosanoid metabolism, will play a key role in understanding *their* physiological importance in many disease states.

REFERENCES

1. Lands, W.E.M. (1979) Ann. Rev. Physiol., 4, 633-652.
2. Yamamoto, S., Ohki, S., Ogino, N., Shimizu, T., Yoshimoto, T., Watanabe, K. and Hayaishi, O. (1978) Adv. Prostagladin Thromboxane Res., 6, 27-34.
3. Samuelsson, B., Ramwell, P.W., and Paoletti, E., eds. (1980) Advances in Prostaglandin and Thromboxane Research, Vols. 6, 7, and 8. New York: Raven Press.
4. Bannister, J.V. and Hill, H.A.O., eds. (1980) Chemical and Biochemical Aspects of Superoxide and Superoxide Dismutase, New York: Elsevier/North-Holland.
5. Bannister, W.J. and Bannister, J.V., eds. (1980) Biological and Clinical Aspects of Superoxide and Superoxide Dismutase, New York: Elsevier/North-Holland.
6. Hammarstrom, S. and Farlardeau, S. (1977) Proc. Natl. Acad. Sci., USA, 74, 3691-3695.
7. Davies, P., Bonney, R.J., Humes, J.L., and Kuehl, F.A., Jr. (1979) Agents Actions, Suppl. 6, 143-149.
8. Ferriera, S.H. (1979) in Chemical Messengers of the Inflammatory Process, Houck, J.C., ed., Amsterdam: Elsevier/North-Holland, pp. 113-151.
9. Rossi, F. and Zalti, M. (1964) Br. J. Exp. Pathol., 298, 659-669.
10. Smith, M.J.H. (1979) Agents Actions, Suppl. 6, 91-103.
11. Brune, K., Kälin, H., Rainsford, K.D., and Wagner, K. (1980) Adv. Prostaglandin Thromboxane Res., 8, 1697-1684.
12. Ford-Hutchinson, A.W., Bray, M.A., Doig, M.V., Shipley, M.E., and Smith, M.J.H. (1980) Nature, 286, 264-265.
13. Bryant, R.W. and Bailey, J.M. (1978) Adv. Prostaglandin Thromboxane Res., 6, 95-99.
14. McGuire, J.G. and Sun, F.F. (1980) Adv. Prostaglandin Thromboxane Res., 8, 1665-1667.
15. Klickstein, L.B., Shapleigh, C., and Goetzl, E.J. (1980) J. Clin. Invest., 66, 1166-1170.
16. McMillan, R.M., Fahey, J.V., Brinckerholt, C.E., and Harris, E.D. (1980) Adv. Prostaglandin Thromboxane Res., 6, 1701-1704.
17. Higg, G.A., Vane, J.R., Hart, F.D., and Wojtulewski, J.A. (1974) in Prostaglandin Synthetase Inhibitors, Robinson, J.H., and Vane, J.R., eds., New York: Raven Press, pp. 165-173.

18. Trang, L.E., Granström, E., and Lovgren, O. Scand. J. Rheumatol., 6, 151-154.
19. Brodie, M.J., Hensby, C.N., Parke, A., and Gordon, D. (1980) Life Sci., 27, 603-608.
20. Kinsella, L.B. (1979) Biochem. J., 184, 701-704.
21. Lewis, G.P. and Piper, P.J. (1975) Nature, 254, 308-311.
22. Gryglewski, R.J., Panczenko, B., Korbut, R., Grodzinska, L., and Ocetkiewics, A. (1975) Prostaglandins, 10, 343-355.
23. Hong, S.-C. and Levine, L. (1976) Proc. Natl. Acad. Sci. USA, 73, 1730-1734.
24. Mentz, P., Giessler, C.H., and Forster, W. (1980) Pharm. Res. Commun., 12, 611-621.
25. Blackwell, G.J., Carnuccio, R., DiRosa, M., Flower, R.J., Parente, L., and Persico, P. (1980) Nature, 287, 147-149.
26. Vigo, C., Lewis, G.P., and Piper, P.J. (1980) Biochem. Pharmacol., 29, 623-627.
27. Bowery, P. and Lewis, G.P. (1973) Br. J. Pharmacol., 47, 305-314.
28. Kaplan, L., Weiss, J. and Elsbach, P. (1978) Proc. Natl. Acad. Sci. USA, 75, 2955-2958.
29. Kaplan-Harris, L. and Elsbach, P. (1980) Biochim. Biophys. Acta, 618, 318-326.
30. Miyamoto, T., Ogino, N., Yamaoto, S., and Hayaishi, O. (1976) J. Biol. Chem. 251, 2629-2636.
31. Van der Ouderaa, F.J., Buytenhek, M., Nugteren, D.H., and Van Dorp, D.A. (1977) Biochim. Biophys. Acta, 487, 315-331.
32. Peterson, D.A. and Gerrard, J.M. (1979) Med. Hypoth., 5, 683-694.
33. Egan, R.W., Paxton, J., and Kuehl, F.A., Jr. (1976) J. Biol. Chem., 251, 7329-7335.
34. Egan, R.W., Gale, P.H., and Kuehl, F.A., Jr. (1979) J. Biol. Chem., 254, 3295-3302.
35. Hamberg, M. and Samuelsson, B. (1967) J. Biol. Chem., 242, 5344-5354.
36. Mason, R.P., Kalyanaraman, B., Tainer, B.E., and Eling, T.E. (1980) J. Biol. Chem., 255, 5019-5022.
37. Hemler, M.E. and Lands, W.E.M. (1980) J. Biol. Chem., 255, 6253-6261.
38. Kuehl, F.A., Jr., Humes, J.L., Torchiana, M.L., Ham, E.A., and Egan, R.W. (1979) Adv. Inflammation Res., 1, 419-430.
39. Kuehl, F.A., Jr., Humes, J.L., Ham, E.A., Egan, R.W., and Dougherty, H.W. (1980) Adv. Prostaglandin Thromboxane, 6, 77-86.
40. Dunford, H.B. and Stillman, J.S. (1976) Coord. Chem. Rev., 19, 187-251.
41. Poulos, T.L. and Kraut, J. (1980) J. Biol. Chem., 255, 8199-8205.
42. Dolphin, D., Forman, A., Borg, D.C., Fajer, J., and Felton, R.H. (1971) Proc. Natl. Acad. Sci. USA, 68, 614-618.
43. Roberts, J.E., Hoffman, B.M., Rutter, R., and Hager, L.P. (1981) J. Biol. Chem., 256, 2118-2121.
44. Chevrier, B., Weiss, R., Lange, M., Chottard, J.-C. and Mansuy, D. (1981) J. Amer. Chem. Soc., 103, 2899-2901.
45. Chin, D.-H., Balch, A.L., and La Mar, G.N. (1980) J. Amer. Chem. Soc., 102, 1446-1448.
46. Chin, D.-H., La Mar, G.N., and Balch, A.L. (1980) J. Amer. Chem. Soc., 102, 5954-5947.
47. Green, M.R., Hill, H.A.O., Okolow-Zubkowska, M.J., and Segal, A.W. (1979) FEBS Lett., 100, 23-26.
48. DiNello, R.K. and Dolphin, D. (1978) Biochem. Biophys. Res. Commun., 80, 698-703.
49. Groves, J.T., Haushalter, R.C., Nakamura, M., Nemo, T.E., and Evans, B.J. J. Amer. Chem. Soc., 103, 2884-2886.
50. Siegel, M.I., McConnell, R.T., and Cuatrecasas, P. (1979) Proc. Natl. Acad. Sci. USA, 76, 3774-3778.
51. Siegel, M.I., McConnell, R.T., Porter, N.A., and Cuatrecasas, P. (1980) Proc. Natl. Acad. Sci. USA, 77, 308-312.
52. Smith, W.L. and Lands, W.E.M. (1971) J. Biol. Chem., 246, 6700-6704.
53. Kuehl, F.A., Jr., Humes, J.L., Egan, R.W., Ham, E.A., Beveridge, R.C., and Van Arman, C.G. (1977) Nature, 265, 170-173.

54. Kuehl, F.A., Jr., Humes, J.L., Beveridge, G.C., Van Arman, C.G., and Egan, R.W. (1977) Inflammation, 2, 285-294.
55. Duggan, D.E., Hooke, K.F., Risley, E.A., Shen, T.Y., and Van Arman, C.G. (1977) J. Pharmacol. Exp. Therap., 201, 8-13.
56. Shen, T.Y. and Winter, C.A.   Adv. Drug Res., 12, 89-245.
57. Marnett, L.J., Bienkowski, M.J., and Pagels, W.R. (1979) J. Biol. Chem., 254, 5077-5082.
58. Marnett, L.J., and Bienkowski, M.J. (1980) Biochem. Biophys. Res. Commun., 96, 639-647.
59. Weiss, S.J., Turk, J., and Needleman, P. (1979) Blood, 53, 1191-1196.
60. Ham, E.A., Egan, R.W., Soderman, D.D., Gale, P.H., and Kuehl, F.A., Jr. (1979) J. Biol. Chem., 254, 2191-2194.
61. O'Brien, P.J. and Hawco, F.J. (1978) Biochem. Soc. Trans., 6, 1169-1171.
62. O'Brien, P.J. and Hulett, L.G. (1980) Prostaglandins, 19, 683-691.
63. Sagone, A.L., Jr., Wells, R.M., and Democko, C. (1980) Inflammation, 4, 65-71.
64. Taylor, R.J. and Salata, J.J. (1976) Biochem. Pharmacol., 25, 2479-2484.
65. Lerner, L.J., Carminati, P., and Schiatti, P. (1975) Proc. Soc. Exp. Biol. Med., 148, 329-332.
66. Ahern, D.G. and Downing, D.I. (1970) Biochim. Biophys. Acta, 210, 456-461.
67. Downing, D.T., Barve, J.A., Gunstone, F.D., Jacobsberg, F.R., and Lie Ken Jie, M. (1972) Biochim. Biophys. Acta, 280, 343-347.
68. Goetz, J.M., Sprecher, H., Cornwell, D.G., and Panganamala, R.V. (1976) Prostaglandins, 12, 187-192.
69. Burnstein, S., Taylor, D., El-Feraly, F.S., and Turner, C. (1976) Biochem. Pharmacol., 25, 2003-2004.
70. Stone, K.J., Mather, S.J., and Gibson, P.P. (1975) Prostaglandins, 10, 241-252.
71. Lee, R.E. (1974) Prostaglandins, 5, 63-68.
72. Ceserani, R., Colombo, M., Robushi, M., and Bianco, S. (1978) Prostaglandins Med., 1, 499-505.
73. Arturson, G. and Johansson, C.E. (1975) Prostaglandins, 10, 941-948.
74. Baumann, J., F.V. Bruchhausen, and Wurm, G. (1980) Prostaglandins, 20, 627-639.
75. Dewhirst, F.E. (1980) Prostaglandins, 20, 209-222.
76. Lands, W.E.M., Le Tellier, P.R., Rome, L.H., and Vanderhoek, J.Y. (1973) Adv. Biosci., 9, 15-28.
77. Gund, P. and Shen, T.Y. (1977) J. Med. Chem., 20, 1146-1152.
78. Appleton, R.A. and Brown, K. (1979) Prostaglandins, 18, 29-34.
79. Salvetti, F., Buttinoni, A., Ceserani, R., and Tosi, C. (1981) Eur. J. Med., Chem., 16, 81-90.
80. Humes, J.L., Winter, C.A., Sadowski, S.J., and Kuehl, F.A., Jr. (1981) Proc. Natl. Acad. Sci., USA, 78, 2053-2056.
81. Beerthuis, R.K., Nugteren, D.H., Pabon, H.J.J., and Van Dorp, D.A. (1968) Rec. Trav. Chim., 87, 461-479.
82. Van Dorp, D.A. and Christ, E.J. (1975) Rec. Trav. Chim., 94, 247-253.
83. Harada, Y., Tanaka, K., and Katori, M. (1980) Jap. J. Pharmacol., 30, 549-557.
84. Roth, G.J., Stanford, N., and Majerus, P.W. (1975) Proc. Natl. Acad. Sci. USA, 72, 3073-3076.
85. Gryglewski, R.J. (1974) in Prostaglandin Synthetase Inhibitors, Robinson, H.J. and Vane, J.R., eds., New York: Raven Press, pp. 32-52.
86. Hamberg, M. and Samuelsson, B. (1974) Biochim. Biophys. Res. Commun., 61, 942-949.
87. Nugteren, D.H. (1970) Biochim. Biophys. Acta, 210, 171-176.
88. Rome, L.H. and Lands, W.E.M. (1975) Proc. Natl. Acad. Sci. USA, 72, 4863-4865.
89. Oates, J.A., Roberts, L.T., Sweatman, B.J., Maas, R.L., Gerkens, J.F., and Taber, F.A. (1980) Adv. Prostaglandin Thromboxane Res., 6, 35-41.
90. Flower, R.J. (1974) Pharmacol. Rev., 26, 33-67.

91. Hansen, H.S. (1974) Prostaglandins, 7, 95-105.
92. Hoult, J.R.S. and Moore, P.K. (1980) Br. J. Pharmacol., 68, 719-730.
93. Hoult, J.R.S. and Moore, P.K. (1978) Br. J. Pharmacol., 64, 6-8.
94. Holma, R.T. (1951) in The Enzymes, first edition, Holman, R.T. and Bergstrom, S., eds., New York: Academic Press.
95. Nugteren, D.H. (1975) Biochim. Biophys. Acta, 380, 299-307.
96. Hemler, M.E., Crawford, C.G., and Lands, W.E.M. (1978) Biochemistry, 17, 1772-1779.
97. Chan, H.W.S. (1973) Biochim. Biophys. Acta, 327, 32-35.
98. Boza, M. and Franke, A. (1973) Biochim. Biophys. Acta, 327, 24-31.
99. Hamberg, M. and Samuelsson, B. (1974) Proc. Natl. Acad. Sci. USA, 71, 3400-3404.
100. Borgeat, P., Hamberg, M. and Samuelsson, B. (1976) J. Biol. Chem., 251, 7816-7820, and correction 252, 8772.
101. Borgeat, P. and Samuelsson, B. (1979) J. Biol. Chem., 254, 7865-7869.
102. Higgs, G.A., Flower, R.J., and Vane, J.R. (1979) Biochem. Pharmacol., 28, 1959-1961.
103. Doig, M.V. and Ford-Hutchinson, A.W. (1980) Prostaglandins, 20, 1007-1019.
104. Samuelsson, B., Borgeat, P., Hammarstron, S., and Murphy, R.C. (1980) Adv. Prostaglandin Thromboxane Res., 6, 1-18.
105. Borgeat, P. and Sirois, P. (1981) J. Med. Chem., 24, 121-126.
106. Jones, R.L. (1979) Agents Actions, Suppl. 6, 19-26.
107. Higgs, G.A., Eakins, K.E., Moncada, S., and Vane, J. (1979) Agents Actions, Suppl. 6, 167-175.
108. Bray, M.A., Ford-Hutchinson, A.W., and Smith, M.J.H. in SRS-A and Leuko-trienes, Piper, P.J., ed., Chichester, U.K.: Research Studies Press, pp. 253-270.
109. Downing, D.T. (1972) Prostaglandins, 1, 437-441.
110. Vanderhoek, J.Y., Bryant, R.W., and Bailey, J.M. (1980) J. Biol. Chem., 255, 5996-5998.
111. Sun, F.F., McGuire, J.C., Morton, D.R., Pike, J.E., and Sprecher, H. (1981) Prostaglandins, 21, 323-332.
112. Wilhelm, T.E., Sankarappa, S.K., Van Rollins, M., and Sprecher, H. (1981) Prostaglandins, 21, 323-332.
113. Bokoch, G.M. and Reed, P.W. (1981) J. Biol. Chem., 256, 4156-4159.
114. Seed, S.A., Drew, M., and Collier, H.O.J. (1980) Eur. J. Pharmacol., 67, 169-170.
115. Kuehl, F.A., Jr., Cirillo, V.J., Ham, E.A., and Humes, J.L. (1973) Adv. Biosci., 9, 155-172.
116. Weissman, G., Smolen, J.E., and Korchak, H. (1980) Adv. Prostaglandin Thromboxane Res., 8, 1637-1654.
117. Weissman, K. (1980) Adv. Prostaglandin Thromoboxane Res., 8, 1655-1665.
118. Greenwald, R.A. (1981) J. Rheumatol., 8, 185-187.
119. McCord, J.M. (1974) Science, 185, 529-531.
120. Kofoed, J.A. and Barcelo, A.C. (1978) Experimentia, 34, 1545-1546.
121. Aronson, N.A., Jr., and Davidson, E.A. (1965) J. Biol. Chem., 240, 3222-3224.
122. Fong, K.L., McCay, P.B., Poyer, J.L., Keele, B.B., and Misra, H. (1973) J. Biol. Chem., 248, 7792-7797.
123. Turner, S.R., Campbell, J.A., and Lynn, W.S. (1975) J. Exp. Med., 141, 1437-1441.
124. Perez, H.D., Weksler, B.B., and Goldstein, I.M. (1980) Inflammation, 4, 313-328.
125. Fridovich, S.E. and Porter, N.A. (1981) J. Biol. Chem., 256, 260-265.
126. Weiss, S.J. and Sagone, A.L., Jr. (1979) Biochim. Biophys. Acta, 585, 620-629.
127. Sagone, A.L., Jr., Wells, R.M., and DeMocko, C. (1980) Inflammation, 4, 65-71.
128. Carp, H. and Janoff, A. (1980) J. Clin. Invest., 66, 987-995.
129. Clark, R.A., Stone, P.J., El Hog, A., Calore, J.D., and Franzblau, C. (1981) J. Biol. Chem., 256, 3348-3353.

130. Petkau, A. (1980) Acta Physiol. Scand., Suppl., 492, 81-90.
131. Klebanoff, S.J. and Rosen, H. (1978) J. Exp. Med., 148, 490-506.
132. Slivka, A., LoBuglio, A.F., and Weiss, S.J. (1980) Blood, 55, 347-350.
133. Yamazaki,
134. Thomson, A.J. (1980) Private communication.
135. Halliwell, B. (1978) FEBS Lett., 96, 238-242.
136. McCord, J.M. and Day, E.D., Jr. (1978) FEBS Lett., 86, 139-142.
137. Ambruso, D.R. and Johnston, R.B., Jr. (1981) J. Clin. Invest.,' 67, 352-360.
138. Wimterbourn, C.C. (1979) Biochem. J., 182, 625-628.
139. Bors, W., Saran, M., Lengfelder, E., Michel, C., Fuchs, C., and Frenzel, C. (1978) Photochem. Photobiol., 28, 629-637.
140. Pasternack, R.F. and Skowronek, W.R., Jr. (1979) J. Inorg. Biochem., 11, 261-267.
141. Pasternack, R.F. and Halliwell, P. (1979) J. Am. Chem. Soc., 101, 1026-1031.
142. Jones, P., Prudhoe, K. and Robson, T. (1973) Biochem. J., 135, 361-365.
143. Weiss, S.J. (1980) J. Biol. Chem., 255, 9912-9917.
144. Tein, M., Svingen, B.A. and Aust, S.D. (1981) Fed. Proc., 40, 179-182.
145. Bors, W., Saran, M., Lengfelder, E., Michel, C., Fuchs, C. and Frenzel, C. (1978) Photochem. Photobiol., 28, 629-637.
146. Buettner, G.R. and Oberley, L.W. (1978) Biochem. Biophys. Res. Commun., 83, 69-74.
147. Walling, C. (1975) Acc. Chem. Res., 8, 125-131.
148. Weiss, S.J., Rustagi, P.K., and LoBuglio, A.F. (1978) J. Exp. Med., 147, 316-323.
149. Repine, J.E., Eaton, J.W., Anders, M.W., Hordal, J.R., and Fox, R.B. (1979) J. Clin. Invst., 64, 1642-1651.
150. Bennett, A., Berstock, D.A., Harris, M., Raja, B., Rowe, D.J.F., Stamford, I.F., and Wright, J.E. (1980) Adv. Prostaglandin Thromboxane Res., 6, 595-600.
151. Fichman, M.P., Telfer, N., Zai, P., Speckart, P., Golub, M., and Rude, R. (1976) Am. J. Med., 60, 785-797.
152. Gill, J.R., Frolich, J.C., Bowden, R.E., Taylor, A.A., Keiser, H.R., Seyberth, H.W., Oates, J.A., and Bartler, J.C. (1976) Am. J. Med., 61, 43-51.
153. Bartler, F.C., Gill, J.R., and Frohlich, J.C. (1978) Adv. Nephrol., 7, 191-198.
154. Zipser, R.D., Rude, R.K., Zai, P.K., and Fichman, M.P. (1979) Am. J. Med., 67, 263-267.
155. Armstrong, J.M., Blackwell, G.J., Flower, R.J., McGiff, J.C., Mullane, K.M. and Vane, J.R. (1976) Nature, 260, 582-586.
156. Romero, J.C. and Strong, C.G. (1977) Mayo Clin. Proc., 52, 462-464.
157. Ahnfelt-Ronne, I. and Arrigoni, Martelli, E. (1977) Biochem. Pharmacol., 26, 485-488.
158. Styles, V.G., Smith, W.L., Reinke, D.A., and Hook, J.B. (1978) Biol. Neonate, 33, 309-313.
159. Sharon, P., Ligumsky, M., Racjmilewitz, D., and Zan, U. (1978) Gastroenterology, 75, 638-640.
160. Harris, D.W., Greenberg, R., Phillips, M.B., Osman, G.H., Jr., and Antonaccio, M.J. (1980) Adv. Prostaglandin Thromboxane Res., 6, 437-441.
161. Collier, H.O.J. (1974) in Prostaglandin Synthetase Inhibitors, Robinson, H.J. and Vane, J.R., eds., New York: Raven Press, pp. 121-133.
162. Collier, H.O.J., McDonald-Gibson, W.J., and Seed, S.A. (1976) Br. J. Pharmacol., 58, 193-199.
163. Pickles, V.R., Hall, H.W., Best, F.A., and Smith, G.M. (1965) J. Obstet. Gynec., 72, 185-192.
164. Verberkmoes, R., Van Damme, B., Clement, J., Amery, A., and Michielsen, P. (1976) Kidney Internal., 9, 302-307.
165. Horton, R. and Zipser, R. (1978) Contr. Nephrol., 14, 87-96.
166. Garin, E.H., Fennell, R.S., Iravani, A., and Richard, G.A. (1980) Am. J. Dis. Child., 134, 258-261.

167. Klotz, U., Maier, K., Gischer, C., and Heinkel, K. (1980) N. Engl. J. Med., 303, 1499-1502.
168. Brocklehurst, W.E. (1960) J. Physiol., 151, 416-435.
169. Adcock, J.J., Garland, L.G., Moncada, S., and Vane, J.R. (1980) Prostaglandins, 16, 179-187.
170. Engineer, D.M., Niederhauser, U., Piper, P.J., and Sirois, P. (1978) Br. J. Pharmacol., 62, 61-66.
171. Goetzl, E.J. (1980) N. Engl. J. Med., 303, 822-825.
172. Dahlen, S.-E., Hedqvist, P., Hammarstrom, S.M., and Samuelsson, B. (1980) Nature, 288, 484-486.
173. Hanna, C.J., Bach, M.K., Parc, P.D., and Schellenberg, R.R. (1981) Nature, 290, 343-344.
174. Burke, J.F. and Garland, L.G. (1977) Br. J. Pharmacol., 67, 23-32.
175. Altounyan, R.E.C. (1967) Acta Allergol., 22, 487-488.
176. Broughton, B.J., Chaplan, P., Knowles, P., Lunt, E., Pain, D.L., Wooldridge, K.R.H., Ford, R., Marshall, S., Walker, J.L., and Maxwell, D.R. (1974) Nature, 251, 650-652.
177. Butchers, P.R., Fullarton, J.R., Skidmore, I.F., Thompson, L.E., Vardley, C.E., and Wheeldon, A. (1979) Br. J. Pharmacol., 67, 23-32.
178. Chard, N. (1979) Agents Actions, 9, 133-140.
179. Dawson, W. and Sweatman, W.J.F. (1980) Br. J. Pharmacol., 71, 387-396.
180. Walker, J.R., Boot, J.R., Cox, B., and Dawson, W. (1980) J. Pharm. Pharmacol., 32, 866-867.
181. Rainsford, K.D. (1979) Agents Actions, Suppl. 6, 193-201.
182. Nair, V., Vietti, D.E., and Cooper, C.S. (1981) J. Am. Chem. Soc., 103, 3030-3036.
183. Benedetti, A., Comporti, M. and Esterbauer, H. (1980) Biochim. Biophys. Acta, 620, 281-296.
184. Benedetti, A., Ferrali, M., Casini, A.F., Pieri, S., and Comportie, M. (1980) Biochem. Pharmacol., 29, 121-124.
185. Brune, K., Rainsford, K.D., Wagner, K., and Peskar, B.A. (1981) Naunyn Schmeidebergs Arch. Pharmacol., 315, 269-276.
186. Egan, R.W., Gale, P.H., VandenHeuval, W.J., and Kuehl, F.A., Jr. (1979) Agents Actions, Suppl., 6, 39-49.
187. Ford-Hutchinson, A.W., Bray, M.A., Cunningham, F.M., Davidson, E.M., and Smith, M.J.H. (1981) Prostaglandins, 21, 143-152.

CHAPTER 6   OXYGEN TOXICITY IN PROKARYOTES

HOSNI M. HASSAN AND IRWIN FRIDOVICH
Department of Food Science, North Carolina State University, Raleigh,
North Carolina 27650; and Department of Biochemistry, Duke University Medical
Center, Durham, North Carolina 27710, USA.

Oxygen, which is exceedingly useful in energy-yielding metabolism and biosynthesi
also constitutes a threat to living cells. The toxicity of oxygen is a well known
phenomenon. Louis Pasteur was apparently the first to appreciate the potential
toxicity of oxygen by finding that certain organisms will not grow in its presence.
It is now recognized that even among the anaerobes there exists a complete spectrum
of oxygen tolerance (Ref. 1). It is difficult to classify the anaerobes according
to their oxygen tolerance, because differences have been noted among strains of
the same species and even within the same organism harvested at different phases
of growth or from different media.

The problem of oxygen toxicity in prokaryotes is multifaceted, and a distinction
should be made between the ability to grow and the ability to survive in presence
of adverse concentrations of oxygen. Thus, *Methanobacterium* AZ stops growing and
producing methane at 0.1 ppm O_2 but survives 7 ppm dissolved oxygen (Ref. 2). The
inability of anaerobic organisms to grow in the presence of oxygen may be due to the
increase in the redox potential (E_h) of the cultures (Ref. 2), and this does not
result in cell death. This bacteriostatic effect of oxygen is usually reversed
upon removal of oxygen. On the other hand, longer exposure of anaerobes to
oxygen could result in death of the cells, unless the organism possesses a defense
against this bacteriocidal effect.

The toxicity of oxygen is a common phenomenon among all organisms. Obligate
anaerobes are sensitive to atmospheric concentrations of oxygen (20%) while facultative anaerobes and aerobes display sensitivity to hyperoxia. During the past
century, several hypotheses have been advanced to explain the mechanism(s) of
oxygen toxicity (for reviews, see Refs. 3-5).

Oxygen is a peculiar oxidant in that its complete four electron reduction to
water, proceeds most readily by a stepwise pathway which generates partially reduced
intermediates (Refs. 6,7). These are the superoxide radical (O_2^-), hydrogen peroxide
(H_2O_2), and the hydroxyl radical ($OH^{\cdot}$); all of which are dangerously reactive. A
rational defense against oxygen toxicity whould thus include enzymes capable of
scavenging both H_2O_2 and O_2^- and antioxidants to minimize free radical chain oxidations. Catalases and peroxidases have long been known to remove H_2O_2 and
superoxide dismutases have more recently been shown to eliminate O_2^- (Ref. 8).
This review will deal with the superoxide theory, which states that superoxide
radical is an important agent of oxygen toxicity, and that superoxide dismutases

provide the primary defense against such toxicity (Ref. 9).

Superoxide radical as a commonplace product of biological oxygen reduction

The superoxide radical is a minor, but not a trivial, product of biological oxygen reduction. Attempts to measure the rates of O_2^- generated inside cells are usually hampered by the ubiquity of superoxide dismutases, which scavenge this radical. However, a recent study in which a specific inhibitory antibody was used to neutralize the activity of superoxide dismutase has demonstrated that 17% of the total oxygen consumed by crude extracts of *Streptococcus faecalis* is channelled *via* a univalent pathway and generates O_2^- (Ref. 10). The quantitatively most significant sources of O_2^- within any type of cell remain unknown. However, we know of many important biological oxidations which produce substantial amounts of O_2^- (for complete survey see Refs. 4,11). It is safe to conclude that the superoxide radical is produced in most living cells that are capable of reducing oxygen.

Cytotoxicity of superoxide

Although the chemistry of O_2^- in aqueous solutions indicates that it is much less reactive than the hydroxyl radical, $OH^{\cdot}$ (Ref. 12), it has been demonstrated over and over again that enzymatically, photochemically, or electrochemically generated fluxes of O_2^- are toxic and destructive to living cells (see Refs. 4 and 11 for complete survey). Furthermore, in a recent study paraquat, which is known to increase the production of O_2^-, was found to be highly mutagenic in the *Salmonella typhimurium* (Ref. 13). In most cases, superoxide dismutase, catalase, or compounds known to scavenge $OH^{\cdot}$, were found to protect against the deleterious effects of O_2^-. These findings led to the proposal that O_2^- and H_2O_2 can interact to produce $OH^{\cdot}$ (Ref. 14), as was originally suggested by Haber and Weiss in 1934 (Ref. 15). Attempts to demonstrate the generation of $OH^{\cdot}$ from the direct interaction between O_2^- and H_2O_2 showed that iron complexes are required as catalysts (Ref. 16). Since the dismutation of O_2^- generated H_2O_2, it is clear that O_2^- production could, in the presence of iron catalysts, lead to $OH^{\cdot}$ formation and cellular damage. Superoxide dismutases and hydroperoxidases protect the cells by lowering the steadystate concentration of both O_2^- and H_2O_2, respectively, at the same time minimizing the likelihood of the production of $OH^{\cdot}$.

Correlation between superoxide dismutase and oxygen tolerance: surveys

The first test of the superoxide theory was a survey of different organisms for their contents of superoxide dismutase and of catalase. It was reasoned that organisms that utilize oxygen must maintain defenses against the toxicity of oxygen, whereas those that never encounter oxygen, and are sensitive to it, could do without such defense. The results were encouraging, thus the aerobes contained more superoxide dismutase and catalase than the aerotolerant organisms, while the anaerobes had none (Ref. 9). The situation with anaerobes turned out to be more complex than was revealed in this first study. This complexity stems from the practice of referring to obligate anaerobes as organisms unable to grow in air, a grouping which includes species with widely differing sensitivities towards oxygen (Ref. 1). Thus, related species of obligately anaerobic bacteria were found to display large differences in their oxygen-tolerance (Ref. 17), and to contain superoxide dismutase (Ref. 18). A positive correlation, however, was found between the degree of aerotolerance of some anaerobes and their content of superoxide dismutase (Ref. 19). Other anaerobes have since been found to contain superoxide dismutase (Refs. 20-26). It would thus appear that mechanisms for the univalent reduction of oxygen do exist in some anaerobes and that superoxide dismutase is then needed to provide protection against oxygen toxicit This should not be surprising, since even obligate anaerobes are frequently, if transiently, exposed to oxygen *en route* from one anaerobic niche to another. Besides some environments, which are traditionally thought to be anaerobic, such as the intestinal tracts of large animals, are not really oxygen free (Ref. 27). Some anaerobes were able to induce higher levels of superoxide dismutase upon exposure to low levels of oxygen (Refs. 26,28,29). Elevated levels of superoxide dismutase in *Bacteroides fragilis* imparted resistance towards 5 Atm oxygen (Ref. 28).

The presence of superoxide dismutases in some anaerobes is not inconsistent with the superoxide theory of oxygen toxicity, since they need a measure of oxygen toler- ance. However, the aerotolerant *Lactobacillus plantarum* did appear to be an embarrassment for this theory since it was reported to be devoid of superoxide dis- mutase and catalase (Ref. 9). A satisfactory explanation for this anomaly was found in the lack of respiration of logarithmic phase cells growing on a glucose containing medium (Ref. 9,30). Thus, it was reasoned that an organism which did not reduce O_2 could not make O_2^- or H_2O_2, and so could afford to dispense with enzymic scavengers of these reactive intermediates. This explanation did not hold up under close scrutiny. Thus, *L. plantarum* consumes oxygen under certain conditions (Ref. 31). Yousten et al (Ref. 32) also noted that respiration increased during the stationary phase in glucose-exhausted media and low levels of SOD were found in extracts of these cells. A thorough re-examination of respiration, oxygen toxicity, and of the scavenging of O_2^- in *L. plantarum* revealed that this organism can respire and generate O_2^-, more- over, it has replaced superoxide dismutase with another scavenger of O_2^- (Ref. 33). This O_2^- scavenger was found to be dialyzable and EDTA-inhibitable, and it turned out to be Mn(II). Thus, while most aerotolerant organisms protect themselves against oxygen toxicity with micromolar levels of superoxide dismutase, *L. plantarum* achieves the same end with millimolar levels of Mn(II) and it exhibits oxygen-intolerance when deprived of Mn(II) (Ref. 33). The reason for choosing this unusual strategy is not known, but it clearly demonstrates that O_2^- is an important agent of oxygen toxicity and that some defense against this radical is needed.

The strategy employed by the strains of *Neisseria gonorrhoeae* that were reported

(Ref. 34) to have no superoxide dismutase activity while possessing relatively higher levels of catalase remains unclear. Further studies are also needed to explain the apparent lack of superoxide dismutase in *Mycoplasma pneumoniae* in spite of its aerobic lifestyle (Ref. 35).

Classes and distribution of superoxide dismutases in prokaryotes

All superoxide dismutases are metalloproteins. The enzymes thus far, isolated from a wide range of microorganisms, fall into two classes depending on the metal found in their active centers. Thus, there are superoxide dismutases that contain iron (FeSOD) or manganese (MnSOD). The Fe- and MnSODs are characteristic of prokaryotes and show a high degree of amino acid sequence homology in their N-terminal regions (Refs. 36,37). On the other hand, no amino acid sequence homology is shared between the Fe- or MnSODs and copper-zinc (CuZn) SODs which are characteristic of eukaryotic cytosols (Refs. 37, 38). The finding of a CuZnSOD in the symbiotic prokaryote, *Photobacterium leiognathi* (Ref. 39), represents an exception to the rule that this class of enzymes are characteristic of eukaryotic cytosols. (See also Ref. 39a which describes a CuZnSOD in the free-living bacterium *Paracoccus denitrificans*.) Amino acid analysis (Ref. 40) strongly endorsed the original proposal that *P. leiognathi* has acquired its CuZn-enzyme from its eukaryotic host, the pony fish, *via* gene transfer (Ref. 41).

In general, there is no correlation between the Gram-reaction and the type of superoxide dismutase (Ref. 10), however, most anaerobes seem to possess the iron-class of enzymes.

Synthesis of superoxide dismutase in *E. coli* in response to atmospheric changes

Aerobically grown *E. coli* contains three distinct isozymes of superoxide dismutase (Ref. 42), one of which contains manganese (Ref. 43), the second, iron (Ref. 44), and the third contains iron, but appears to be a hybrid containing one subunit from each of the other isozymes (Ref. 45). Anaerobically grown cells, in contrast, contain only FeSOD. Thus the synthesis of MnSOD in *E. coli* seems to be under rigorous control. The cells are also able to efficiently modulate the level of this enzyme to meet their defense requirements. The constitutive FeSOD of *E. coli* provides a backup defense against oxygen toxicity during sudden exposures to oxygen and represents a compromise between the expense of maintaining a large standing level of defensive enzyme and the damage sustained during the delay inherent in induction.

Induction of Superoxide Dismutase

The substrate for superoxide dismutase, O_2^-, can only be made in the presence of oxygen. The induction of the biosynthesis of an enzyme by its substrate is probably the surest indication that its in vivo function is to act upon that substrate or upon metabolic derivatives thereof. This led to the prediction that exposure to higher levels of oxygen might induce higher levels of the enzyme(s) needed for protection against oxygen toxicity. This has been seen. Thus, exposure of E. *coli* (Ref. 46), *Streptococcus faecalis* (Ref. 47), B. *fragilis* (Ref. 28), and numerous other organisms to oxygen resulted in increased intracellular levels of superoxide dismutase. These increased levels of superoxide dismutase, achieved by oxygen exposure, correlated with increased resistance towards oxygen toxicity (Refs. 46-48), and towards the oxygen enhancement of the toxicity of streptonigrin (Ref. 48). These results support the superoxide theory of oxygen toxicity, but suffer from the circularity involved in inducing the enzyme with oxygen and then noting a gain in the resistance of the cells towards this same stress. Our argument would be better served if we could manipulate the level of superoxide dismutase without changing pO_2 and then see a correlation between the enzyme level and oxygen tolerance. This has been achieved in E. *coli* by several different strategies.

Chemostat culture: superoxide dismutase as a function of growth rate

When the specific growth rate of E. *coli* was manipulated by changing the dilution rate in a glucose-limited chemostat culture, while maintaining constant and abundant aeration, the concentration of superoxide dismutase varied in proportion to the specific growth rate and to the rate of respiration (Ref. 49). Increased levels of superoxide dismutase, achieved under this condition of constant aeration, correlated with resistance of the cells towards the lethality of hyperbaric oxygen. In this case, there was no circularity in the correlation between superoxide dismutase levels and resistance to oxygen toxicity since the pO_2 was constant.

These experiments also provided the first clue that the inducer for superoxide dismutase is not molecular oxygen *per se* but rather a product of its metabolism Thus, if we assume that a constant fraction of the total oxygen metabolized by the cells is reduced *via* the univalent pathway, then low growth rate and low respiration rate must be associated with a low intracellular production of O_2^- and a correspondingly low level of superoxide dismutase, which suffices to scavenge this low level of O_2^-. Increased growth rates would be accompanied by increased respiration, O_2^- production, and superoxide dismutase level. The results of these experiments promoted the hypothesis that the level of superoxide dismutase within the cell is in line with the intracellular level of O_2^- generated during growth in the presence of oxygen.

The glucose effect and superoxide dismutase levels

E. *coli* grown in minimal medium with glucose as the sole source of carbon, contained lower levels of superoxide dismutase than cells grown on succinate or lactate (Ref. 50). The level of superoxide dismutase was not a simple function of growth rate, as was the case in the glucose-limited chemostat culture mentioned above, since cells placed in media containing succinate or lactate grew at much slower rates and contained higher levels of superoxide dismutase than did cells grown on glucose. A kinetic study of superoxide dismutase synthesis, during a growth cycle on trypticase soy-yeast extract (TSY) medium, which contained a limited amount of glucose (0.25%), revealed the complexity of this glucose effect (Ref. 50). The data clearly showed that superoxide dismutase content declined to a minimum early in the growth cycle and then increased again (Ref. 50). The decline in superoxide dismutase level coincided with a decline in the glucose content and the pH of the medium, which suggested glucose fermentation. The rise in superoxide dismutase level began when glucose was exhausted and the pH of the medium began to rise, which indicated a utilization of the accumulated organic acids and amino acids. Furthermore, when cells were shifted from a glucose-minimal medium to a rich medium (TSY) the cells' content of superoxide dismutase remained constant (at the level characteristic of glucose grown cells), while glucose was being utilized, and then increased abruptly as glucose was exhausted to reach a level of superoxide dismutase characteristic of late growth cycle cells in the TSY medium (Ref. 50). However, when the TSY medium was prepared free of glucose, superoxide dismutase synthesis increased in the outset. This effect of glucose was not due to classical catabolite repression, since cyclic AMP had no effect on the variation of superoxide dismutase content during growth cycle in TSY medium. Furthermore, α-methyl glucoside, which mimics glucose in causing catabolite repression, was without effect on the synthesis of superoxide dismutase in TSY medium devoid of glucose (Ref. 50). These results, led us to conclude that the rate of O_2^- production in the cells was low during glucose utilization, but increased during the oxidative phase of metabolism and that the cells modulated the level of superoxide dismutase to meet their changing needs for the scavenging of O_2^-. This supposition was tested by artificially increasing the intracellular production of O_2^- with methyl viologen (paraquat). When this was done there was a profound induction of superoxide dismutase, which was seen even in fresh TSY medium containing glucose (Ref. 50).

Induction of superoxide dismutase by paraquat and related compounds

Some redox active compounds can enter E. coli and other cells and divert electron flow from the water-producing cytochrome pathway to an O_2^--producing pathway. These compounds are rapidly reduced by diaphorases present in the cells, yielding reduced forms which are rapidly reoxidized by oxygen to yield O_2^-. Paraquat, pyocyanine, streptonigrin, juglone, plumbagin and menadione are among the compounds which function in this way. They all act catalytically to increase O_2^- production and to increase cyanide-resistant respiration, since they provide a cytochrome-independent pathway to oxygen (Ref. 51-54). These compounds exhibit an oxygen-dependent toxicity, and in a real sense they exacerbate the toxicity of oxygen. The toxicity of these compounds was dependent upon the presence of oxygen and of a rapidly metabolizable substrate that can provide electrons (Ref. 52).

E. coli were found to be much more tolerant to paraquat when grown in rich medium, such as TSY, than in a glucose-salts medium (Ref. 52). This was due to the rapid induction of superoxide dismutase in the rich medium, which was not possible in the minimal medium. When rapid induction of superoxide dismutase was prevented by adding inhibitors of protein synthesis (i.e., puromycin or chloramphenicol), the protective effect of the rich medium was eliminated. Kinetic analysis of superoxide dismutase induction, showed that addition of 0.5 mM paraquat to an aerobically growing culture of E. coli resulted, after a brief lag, in a rapid linear increase in superoxide dismutase. Removal of paraquat from the growth medium caused a sharp decline in the rate of superoxide dismutase synthesis. These results indicated that increased synthesis of superoxide dismutase in response to paraquat was due to true induction rather than selection by paraquat of some super producers of superoxide dismutase (Ref 51). Disc gel electrophoresis, activity staining, and linear scanning densitometry demonstrated that paraquat, as well as the other redox active compounds that were capable of increasing the flux of intracellular O_2^-, induced the Mn- but not the FeSOD (Refs. 51,53). This increase in the biosynthesis of the MnSOD by paraquat was prevented by inhibitors of transcription or translation, but not by inhibitors of replication (Ref. 53). Thus, the increase in MnSOD biosynthesis in response to increases in intracellular O_2^-, as caused by paraquat, was due to *de novo* enzyme synthesis activated at the level of transcription, and O_2^-, or a unique product derived therefrom, was the effector. Induction of superoxide dismutase by one of the redox active compounds was found to impart resistance toward the others, which pointed out the similarity of their mechanism of action and the protective role of superoxide dismutase against O_2^--mediated oxygen toxicity.

The components of the electron transport chain are not readily autoxidized. Nevertheless they do autoxidize to some degree, which accounts for the small production of O_2^- and of H_2O_2 by submitochondrial particles (Refs. 55-62), and probably by respiring prokaryotes. Blocking cytochrome oxidase with cyanide or azide should increase the degree of steady-state reduction of these electron carriers and should therefore increase the rate at which they reduce O_2 to O_2^-. This led to the expectation and the finding that CN^- or N_3^- induces MnSOD in E. coli (Ref. 53).

Effects of extracellular superoxide radical

Extracellularly generated O_2^- did not cause induction of superoxide dismutase, and evidence has been presented showing that O_2^- does not cross the E. coli cell envelope (Ref. 63). However, there have been several reports on the lethality of exogenous O_2^- Thus, part of the lethal effect of paraquat is due to extracellular generation of O_2^- *via* the reoxidation of the reduced paraquat radical that diffuses from the cells when the intracellular O_2 concentration is depleted by active respiration. The extracellular aerobic reoxidation of the reduced paraquat radical generates O_2^- which can dismute to generate H_2O_2, and under these conditions some protection is afforded by superoxide dismutase and by catalase, added to the suspending medium (Ref. 63). E. coli grown in an iron-deficient medium, were killed by photochemically as well as by enzymically generated O_2^-, and superoxide dismutase added to the suspending medium provided complete protection (Ref. 46). Protection by both superoxide dismutase and by catalase against killing by a photochemical source of O_2^- was noted in L. plantarum (Ref. 30). There have also been conflicting reports. Both E. coli and Staphylococcus epidermidis were killed by the O_2^- generated by the xanthine oxidase reaction. S. epidermidis was protected by both superoxide dismutase and by catalase, while E. coli was protected only by catalase (Ref. 64). Catalase protected Neisseria gonorrhoeae against the lethality of the xanthine oxidase reaction while superoxide dismutase did not (Ref. 65).

In some of these studies, O_2^- appears to have been the major lethal agent, while in others both O_2^- and H_2O_2 were involved and still in others H_2O_2 was the important agent. Some of these apparent conflicts may be explained on the basis of differences in the test organism or in the O_2^--generating system. Recently, Rosen and Klebanoff (Ref. 66) have carefully studied the effect of some of these factors on the bacteriocidal activity of O_2^-. Exposure to the xanthine oxidase reaction killed Staphylococcus aureus and Sarcina lutea and both superoxide dismutase and catalase protected, which suggested that both O_2^- and H_2O_2 were involved (Ref. 66). There were strain differences, thus a non-pigmented strain of S. lutea was more susceptible than a yellow strain. There were also differences based on the O_2^--generating system, in that the lethality was greater when acetaldehyde was used in place of xanthine in the xanthine oxidase reaction. This was apparently the case because xanthine and the product of the reaction, urate, protected the cells. Finally, if myeloperoxidase plus a halide were also present the lethality of the reaction mixture was greatly augmented and depended primarily upon H_2O_2.

Superoxide dismutase was also seen to protect against O_2^- generated by ionizing radiation. Thus, in suspensions of E. coli exposed to X-irradiation the lethality was enhanced by the presence of oxygen and both superoxide dismutase and catalase decreased this oxygen enhancement (Refs. 67-69). It is clear, therefore, that exogenous O_2^- can exert marked deleterious effect on bacteria as well as on other biological systems and that superoxide dismutase protects.

Oxygen-sensitive mutants of E. coli

The physiological roles of superoxide dismutase and catalase in protecting E. coli against the toxic effects of oxygen were further explored by selecting mutants lacking these enzymes (Ref. 70,71). E. coli K12 was mutagenized with N-methyl-N'-nitro-N-nitrosoguanidine and a replica plating technique was used to select mutants with a temperature-dependent intolerance for oxygen. One of these mutants exhibited a temperature-dependent decline in its content of superoxide dismutase, which parallel its intolerance for oxygen (Ref. 70). In a more recent study, oxygen sensitive mutants of E. coli were isolated and found to fall into two groups (Ref. 71). One group had lost the ability to induce both catalase and peroxidase, when exposed to oxygen, but retained their ability to induce MnSOD. The second group of mutants had

136

lost the ability to induce all three enzymes. Oxygen was lethal to both groups. When a member of the first group of mutants was prevented from inducing MnSOD by adding puromycin, the lethal effect of oxygen was greatly increased. These results indicated that enzymic scavenging of both O_2^- and H_2O_2 provides the ultimate defense against oxygen toxicity. The mutants were found to revert to wild type phenotype (oxygen-tolerance) at a frequency of 1 in 10^5 cells to 1 in 10^4 cells, which is much higher than the normal spontaneous rate expected for single mutations. This pointed to the possibility that the unscavenged fluxes of O_2^- and H_2O_2 might be mutagenic agents. This prediction has recently been confirmed (Ref. 13), by showing that paraquat is mutagenic to Ames tester strains and that this mutagenic effect was oxygen dependent.

Summary

The data strongly supported the notion that O_2^- can be generated within respiring cells, and it is an important agent of the toxicity of oxygen, paraquat, pyocyanine, and several redox-active compounds and that superoxide dismutase is the primary defense against the deleterious effects of this radical. Increasing the rate of intracellular O_2^- production, by different means, leads to an adaptive increase in the synthesis of superoxide dismutase. Blocking this adaptive response with inhibitors of protein biosynthesis or with a nutritionally restricted medium, causes the cells to die.

The presence of superoxide dismutase in some anaerobes, and the presence of constitutive FeSOD in E. coli represents an evolutionary response to the toxicity of oxygen that ensure their continual survival.

REFERENCES

1. Loesche, W.J. (1969) Appl. Microbiol., 18, 723-727.
2. Morris, J.G. (1979) in Strategies of Microbial Life in Extreme Environments, Shilo, M., ed., Dahlem Konferenzen, Verlag Chemie, Weinheim, pp. 149-162.
3. Haugaard, N. (1968) Physiol. Rev., 48, 311-373.
4. Fridovich, I. (1975) Ann. Rev. Biochem., 44, 147-159.
5. Morris, J.G. (1975) in Advances in Microbial Physiology, Vol. 12, Rose, A.H. and Tempest, D.W., eds., New York: Academic Press, pp. 169-246.
6. Taube, H. (1965) J. Gen. Physiol., 49 (Suppl.), 29-52.
7. Hamilton, G.A. (1974) in Molecular Mechanisms of Oxygen Activation, Hayaishi, O., ed., New York: Academic Press, pp. 405-451.
8. McCord, J.M. and Fridovich, I. (1969) J. Biol. Chem., 244, 6049-6055.
9. McCord, J.M., Keele, B.B., Jr., and Fridovich, I. (1971) Proc. Natl. Acad. Sci. USA, 68, 1024-1027.
10. Britton, L., Malinowski, D.P., and Fridovich, I. (1978) J. Bacteriol., 134, 229-236.
11. Fridovich, I. (1979) in Advances in Inorganic Biochemistry, Eichhorn, G.L. and Marzilli, D.L., eds., New York: Elsevier-North Holland, pp. 67-90.
12. Bielski, B.H.J. and Richter, H.W. (1977) J. Am. Chem. Soc., 99, 3019-3023.
13. Hassan, H.M. and Fein, J.E. (1982) for publication.

14. Beauchamp, C.O. and Fridovich, I. (1970) J. Biol. Chem., 245, 4641-4646.
15. Haber, F. and Weiss, J. (1934) Proc. Roy. Soc. Lond. A, 147, 332-351.
16. McCord, J.M. and Day, E.D., Jr. (1978) FEBS Lett., 86, 139-142.
17. O'Brien, R.W. and Morris, J.G. (1971) J. Gen. Microbiol., 68, 307-318.
18. Hewitt, J. and Morris, J.G. (1975) FEBS Lett., 50, 315-318.
19. Tally, F.P., Goldin, H.R., Jacobus, N.V., and Gerbach, S.L. (1977) Infect. Immun., 16, 20-25.
20. Lindmark, D.G. and Müller, M. (1974) J. Biol. Chem., 249, 4634-4637.
21. Gregory, E.M., Kowalski, J.B., and Holdeman, L.V. (1977) J. Bacteriol., 129, 1298-1302.
22. Hatchikian, E.C. and Henry, Y.A. (1977) Biochimie, 59, 153-161.
23. Gregory, E.M., Moore, W.E.C., and Holdeman, L.V. (1978) Appl. Environ. Microbiol., 35, 988-991.
24. Vesugi, I. and Yajima, M. (1978) Ziet. F. Allg. Microbiol., 18, 593-601.
25. Kanematsu, S. and Asada, K. (1978) Arch. Biochem. Biophys., 185, 473-482.
26. Wimpenny, J.W.T. and Samah, O.A. (1978) J. Gen. Microbiol., 108, 329-332.
27. Levitt, M.D. and Bond, J.H., Jr. (1970) Gastroenterology, 59, 921-929.
28. Privalle, C.T. and Gregory, E.M. (1979) J. Bacteriol., 138, 139-145.
29. Pritchard, G.G., Wimpenny, J.W.T., Morris, H.A., Lewis, M.W.A., and Hughes, D.E. (1977) J. Gen. Microbiol., 102, 223-233.
30. Gregory, E. M. and Fricovich, I. (1974) J. Bacteriol., 117, 166-169.
31. Strittmatter, C.F. (1959) J. Biol. Chem., 234, 2789-2793.
32. Yousten, A. A., Johnson, J.L., and Salin, M. (1975) J. Bacteriol., 123, 242-247.
33. Archibald, F.S. and Fridovich, I. (1981) J. Bacteriol., 145, 442-451.
34. Norrod, P. and Morse, S.A. (1979) Biochem. Biophys. Res. Commun., 90, 1287-1294.
35. Lynch, R.E. and Cole, B.C. (1980) in Biological and Clinical Aspects of Superoxide and Superoxide Dismutase, Bannister, W.H. and Bannister, J.V., eds., New York: Elsevier-North Holland, pp. 49-56.
36. Steinman, H.M. and Hill, R.L. (1973) Proc. Natl. Acad. Sci. USA, 70, 3725-3729.
37. Harris, J.I. and Steinman, H.M. (1977) in Superoxide and Superoxide Dismutases, Michelson, A.M., McCord, J.M., and Fridovich, I., eds., New York: Academic Press, pp. 225-230.
38. Steinman, H.M. (1978) J. Biol. Chem., 253, 8708-8720.
39. Puget, K. and Michelson, A.M. (1974) Biochem. Biophys. Res. Commun., 58, 830-838.
39a Vignais, P.M., Henry, M.-F., Terech, A. and Chabert, J. (1980) in Chemical and Biological Aspects of Superoxide and Superoxide Dismutase, Bannister, J.V. and Hill, H.A.O., eds., New York: Elsevier-North Holland, pp. 154-159; Terech, A. and Vignais, P.M. (1981) Biochim. Biophys. Acta, 657, 411-424.
40. Martin, J.P. and Fridovich, I. (1980) J. Biol. Chem., 256, 6080-6089.
41. Fridovich, I. (1978) Science, 201, 875-880.
42. Hassan, H.M. and Fridovich, I. (1977) J. Bacteriol., 129, 1574-1583.
43. Keele, B.B., Jr., McCord, J.M., and Fridovich, I. (1970) J. Biol. Chem., 245, 6176-6181.
44. Yost, F. J., Jr. and Fridovich, I. (1973) J. Biol. Chem., 248, 4905-4908.
45. Dougherty, H. W., Sadowski, S.J., and Baker, E.E. (1978) J. Biol. Chem., 253, 5220-5223.
46. Gregory, E.M., Yost, F.J., Jr., and Fridovich, I. (1973) J. Bacteriol., 115, 987-991.
47. Gregory, E.M. and Fridovich, I. (1973) J. Bacteriol., 114, 543-548.
48. Gregory, E.M. and Fridovich, I. (1973) J. Bacteriol., 114, 1193-1197.
49. Hassan, H.M. and Fridovich, I. (1977) J. Bacteriol., 130, 805-811.
50. Hassan, H.M. and Fridovich, I. (1977) J. Bacteriol., 132, 505-510.
51. Hassan, H.M. and Fridovich, I. (1977) J. Biol. Chem., 252, 7667-7672.
52. Hassan, H.M. and Fridovich, I. (1978) J. Biol. Chem., 253, 8143-8148.
53. Hassan, H.M. and Fridovich, I. (1979) Arch. Biochem. Biophys., 196, 385-395.
54. Hassan, H.M. and Fridovich, I. (1980) J. Bacteriol., 141, 156-163.
55. Boveris, A. and Chance, B. (1973) Biochem. J., 134, 707-716.
56. Forman, H.J. and Kennedy, J.A. (1974) Biochem. Biophys. Res. Commun., 60, 1044-1050.

138

57. Loschen, G., Azzi, A., Richler, C., and Flohé, L. (1974) FEBS Lett., 42, 68-72.
58. Tyler, D.D. (1975) Biochim. Biophys. Acta, 396, 335-346.
59. Boveris, A. and Cadenas, E. (1975) FEBS Lett., 54, 311-314.
60. Boveris, A. (1977) Adv. Exptl. Med. Biol., 78, 67-82.
61. Boveris, A., Sanchez, R.A., and Beconi, M.T. (1978) FEBS Lett., 92, 333-338.
62. Takeshige, K. and Minakami, S. (1979) Biochem. J., 180, 129-135.
63. Hassan, H.M. and Fridovich, I. (1979) J. Biol. Chem., 254, 10846-10852.
64. Babior, B., Curnutte, J.T. and Kipnes, R.S. (1975) J. Lab. Clin. Med., 85, 235-244.
65. Ismail, G., Sawyer, W.D., and Wegener, W.S. (1977) Proc. Soc. Exptl. Biol. Med., 155, 264-269.
66. Rosen, H. and Klebanoff, S.J. (1979) J. Exp. Med., 149, 27-30.
67. Misra, H.P. and Fridovich, I. (1976) Arch. Biochem. Biophys., 176, 577-581.
68. Oberly, L.W., Lindgren, A.L., Baker, S.A., and Stevens, R.H. (1976) Radiat. Res., 68, 320-328.
69. Niva, T., Yamaguchi, H., and Yano, K. (1977) in Biochemical and Medical Aspects of Active Oxygens, Hayaishi, O. and Asada, K., eds., Tokyo: Univ. Tokyo Press, pp. 209-225.
70. McCord, J.M., Beauchamp, C.O., Goscin, S., Misra, H.P., and Fridovich, I. (1973) in Oxidases and Related Redox Systems, King, T.E., Mason, H.S., and Morrison, M., eds., Baltimore: University Park Press, pp. 66-73.
71. Hassan, H.M. and Fridovich, I. (1979) Rev. Infect. Dis., 1, 357-367.

CHAPTER 7   OXYGEN TOXICITY IN EUKARYOTES

ANNE P. AUTOR
Department of Pharmacology, University of Iowa, Iowa City, Iowa 52240, USA

Introduction

The toxic potential of oxygen was recognized at the time of its discovery and molecular identification over two hundred years ago. Its pathophysiological effects when breathed at high tensions were studied by the great physiologist, J.L. Smith, before the beginning of the 20th century (Ref. 1). Renewed interest in the nature of oxygen toxicity arose in conjunction with the advances in the technology of high altitude flying and in deep sea diving which began in the mid-1940s. The necessity of understanding the physiological consequences from alterations in oxygen tensions provided an impetus for the renewed study of hyperoxia. The ramifications of oxygen-associated pathology have, however, only been revealed in the past fifteen years.

Clinicians became directly acquainted with oxygen toxicity when retrolental fibroplasia, a pathology of premature infants, was traced to the hyperoxia therapy administered to alleviate pulmonary insufficiency or respiratory distress syndrome associated with premature birth (Ref. 2). Improved techniques of oxygen delivery dramatically lowered the incidence of retrolental fibroplasia in premature babies. Nevertheless, pulmonary pathology associated with hyperoxia has persisted. This includes bronchopulmonary dysplasia of infants and acute pulmonary edema followed by atelectasis and fibrin formation in the lungs of adults consequent to prolonged hyperoxic therapy (Refs. 3,4).

Basic research on oxygen poisoning has accelerated since the mid-1960s and has provided a much clearer understanding of the molecular mechanisms associated with oxygen-provoked toxicity. From these investigations, two important processes have been described and substantiated by experimental data. One of these is that oxygen manifests its toxicity through the generation of oxygen free radicals or reduction products. Furthermore, these free radicals are produced, albeit at a low level, even at the relatively low extra- and intracellular oxygen content of air-breathing organisms. As a result, a constant flow of chemically reactive, and therefore, potentially damaging free radicals occurs even with normal, aerobic metabolism. The second proposal elaborated from the first is that intrinsic protective mechanisms against oxygen-derived free radicals must be present in aerobic cells.

The elaboration of these proposals and the subsequent experimental confirmation emanated from various investigators, both clinical and basic scientists. Two pioneers who were instrumental in developing an understanding of the importance of oxygen-derived free radicals in biological systems were Leonor Michaelis and Rebecca S. Gerschman. Professor Michaelis, in the 1930s, elaborated the theoretical framework which explained the biological generation of free radicals (Ref. 5) and elegantly described the quinone reduction cycle as a free radical reaction. Two decades later, as a consequence of her efforts towards understanding the fundamental mechanism of oxygen poisoning and her insight that very possibly its mechanism resembled X-radiation-induced toxicity, Dr. Gerschman proposed that oxygen radical generation is the basis of oxygen toxicity (Ref. 6). The current understanding of oxygen toxicity expressed via partially reduced free radical metabolites of oxygen has consequently been built from these theoretical and experimental foundations. Furthermore, we now know that oxygen radical toxicity encompasses more than the side effects of therapeutic or occupational hyperoxia. Inflammatory conditions associated with bacterial infection (Ref. 7), arthritis (Refs. 8,9), brain edema (Ref. 10), radiation toxicity (Ref. 11 and prostaglandin synthesis (Ref. 12) are related to or as a consequence of oxygen radicals. The toxic side effects of many drugs, particularly the quinone-containing anti-tumor agents (Ref. 13) are now attributed to oxygen radicals. Toxic effects of environmental pollutants such as ozone and nitrous oxide (and other nitrogen oxides) have also been traced to oxygen-derived free radicals. Oxygen metabolites are implicated in aging (Ref. 14) and carcinogenesis (Ref. 15) according to recent evidence.

Concomitant with the understanding of the oxygen radical mechanisms of cytotoxicity there has been a growing knowledge of the endogenous means by which aerobic cells mount protection against oxygen radical toxicity. The first important contribution came from McCord and Fridovich (Ref. 16) who discovered the enzyme superoxide dismutase. It has been well documented by the work of Tyler (Ref. 17) and Boveris (Ref. 18) that superoxide radicals and hydrogen peroxide are generated from the electron transport chain and from intact mitochondria during oxidative metabolism. Superoxide dismutase is therefore to be considered the first line of defense against oxygen toxicity. The pathology of oxygen has recently been documented (Ref. 19). The mitochondrial form of superoxide dismutase has been shown to be elevated during enhanced oxygen and hydrogen peroxide generation (Ref. 20). Defense against hydrogen peroxide comes from catalase and glutathione peroxidase (Ref. 21).

Finally the production of a third oxygen centered species has to be considered. This is the hydroxyl radical which can be generated through a Fenton-catalyzed Haber-Weiss reaction. The non-heme iron containing proteins, lactoferrin and transferrin have been proposed as catalysts for this reaction (Refs. 22,23,24).

Of the three partially reduced oxygen moieties, the hydroxyl radical OH$^\bullet$, a powerful oxidizing agent, is the most reactive. The role of superoxide radicals and hydrogen peroxide, common products of cellular oxygen metabolism, in toxic oxidative stress therefore appears to be as precursors of OH$^\bullet$. In normal aerobic metabolism superoxide dismutase, glutathione peroxidase, catalase and the small molecular weight radical scavengers (ascorbate, α-tocophenol and β-carotene) are adequate to remove these reactive intermediates. When the steady state levels of either or both reactants is elevated due to metabolism in hyperoxia (Refs. 18, 25) or the presence of oxygen radical generators, the protective capacity of these cell components appears to be inadequate to prevent the consequences of destructive oxidizing reactions initiated by OH$^\bullet$. Although the precise nature and sequence of these reactions in cells is not known, the action of OH$^\bullet$ on isolated biomacromolecules has been described. Hydroxyl radicals have been shown to cleave DNA (Ref. 26), initiate lipid peroxidation of polyunsaturated fatty acids (Ref. 27) and oxidizes sulfhydryl-containing amino acids in proteins (Ref. 28). Whole cells are destroyed in a rapid, time dependent manner when exposed to chemical systems which generate OH$^\bullet$ (as demonstrated by electron spin resonance spin-trapping) (Ref. 29).

Simple eukaryotes

Oxygen toxicity in eukaryotic organisms has been studied in two general ways. One method has used the known effect of hyperoxic induction of superoxide dismutase and catalase. In this way, the cellular content of enzymes which remove oxygen radicals can be manipulated and the response of the altered cells to hyperoxia observed. This approach works well with unicellular organisms and has been successfully used with the simple eukaryotic yeast *Saccharomyces cerevisiae*. When grown in 100% oxygen (1 atm.) *S. cerevisiae* induced superoxide dismutase and catalase six-fold and two-fold, respectively. Increased endogenous superoxide dismutase was associated with increased resistance to lethality consequent to hyperbaric oxygen or irradiation (Ref. 30). Conversely yeast grown strictly anaerobically contain no active superoxide dismutase (Ref. 31) or catalase (Ref. 32). A constant rate of superoxide radical generation was detected in the cell contents of anaerobically grown yeast which was not present in aerobically grown organisms which contain active superoxide dismutase (Ref. 31). Anaerobically grown yeast are incapable of growing in air (21% oxygen) unless they are allowed to adapt, a process which involves the *de novo* synthesis of superoxide dismutase and catalase. The oxygen free radical mechanisms of oxygen poisoning would predict this result. Other cell components, such as cytochromes and cell membrane constituents are altered or restored when facultative anaerobes undergo respiratory adaptation (Ref. 33) but a systematic study of this alteration with respect to oxygen toxicity has not been done.

142

The second method of studying oxygen poisoning via oxygen free radicals has
been to study the consequences to cells exposed to generated superoxide and
hydroxyl radicals and hydrogen peroxide. Most of these studies have been
conducted with prokaryotes or with complex eukaryotes.

Complex eukaryotes

In air breathing animals, the lung is the primary target of oxygen poisoning
in a normabaric atmosphere which contains toxic concentrations of oxygen (> 70%).
Many factors influence the time of exposure to hyperoxia which results in pulmonary failure and death. These include age, nutritional states, species and pre-
existing pathological conditions (Ref. 34). Nevertheless, the ultimate effect on
lung tissue is similar (Table 1). Oxygen toxicity in complex eukaryotes has been

TABLE 1

Pathologic Manifestations of Pulmonary Oxygen Toxicity

Edema	Accumulation of fluid in the airspaces and the interstitium (basement membrane)
Congestion	Accumulation of fluid in the perivascular and peribronchial regions. Constriction of venules and arterioles.
Atelectasis	Collapse of the normally expanded terminal airways (alveoli)
Hyaline membrane formation	Accumulation of fibrin strands and cell debris which deposit in the septa of the alveoli and the terminal bronchioles.

commonly studied, therefore, by the examination of oxygen-induced damage to lung
tissue. These studies have encompassed exposure of whole animals, isolated
perfused lungs or cultured lung cells either to high oxygen concentrations or to
oxygen radical generating systems and the morphological, functional and biochemical
results examined. In the intact animal exposed to oxidative stress, oxygen
radicals originate from three sources which can be described as metabolic, cellular and chemical. Metabolically generated free radicals occurring as substrates
are oxidized by enzymes in the mitochondria, endoplasmic reticulum and cytosol
and oxygen is concomitantly reduced. Oxygen radicals normally low at 21% oxygen
are generated at a higher rate as the ambient oxygen concentration is elevated
to 100%. Cellular generation of oxygen radicals emanates from stimulated phagocytic cells, primarily leukocytes and pulmonary macrophages, by the action of
an NADPH-dependent, membrane bound oxidase. The activity of the oxidase is expressed when phagocytes are stimulated by particulate or soluble factors (Ref. 7).
Chemical generation of oxygen radicals involves the activation, generally by
univalent reduction of drugs, xenobiotics or toxic chemicals and a consequent
autoxidation of the reduced chemical according to the following general
reactions:

$$2R + NADPH \xrightarrow{\text{reductase}} 2R^{\bullet} + NADP^{+} + H^{+}$$

$$2R^{\bullet} + 2O_2 \longrightarrow 2R + 2O_2^{-}$$

NADPH-cytochrome P-450 reductase, one of the enzymatic components of the drug-metabolizing mixed function oxidase system of endoplasmic reticulum is commonly associated with this process. Chemical sources of oxygen radicals through these means include the quinone containing drugs and nitrofurantoin and the herbicide paraquat (Ref. 35).

The process of oxygen-induced pulmonary injury begins by initiation with metabolically generated radicals. Structural damage to the alveolar septa which is typical of this process is seen in scanning electron micrographs of lung

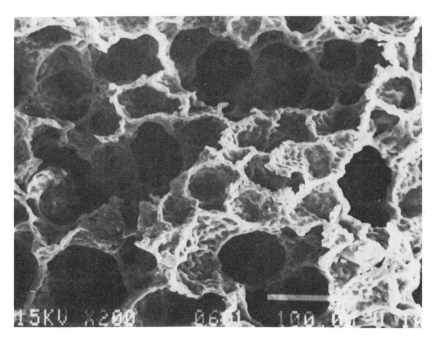

Fig. 1A. Scanning electron micrograph of a normal rat lung after tracheal fixation. The bar in the lower right corner = 100 microns. (Courtesy of Dr. Geoffrey McLennan)

After prolonged hyperoxia the septa show attenuation of membranes, thickening due to edema and pits or holes in the membrane. Detailed morphological analysis of oxygen induced lung damage identified pulmonary capillaries as the first site of lung injury and the consequent pulmonary edema as the initial observable cytopathology. Capillary injury was seen as the destruction of endothelial cells lining the capillaries (Refs. 36-38).

144

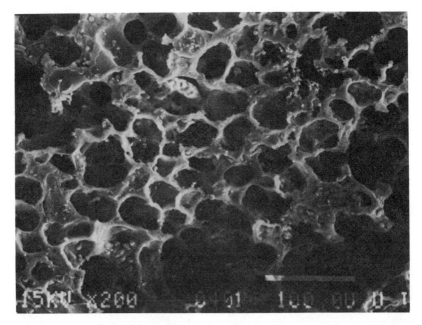

Fig. 1B. Scanning electron micrograph of a rat lung after maintenance of the animal in 95-100% oxygen at one atmosphere for 72 hours. The bar in the lower right corner = 100 microns. (Courtesy of Dr. Geoffrey McLennan)

REFERENCES

1. Smith, J.L. (1899) J. Physiol. (London) 24, 19-35.
2. Kinsey, V.E. (1956) Arch. Ophthalmol., 56, 481.
3. Shanklin, D.R. and Wolfson, S.L. (1967) N. Engl. J. Med., 277, 833-837.
4. Rowland, R. and Newman, C.G.H. (1969) J. Clin. Pathol., 22, 192-198.
5. Michaelis, L. (1940) Ann. N.Y. Acad. Sci., 40, 39.
6. Gersham, R., Gilbert, D.L., Nye, S.W., Dwyer, P., and Fenn, W.O. (1954) Science, 119, 623-627.
7. Babior, B.M. (1978) N. Engl. J. Med., 298, 721-725.
8. Greenwald, R.A. and Moy, W.W. (1979) Arthritis Rheum., 22, 251-259.
9. Flohé, L., Biehl, O., Hofer, H., Kadrnka, F., and Puhl, W. (1980) in Biological and Clinical Aspects of Superoxide and Superoxide Dismutase, Bannister, W.H. and Bannister, J.V., eds., New York: Elsevier-North Holland, pp. 424-430.
10. Flamm, E.S., Demopoulos, H.B., Seligman, M.L., Poser, G.R., and Ransohoff, J. (1978) Stroke, 9, 445.
11. McLennan, G., Oberley, L.W., and Autor, A.P. (1980) Rad. Res., 84, 122-132.
12. Hemler, M.E. and Lands, W.E.M. (1980) J. Biol. Chem., 255, 6253-6261.
13. Lund, C., Hochstein, P., and Ernster, L. (1982) Arch. Biochem. Biophys., 216, 178-185.
14. Tolmasoff, J.M., Ono, T., and Cutler, R.G., Proc. Natl. Acad. Sci., 77, 2777-2781.
15. Peto, R., Doll, R., Buckley, J.D., and Sporn, M.B. (1981) Nature, 290, 201-208.
16. McCord, J.M. and Fridovich, I. (1969) J. Biol. Chem., 244, 6049-6055.
17. Tyler, D.D. (1975) Biochim. Biophys. Acta, 396, 335-346.
18. Boveris, A. (1977) Advan. Exptl. Med. Biol., 78, 67-82.

19. Autor, A.P., ed. (1982) Pathology of Oxygen, New York: Academic Press,
20. Autor, A.P. and Stevens, J.B. (1980) in Chemical and Biochemical Aspects of Superoxide and Superoxide Dismutase, Bannister, J.V. and Hill, H.A.O., eds., New York: Elsevier-North Holland, pp. 104-115.
21. Cohen, G. and Hochstein, P. (1963) Biochemistry, 2, 1420.
22. Ambruso, D.R. and Johnston, R.D. (1981) J. Clin. Invest., 67, 352-360.
23. Bannister, J.V., Bannister, W.H., Hill, H.A.O., and Thornalley, P.J. (1982) Biochim. Biophys. Acta, 716, 116-120.
24. McCord, J.M. and Day, E. (1978) FEBS Letts., 86, 139-142.
25. Turrens, J.F., Freeman, B.A., and Crapo, J.D., (1979) Arch. Biochem. Biophys., 217, 411-421.
26. Brawn, K. and Fridovich, I. (1980) Acta Physiol. Scand., 492 (Suppl.), 9-18.
27. Fong, K., McCoy, P.B., Pover, J.L., Keele, B.B., and Misra, H. (1973) J. Biol. Chem., 248, 7792-7797.
28. Adams, G.E., Bishop, R.H., Cundall, R.B., Redpath, J.L., and Willson, R.L. (1972) Radiat. Res., 49, 290-299.
29. Autor, A.P., McLennan, G., and Fox, A.W. (1980) in Molecular Basis of Environmental Toxicology, Bhatnager, R.S., ed., Ann Arbor Sciences.
30. Gregory, E.M., Gascin, S.A., and Fridovich, I. (1974) J. Bacteriol., 117, 456-460.
31. Autor, A.P. (1982) J. Biol. Chem., 257, 2713-2718.
32. Zimniak, P., Harter, E., Woloszczuk, W., and Ruis, H. (1976) Eur. J. Biochem. 71, 393-398.
33. Woodrow, G. and Schatz, G. (1979) J. Biol. Chem., 254, 6088-6093.
34. Clark, J.M. and Lamberton, C.J. (1971) Pharmacol. Rev., 23, 37-47.
35. Kappus, H. and Sies, H. (1981) Experientia, 37, 1233-1240.
36. Kistler, G.S., Caldwell, P.R.B., and Wiebel, E.R. (1967) J. Cell. Biol., 33, 605-628.
37. Kapanci, Y., Weibel, E.R., Kaplan, H.P., and Robinson, F.R. (1969) Lab. Invest., 20, 101-118.
38. Gould, V.E., Tosco, R., Wheelis, R.F., Gould, N.S., and Kapanci, Y. (1972) Lab. Invest., 26, 499-508.

CHAPTER 8   A DECADE OF SUPEROXIDE DISMUTASE ACTIVITY

J. V. BANNISTER[*] AND G. ROTILIO[+]
[*]Inorganic Chemistry Department, University of Oxford, Oxford OX1 3QR, England;
and [+]Institute of Biological Chemistry and C.N.R. Centre for Molecular Biology,
University of Rome, Rome 00185, Italy.

Introduction

   Although the enzyme superoxide dismutase (EC 1.15.1.1) has been with us for
over a decade, the protein had been known from over three decades ago. It was
first isolated as a green copper protein from bovine erythrocytes and liver by
Mann and Keilin in 1939 (Ref. 1). The isolated proteins were appropriately named
hemocuprein (=erythrocuprein) and hepatocuprein, respectively. However, twenty
years were to elapse before it was realized that a whole family of cupreins was
present in various organs. Hepatocuprein was also isolated from horse liver
(Ref. 2) and cerebrocuprein from bovine (Ref. 3) and human (Ref. 4) brain. The
isolation and characterization of erythrocuprein from human erythrocytes was
carried out by Markowitz et al. (Ref. 5) and Kimmel et al. (Ref. 6) and it is large
to the credit of these workers that much of the earlier properties of the protein
became known. These results indicated similarities between the various cupreins--
all contained copper and had an identical molecular weight. The identity of all
the cupreins was proved beyond doubt by Carrico and Deutsch (Ref. 7), whilst McCord
and Fridovich (Ref. 8) assigned a function to erythrocuprein. Carrico and Deutsch
(Ref. 7) found that erythrocuprein, hepatocuprein and cerebrocuprein gave identical
maps and suggested that they should all be called cytocuprein. The same workers
further reported the presence of zinc in cytocuprein (Ref. 9). The name cuprein,
however, appeared to be not a true descriptive name for the protein since McCord
and Fridovich (Ref.8) had discovered an enzyme activity that might reflect the biological function of the protein. As a result of various observations carried out
at Duke University on the reduction of cytochrome c by xanthine-xanthine oxidase
reaction, erythrocuprein was identified as superoxide dismutase. The historical
events leading to this discovery are documented by McCord and Fridovich (Ref. 10).
   The reduction of cytochrome c was shown to be mediated by univalently reduced
oxygen (the superoxide radical) which is produced by the xanthine-xanthine oxidase
reaction and liberated into free solution (Ref. 11). The fact that a protein
existed which was a competitive inhibitor of the reduction of cytochrome c by the
xantine-xanthine oxidase reaction was first observed in 1962 (Ref. 12). The obser-

vation that erythrocuprein could scavenge superoxide radicals caused a great
deal of scientific activity. Over 1000 publications have appeared over the
last decade dealing not only with the isolation, characterization and enzymatic
activity of superoxide dismutase but also, as documented in Chapter 10 on
the clinical aspects of the enzyme. The enzyme has already been the subject of
four books published as a result of scientific meetings and numerous reviews
have also been published (Refs. 13-16).

Investigations on superoxide dismutase did not stop with the discovery of the
copper/zinc enzyme. Fridovich and collaborators isolated other proteins possessing
superoxide dismutase activity. These proteins were found to contain either manganese (Ref. 17) or iron (Ref. 18) rather than copper and zinc. The iron and manganese
enzymes have been shown to have various similarities in composition and are considered to belong to a class of superoxide dismutase which is totally different
from the copper/zinc class of the enzyme.

Assays for superoxide dismutase

Enzymes being catalysts of biochemical reactions are ordinarily assayed in terms
of their ability to accelerate the specific reaction that they catalyze. Such
assays usually involve the monitoring of the disappearance of the substrate or
the appearance of the product. Such assays are termed direct assays and allow
an extimation of the kinetic parameters of the enzyme catalyzed reaction. A direct
assay is not always conveniently possible for superoxide dismutase because of the
peculiar properties of the substrate (Ref. 19) and the enzyme activity has to be
measured by indirect inexpensive methods. Convenient assays for superoxide dismutase have necessarily been of the indirect type, in which the enzyme decreases
the rate of some reasonable reaction mediated by superoxide. The first assay of
this type was developed by McCord and Fridovich (Ref. 8). In this assay superoxide
dismutase is quantitated in terms of its ability to inhibit the reduction of cytochrome c by superoxide generated by the xanthine-xanthine oxidase reaction. One
unit of superoxide dismutase was defined as the amount that causes 50% inhibition
of the rate of reduction of cytochrome c. This assay, however, cannot be used
with homogenates as agents capable of the oxidation of ferrocytochrome c interfered. It could not, therefore, be easily applied to crude extracts that might
contain cytochrome oxidase or cytochrome c peroxidase activities. Acetylation of
cytochrome c diminishes its ability to react with both cytochrome c reductase and
oxidase but has little effect on its reactivity with superoxide radicals. This
fact has been exploited in minimizing interference with the assay for superoxide
dismutase (Refs. 20,21) and Beauchamp and Fridovich (Ref. 22) overcame this problem
by substituting cytochrome c with nitroblue tetrazolium (NBT). Superoxide radicals
were known to reduce nitroblue tetrazolium to formazan (Refs. 23,24).

Nitroblue tetrazolium has proved to be a useful detector of superoxide radicals
generated by the xanthine-xanthine oxidase reaction although some caution has been

advised by Auclair (Ref. 25). The dye provided the basis for an assay which
was free of interference by other catalytic activities and which could be used
for measuring superoxide dismutase activities in crude extracts. The assay was
applied during the purification of superoxide dismutase from two fungal species
(Ref. 26). The use of nitroblue tetrazolium was also applied for the detection of
superoxide dismutase activity on polyacrylamide gels (Ref. 22). However, instead
of using the xanthine-xanthine oxidase reaction for the generation of superoxide
radicals, the observation that photochemically reduced flavins generate superoxide radicals upon reoxidation in air (Ref. 27), was applied. When the reaction
was performed on acrylamide gels, using photo-oxidation of riboflavin, the localization of superoxide dismutase activity was evident from the formation of achromatic zones, whilst the rest of the gel was uniformly blue.

A simple and rapid spectrophotometric assay for superoxide dismutase was reporte
by Misra and Fridovich (Ref. 28). This assay is based on the ability of superoxide
dismutase to inhibit the autoxidation of epinephrine at alkaline pH. Since the
oxidation of epinephrine leads to the formation of pink colored adrenochrome,
the rate of increase of the absorbance at 480 nm, which represents the rate of
autoxidation of epinephrine, can be conveniently followed. Superoxide dismutase
was found to inhibit the radical-mediated chain process involved in the autoidation
of epinephrine. Sun and Zigman (Ref. 29) suggested that the absorbance change
should be monitored at 420 nm as at this wavelength the absorption was found to
be 6 to 10 times higher and also more consistent than that measured at 480 nm.
The absorption of adrenochrome at 480 nm corresponds to a relatively weak and
broad absorption band with a molar extinction coefficient at about 4000 $M^{-1}cm^{-1}$
(Ref. 30). It should also be pointed out that epinephrine is not the direct precursor of adrenochrome (Ref. 31). A similar type of assay involves the inhibition
of the oxidation of hydroxylamine. At neutral pH hydroxylamine is oxidized to
nitrite by superoxide and the nitrite formed is determined with α-napthylamine
at 580 nm (Refs. 32,33). Kono (Ref. 34) linked the assay to nitroblue tetrazolium
and added Triton X-100 to the assay mixture as this brings about a stabilization
of the colloidal product (Ref. 35).

Other indirect assays have utilized the autoxidation of 6-hydroxydopamine
(Ref. 36) measured at 480 nm and the oxidation of pyrogallol (Ref. 37) followed at
420 nm. The use of pyrogallol oxidation as an assay for superoxide dismutase has,
however, a few limitations. Trace amounts of iron were found to accelerate pyrogallol oxidation in spite of the presence of EDTA in the assay buffer. DTPA has
been suggested as an alternative chelator. Peroxidases were also found to interfere by accelerating the reaction.

The inhibition of superoxide-dependent oxidation of sulphite, first described
by McCord and Fridovich (Ref. 38), was utilized by Tyler (Ref. 39). Sulphite was
measured polarographically during oxidation carried out by superoxide, generated

by the xanthine-xanthine oxidase reaction. A reciprocal plot of sulphite oxidation rate against various amounts of either a rat liver fraction or purified erythrocyte superoxide dismutase, added to the system, indicated that the inhibition of sulphite oxidation by superoxide dismutase was strictly competitive. A similar result was obtained for the inhibition of the autoxidation of epinephrine (Ref. 28). A positive indirect assay utilizing o-dianisidine was reported (Refs. 40,41). However, this assay is rather laborious to set up and the dye formed is not easily cleaned from the cuvettes.

The assay methods so far described are based on a series of consecutive and parallel reactions and do not permit a direct determination of the true kinetic parameters for superoxide dismutase. They do not give a linear response to increasing enzyme concentrations and produce superoxide radicals at a very low steady-state concentration. They are not suited for mechanistic studies, although correct determinations of the catalytic constants can be carried out by comparative procedures (Refs. 42,43). Direct methods, however, give the rate constants for the overall process and can be used for studies to determine the mechanisms of dismutation. These methods often require the use of specialized techniques, such as electron spin resonance (Ref. 44), pulse radiolysis (Refs. 44-49), polarography (Ref. 50) or stopped-flow spectrophotometry (Ref. 51). The simplest direct assay was described by Marklund (Ref. 52). This assay follows the decay of superoxide radicals at 250 nm ($\varepsilon_{M-1} = 2000$ $M^{-1}cm^{-1}$ for superoxide radicals). Superoxide radicals are generated from potassium superoxide dissolved in DMSO containing DTPA, as commercial preparations of potassium superoxide appear to be heavily contaminated with iron. The results obtained were found to be in full agreement with previously published pulse radiolysis data.

The pulse radiolysis assay involves the generation of superoxide radicals in aqueous oxygenated solutions in the presence of a hydroxyl radical scavenger, usually ethanol. The decrease in the ultraviolet absorbance of the superoxide radical is monitored at 250 nm. This method is the most useful for studies on the mechanism of action of superoxide dismutase, being the only one that allows the measurement of independent rate constants of the dismutation reaction. It is, however, too cumbersome for a routine assay and the apparatus is not only too expensive to obtain, but also to operate. In the polarographic method, described by Rigo et al. (Ref. 50), the reduction of oxygen at a dropping mercury electrode coated with triphenylphosphine oxide, a univalent process producing a rather high steady state concentration of superoxide is utilized. Superoxide dismutase was found to increase the height of the polarographic oxygen reduction wave by dismuting superoxide to oxygen and hydrogen peroxide. This is a very sensitive assay but its application to mechanistic studies is limited because the reaction can only be observed at pH values greater than 9. Another electrochemical assay involves the use of a rotating disc electrode; although less sensitive this

method permits determinations at pH values as low as pH 7.5 (Ref. 53). Rigo et al.
(Ref. 54) have also developed an assay which utilizes nuclear magnetic resonance.
This assay can also be used below pH 9.0 although it is less sensitive than the
polarographic assay. The assay does not involve the measurement of the catalytic
activity but is based on a spectroscopic property of the active site. It appears
to be absolutely specific and free of interferences. It utilizes the fact that
the ^{19}F longitudinal nuclear magnetic relaxation rate (T_{Ip}^{-1}) of fluoride solutions
is greatly enhanced by the copper/zinc or manganese superoxide dismutase, while
it is practically unaffected by the presence of other metalloproteins including the
iron form of superoxide dismutase. The method is not limited to pulse nuclear
magnetic resonance equipment but is also accessible to high resolution nuclear
magnetic resonance spectrometers. In fact ^{19}F transverse nuclear relaxation time
(T_2) was found to be more sensitive than T_1 measurement at low concentrations of
the copper/zinc superoxide dismutase (Ref. 55) and T_2 can easily be evaluated by
^{19}F line measurements.

Radio-immunoassays using either ^{125}I or ^{57}Co or ^{60}Co as the radiotracer has
been developed for the copper/zinc (Refs. 56-59) and the manganese superoxide
dismutases (Ref. 59,60). The assays have proved to be very accurate and sensitive
and have been applied to the study of superoxide dismutase levels in trisomy 21
patients (Refs. 57,60).

Distribution of superoxide dismutases

(i) Bacteria, animals and plants. The distribution of the three types of
superoxide dismutase in organisms is considered to be a characteristic of the
evolutionary stage of the organism and also of the cell organelle with which it
is associated. If the distribution is linked to the evolutionary history of the
organism, then the distribution of the various superoxide dismutases has to be
considered in the light of the acquisition of a permanent defense against any
form of toxicity arising from the increase, by photosynthetic organisms, of
atmospheric oxygen.

The distribution of the three types of superoxide dismutase has been established
by their isolation and characterization. However, a combination of sensitivities
and insensitivities of the three enzymes to cyanide and hydrogen peroxide have
allowed a determination of the prosthetic metal of the superoxide dismutase in a
crude extract. Cyanide only inhibits the copper/zinc enzyme, whilst the iron
enzyme and the copper/zinc enzyme are inhibited by hydrogen peroxide. These
inhibition studies have been applied to various bacterial extracts (Refs. 62-64.
The three enzymes also exhibit varying degrees of inhibition by azide (Ref. 65).
Most of the work on the distribution of superoxide dismutase has been due to
Kozi Asada and his co-workers of Kyoto University, Japan. These workers have not
only demonstrated the form of superoxide dismutase present in a variety of species

but have also isolated and characterized the protein from a number of species as well.

In general terms the distribution of superoxide dismutase can be stated to be that the copper/zinc enzyme is essentially an eukaryotic enzyme and the iron enzyme is essentially a prokaryotic enzyme. The manganese enzyme can also be considered to be a prokaryotic enzyme. It is, however, also found in the mitochondria of eukaryotes. Whilst certain species of bacteria have one form of superoxide dismutase, i.e., either the iron or the manganese form, there are species with both forms as well. All eukaryotic species have the copper/zinc and manganese forms of the enzyme. The eukaryotic copper/zinc enzyme has been isolated and characterized from two species of bacteria (Refs. 66,67), whilst the seeds of the mustard plant, *Brassica campestris* (Ref. 68), and bovine chromaffin granules (Ref. 69) have been shown to have an iron enzyme.

The most primitive form of superoxide dismutase is considered to be the iron enzyme. The presence of superoxide dismutase in photosynthetic anaerobes, sulphate-reducing bacteria and fermentative anaerobic bacteria was first reported by Hewitt and Morris (Ref. 70), after it had been reported to be absent in obligate anaerobic bacteria, i.e., species which exhibit sensitivity to oxygen at 0.2 atmospheres of less (Ref. 71). A list of anaerobic bacterial species, in which superoxide dismutase activity was demonstrated, is given in Table 1. The enzyme in a partially purified fraction of *Clostridium perfringens* was found to be cyanide insensitive, probably indicating the presence of the iron enzyme.

TABLE 1

Presence of Superoxide Dismutase Activity in Anaerobic Bacterial Species[*]

Photosynthetic anaerobes

    Chlorobium thiosulfatophilium NCIB 8346
    Chromatin sp. NCIB 8346

Sulphate reducers

    Desulfotomaculum nigrificans NCIB 8395
    Desolfovibrio desulfuricans NCIB 8307

Fermentative anaerobes

    Clostridium acetobutylicum NCIB 6445, 8049, 8052
    Clostridium beijerinckii NCIB 4362
    Clostridium bifermentans NCIB 506
    Clostridium butyricum SA1, SA11, CNRZ 528, 531
    Clostridium pasteurianum ATCC 6013
    Clostridium perfringens type A NCIB 11105
    Clostridium sporogenes NCIB 532

---

[*] (Taken from Hewitt & Morris (1975) FEBS Letts., 50, 315-318.)

Since the work of Hewitt and Morris, the enzyme has been reported in other anaerobes (Refs. 72-81). The enzyme has been characterized to be the iron form in the strict anaerobe *Desulfovibrio desulfuricans* (Norway 4) (Ref. 75). In contrast to anaerobic bacteria, aerobic and facultative anaerobic species contain the iron or manganese enzyme or both. The only exceptions to this rule are *Photobacterium leiognathi* (Ref. 66) and *Paracoccus denitrificans* (Ref. 67). Both species were found to have in addition to the iron enzyme, the eukaryotic-type copper/zinc enzyme. The reason for this is as yet unknown. A close relationship exists between the amino acid compositions of *Photobacterium leiognathi* copper/zinc superoxide dismutase, aptly called bacteriocuprein by Puget and Michelson (Ref. 66), and the copper/zinc superoxide dismutase from teleost fish (Ref. 82). The physico-chemical properties of the enzymes were also found to be very similar. The similarities between *Photobacterium leiognathi* copper/zinc superoxide dismutase and the same type of enzyme from its teleost host suggests that gene transfer has taken place from the fish to the bacterium during their coevolutionary history. Investigations demonstrating gene transfer at the molecular level are currently being carried out. The bacteroid from soy bean root-nodules *Rhizobium japonicum* only contains the iron enzyme whilst the superoxide dismutase in the host cells of the nodules is mainly the copper/zinc enzyme (Ref. 83). Not all symbionts, therefore, can gain access to the genetic information contained in the host cells. The reason for the presence of a copper/zinc superoxide dismutase in *Paracoccus denitrificans* is not entirely clear and no predictions of gene transfer can be made as this species is a free-living prokaryote.

Facultative anaerobic bacteria such as *Escherichia coli* contain only the iron enzyme when cultured under anaerobic conditions. However, biosynthesis of the manganese enzyme and of a hybrid iron form of superoxide dismutase (Ref. 84) has been demonstrated to be induced by oxygen (Ref. 85) or superoxide radicals (Ref. 86). Aerobic diazotrophs should only contain the iron enzyme and this has been found to be the case in *Azobacter* and *Rhizobium* (Ref. 87). A very high content of iron superoxide dismutase has been reported in nitrogen fixing bacteria (Ref. 88). These species probably require a high content of superoxide dismutase to protect nitrogenase against oxygen and superoxide radicals. An iron enzyme has been purified from *Escherichia coli* (Refs. 18,89), *Mycobacterium* species (Refs. 90,91), *Pseudomonas ovalis* (Ref. 92), *Bacillus megaterium* (Ref. 93) and *Photobacterium* species (Ref. 94), whilst a manganese superoxide dismutase has been isolated from *Escherichia coli* (Ref. 17), *Streptococcus mutans* (Ref. 95), *Mycobacterium phlei* (Ref. 96), *Mycobacterium* species (Ref. 91), *Rhodopseudomonas spheroides* (Ref. 97), *Mycobacterium lepraemium* (Ref. 98), *Bacillus stearothermophilus* (Ref. 99), *Thermus aquaticus* (Ref. 100), *Streptococcus faecalis* (Ref. 63), and *Thermus thermophilus* (Ref. 101). The enzyme content of *Mycobacterium lepraemium* is the highest in any of the bacterial species so far investigated. The manganese enzyme constitutes about 6% of the soluble proteins. Whilst it is implied that the presence of an iron or manganese enzyme depends on the level of oxygen, this has only been demonstrated in *Escherichia coli*. *Bacillus megaterium* has, in contrast to its iron enzyme, also been shown to possess a manganese form of the enzyme (Ref. 102), whilst Terech and Vignais (Ref. 103) have described the presence of a manganese enzyme in *Paracoccus denitrificans* in contrast to an earlier report demonstrating the presence of an iron form of the enzyme (Ref. 67). Whether the two forms of the enzyme are present in these species or whether the presence of a manganese or iron enzyme depends, for instance, on the growth conditions, remains to be investigated.

No cyanide sensitive activity has been detected in the blue-green algae (cyano-phytes) which may be classified as prokaryotic species rather than eukaryotic. Eukaryotic algae possess either the iron and/or the manganese superoxide dismutase (Refs. 62,73,104-110). The iron and manganese superoxide dismutase have been purified from *Euglena gracilis* (Ref. 111) and the manganese superoxide dismutase from the red algae *Porphyridium cruentum* (Ref. 108) and *Porphyra tenura* (Ref. 112) has been isolated and characterized. The major superoxide dismutase in the prokaryotic blue green algae is the iron-containing enzyme. This form of the enzyme has been purified from *Plectonema boryanum* (Ref. 62,107), *Spirulina platensis* (Ref. 97) and *Anacystis nidulans* (Ref. 110).

A copper/zinc enzyme also appears to be lacking in protozoa. The facultative anaerobic flagellate, *Tritrichomonas foetus* and *Monoceromonas* sp. have been found to possess two cyanide-insensitive bands, with superoxide dismutase activity, on polyacrylamide gels. The two activity bands are probably the iron and mangan-ese enzymes as the two forms could be separated subcellularly (Ref. 113). A similar finding is reported for the aerobic ciliate, *Tetrahymena pyriformis* (Ref. 113) and *Critida fasciculata* (Ref. 105).

The fungi and slime molds have the copper/zinc enzyme. Asada and Kanematsu (Ref. 106) report testing for superoxide dismutase activity in two species of *Myxomyceta* (slime molds) and 43 species of *Eumycota* (fungi). In all the species the presence of the cyanide-sensitive copper/zinc superoxide dismutase was detected as also cyanide-insensitive activity which could be either the iron or manganese form of the enzyme. A manganese superoxide dismutase has been isolated from *Saccharomyces cerevisiae* (Ref. 114) and from the luminescent fungus *Pleurotus olearius* (Ref. 115). The copper/zinc superoxide has been isolated from *Saccharo-myces cerevisiae* (Refs. 116,117), *Neurospora crassa* (Ref. 118) and *Dactylium den-droides* (Ref. 119).

All the remaining animal and plant species can be considered to contain the copper/zinc and the manganese enzyme although the distribution of these forms has not been extensively investigated in eukaryotes. There is one evidence of the presence of the iron enzyme in high animals (Ref. 69) whilst following the report on the isolation and characterization of the iron superoxide dismutase in mustard seeds (Ref. 68) this form of the enzyme has been detected in only three plant families (Ref. 120). Nalbandyan and Gregoryan (Ref. 69) reported the presence of an iron superoxide dismutase in bovine chromaffin granules. This protein was purified to homogeneity (evidence from polyacrylamide gel electrophoresis). Although this superoxide dismutase was found to have spectral properties similar to the iron form of the enzyme, it was found to be cyanide-sensitive which is a behavior ascribed only to the copper/zinc enzyme. Furthermore its subunit molecular weight was found to be 18,000 which is intermediate between the subunit molecular weight of 16,000 for the copper/zinc superoxide dismutase and 20,000 for the iron superoxide dismutase. The iron content was found to be 1.3 atoms per 40,000. A reinvestigation of this enzyme is warranted. The report on the isolation and characterization of the iron superoxide dismutase in mustard seeds is more consistent although the yields are extremely low. It is quite possible that the iron form of the enzyme may not have disappeared at all in higher species but that its concentration is so low that it is not being detected at all.

Bryophytes (mosses), pteridophytes (ferns), gymnosperms and angiosperms (both seed plants) have been demonstrated to contain the copper/zinc enzyme in addition to a cyanide-insensitive form of the enzyme (Refs. 77,104). The copper/zinc enzyme has been purified from green peas (Ref. 121), wheat germ (Ref. 122), spinach leaves (Ref. 123), kidney bean (Ref. 124), and tomato fruit (Ref. 125). Its presence has also been demonstrated in various extracts from plant material (Refs. 120,126). A cyanide-insensitive superoxide dismutase has been detected in extracts from wheat germ (Ref. 122), corn (Ref. 127), green peas (Ref. 128), Jerusalem artichoke (Ref. 129), kidney bean (Ref. 124), and spinach and tea leaves (Ref. 130). In all cases the activity present has been assumed to be due to the presence of the manganese form of the enzyme. A manganese enzyme appears to have been purified only from green peas (Ref. 131) and maize (Ref. 132).

In invertebrate species, superoxide dismutase activity has been poorly studied as also in lower vertebrates. Superoxide dismutase activity has been detected in the hemerythrocytes of sipunculids (Ref. 133), in the sea anemone (Ref. 134), and in the cephalochordate *Amphioxus lanceolatus* (Ref. 135). However, no determination of the type of enzymes present has been made. Asada et al. (Ref. 83) report cyanide-sensitive and cyanide-insensitive superoxide dismutase activity. The copper/zinc enzyme has been isolated from the hepatopancreas of the lamellibranch mollusc *Mytilus galloprovincialis* (Ref. 136) and partially purified from the branchial gland of the cephaloped mollusc *Sepia officinalis* (Ref. 137). The presence of the copper/zinc and manganese superoxide dismutase has been reported in the fruit fly *Ceratitis capitata* by Fernandez-Sousa and Michelson (Ref. 138) and in *Drosophila melanogaster* (Refs. 139,140). Lee et al. (Ref. 141) purified the copper/zinc enzyme from *D. melanogaster*.

A survey of the distribution of the copper/zinc and manganese enzyme activities in vertebrates has been carried out (Refs. 142,143). Enzyme activity has been detected in the fish *Opsanus tau* (Ref. 144). The copper/zinc superoxide dismutase has been isolated from the liver of the swordfish, *Xiphias gladius* (Ref. 145) and from various teleost fish (Ref. 82), whilst among mammalian species no special mention need be given to the enzyme from bovine and human erythrocytes. The enzyme has also been purified from chicken liver (Ref. 146) and pig liver (Ref. 147). Enzyme activity was reported in bovine ocular tissues (Ref. 148), bovine and human milk (Refs. 149-152), and chicken and turkey spermatozoa (Ref. 153).

(ii) <u>Subcellular distribution</u>. Copper/zinc superoxide dismutase was first localized exclusively in the soluble fraction of rat liver homogenates by Rotilio et al. (Ref. 154). Fresh chicken liver was, however, found to contain the two types of superoxide dismutase activity present in eukaryotes. The manganese enzyme was found to be localized in the mitochondria whilst the copper/zinc enzyme was found to be present in the cytosol (Ref. 146). This was the first evidence of compartmentalization of the eukaryotic superoxide dismutases. However, when intact mitochondria were isolated from chicken liver and then separated into fractions containing the outer membrane, the soluble components of the intermembrane space, the inner membrane and the soluble enzymes of the matrix space, the manganese superoxide dismutase activity was found primarily in the matrix space whereas the copper/zinc superoxide dismutase activity previously thought to be completely localized in the cytosol was found in the intermembrane space (Ref. 155). No superoxide dismutase activity was found to be associated with the other subcellular fractions. A strain of petite mutants of *Saccharomyces cerevisiase* which lack mitochondrial DNA was examined for subcellular distribution of superoxide dismutase. The strain was found to contain both the copper/zinc and manganese forms of the enzyme. The results indicate that the manganese superoxide dismutase, although localized in the mitochondrial matrix is actually synthesized under the direction of the nuclear genome. Its synthesis probably takes place in the cytosol.

A similar subcellular distribution of the two enzymes has been reported in mitochondria isolated from rat liver by Tyler (41), Peeters-Joris et al. (156), and Panchenko et al. (157), and in human neutrophils (158). An apparent superoxide dismutase activity observed in neutrophil azurophil granules was attributable not to true superoxide dismutase but to myeloperoxidase. Examination of the subcellular distribution of manganese superoxide dismutase in human liver by McCord et al (159) produced a rather unexpected and surprising observation. Human liver was found to contain twenty times more manganese superoxide dismutase than an equivalent weight of rat liver. The enzyme was found mainly in the soluble fraction. The possibility that mitochondrial rupture may have occurred between time of death and autopsy could not be discounted. However, when the subcellular

distribution of manganese superoxide dismutase in fresh liver obtained from a
primate, the baboon *Papio ursinus*, a similar result was obtained. The reason for
this observation is still unexplained.

In bacteria, superoxide dismutase activity has been shown to be entirely
localized in the cell matrix. A report that the iron superoxide dismutase of
Escherichia coli is a periplasmic enzyme (160) is now seen to be in error (161).
In plants and blue-green algae, the manganese superoxide dismutase is associated
with thylakoids. Okada et al. (162) found that in three species of blue-green
algae, *Plectonema boryanum*, *Anabaena variabilis*, and *Anacystis nidulans*, the
manganese superoxide dismutase is localized in the thylakoids and the iron
superoxide dismutase in the cytosol (Fig. 1).

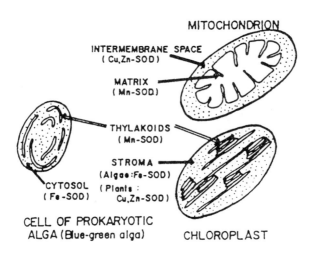

Fig. 1. Subcellular distribution of superoxide dismutases (reproduced from
Asada et al. (1980) in Ref. 14, p. 149).

In higher plants, copper/zinc superoxide dismutase was found in spinach leaf
chloroplasts (123). Manganese superoxide dismutase activity was not detected in
spinach leaf chloroplasts. These were, however, tested with organic solvents.
Such treatment is known to inhibit the activity of the manganese superoxide
dismutase. Some workers have reported that chloroplasts contain the manganese
enzyme (124,163) whilst others have disagreed with this finding (164). Jackson
et al. (165) investigated the subcellular distribution of superoxide dismutase
in the leaves of spinach and other C_3 plants. Intact chloroplast fractions

were found to contain a cyanide-insensitive superoxide dismutase activity pre-
sumed to be the manganese enzyme but according to these workers this activity
is located on the outside of the chloroplast and may be adsorbed during the
preparation. Salin and Bridges (166) however identified the cyanide-insensitive
activity present in the stroma of chloroplasts isolated from *Brassica campetsris*
(mustard) leaves to be the iron-containing superoxide dismutase. Mitochondria
isolated from the same species were found to contain the manganese enzyme in
the matrix and the copper/zinc enzyme in the intermembrane space as in mammalian
species (167).

Purification of superoxide dismutase

   (i) <u>Copper/zinc superoxide dismutase</u>. About thirty years before the discovery
of the superoxide dismutase activity of erythrocuprein, Mann and Keilin (1) had
already isolated the protein from bovine erythrocytes and liver. Essentially
the main problem in the purification procedure was the removal of hemoglobin
and this was achieved by denaturation with a mixture of ethanol/chloroform, the
so-called Tsuchihashi procedure. The organic reagent mixture precipitates the
hemoglobin whilst erythrocuprein remains in solution from which it can be
precipitated with lead acetate and solubilized in 0.3 M potassium phosphate.
Further purification was achieved by acetone precipitation, tricalcium phosphate
and alumina gel. Porter and Folch (3) prepared cerebrocuprein utilizing
chloroform/methanol extraction whilst Markowitz et al. (5) purified erythrocuprein from human erythrocytes utilizing essentially the same procedure as
Mann and Keilin (1) used for bovine erythrocytes. Kimmel et al. (6) increased
the quantity of protein that could be prepared by Markowitz et al. (5) by introducing flow ionophoresis, whilst Nyman (168) further modified the purification
procedure of Markowitz et al. (5) and Kimmel et al. (6) by introducing ion-
exchange chromatography using diethylaminoethyl-cellulose. The lead acetate
extract was applied to an ion-exchange column equilibrated with 5 mM Tris-HCl,
pH 7.4, and elutes with a final gradient concentration of 50 mM Tris-HCl, pH
7.4, containing 166 mM sodium chloride. Rechromatography was carried out. The
purified protein was found to be similar to the protein prepared by Markowitz
et al. (5) and Kimmel et al. (6). The procedure was claimed to give a high
degree of homogeneity. Using a similar procedure Porter et al. (169) isolated
the protein from normal adult human liver. Shields et al. (1970) also purified
erythrocuprein by chromatography on diethylaminoethyl-cellulose after the
Tsuchihashi procedure. They showed that the original erythrocuprein preparation
of Markowitz et al. (5) contained a small amount of a highly antigenic copper-
free impurity which was removed by chromatography on diethylaminoethyl-cellulose.

   The main problem with the purification of erythrocuprein has been the use of
organic solvents. This is admittedly an extremely drastic procedure for enzyme
isolation. However, Porter and Folch (3) claim the chloroform/methanol treatment

had no effect on cerebrocuprein because a similar sedimentation constant and absorption spectral properties were obtained when cerebrocuprein was prepared by a method in which the only organic solvent employed was acetone and the temperature of the acetone/water mixture was maintained at -10°C. Also Markowitz et al. (5) observed that erythrocuprein isolated with the chloroform/ethanol procedure was immunologically identical with the protein in erythrocyte hemolysates. According to Markowitz et al. (5) the appearance of several precipitation bands or an indication of some degree of cross reaction would have been obtained had the protein been altered during the purification procedure.

Stansell and Deutsch (141,172) purified human erythrocuprein by chromatography on diethylaminoethyl-cellulose and gel filtration on Sephadex G-100 followed by rechromatography on diethylaminoethyl-cellulose and carboxymethyl-cellulose and crystallization from 45% saturated ammonium sulphate solution in 50 mM acetate, pH 5.5. These workers were concerned to show that chloroform/ethanol treatment of erythrocuprein, as in the Tsuchihashi procedure, altered the properties of the protein. Protein treated with organic solvents was found to have 10% less copper and showed a 10% decrease in absorbance at 655 nm compared with the untreated protein. Treated protein was also found to have a sedimentation coefficient that was about 9% higher and intrinsic viscosity that was 65% lower than the values obtained for the untreated protein. It was therefore suggested that the axial ratio had decreased. Also an increase in net charge and electrophoretic mobility together with an increased heterogeneity were obtained on starch and polyacrylamide gel electrophoresis. The absorbance of the treated protein decreased by 83% at 190 nm. This suggested an increase in helical content. The protein also failed to crystallize.

Hartz and Deutsch (173) also purified human erythrocuprein by chromatography. A different strategy from that employed by Standsell and Deutsch (171,172) was adopted. The purification involved batch adsorption of the red cell lysate on diethyaminoethyl-cellulose, gel filtration on Sephadex G-75, chromatography on diethylaminoethyl-cellulose at pH 8.0, followed by chromatography at pH 5.5, and a final gel filtration step on Sephadex G-75. Purified protein was found to be heterogeneous in electrophoresis on cellulose acetate and starch gel. Isoelectric focusing showed a major component with a pI of 4.75 and three other minor components with lower isoelectric points. The amino acid composition was in agreement with that reported by Stansell and Deutsch (1972). The exact significance of these findings is not clear. Erythrocuprein prepared by Bannister and Wood (174), behaved as a single component in isoelectric focusing but showed two components on polyacrylamide gel electrophoresis, a major and minor faster migrating band. The mobility of these two bands indicated that they were size isomers. Similar observations have been made using bovine erythrocuprein (175).

Bannister et al. (176) obtained crude human erythrocuprein by the Tsuchihashi procedure and purified the protein by chromatography on diethylaminoethyl-cellulose and gel filtration on Sephadex G-75. Purified protein had a pI of 4.75 which is identical to the value obtained by Hartz and Deutsch (173). Also polyacrylamide gel electrophoresis revealed a small component which moved faster than the main component. The epr spectrum of human erythrocuprein which had been subjected to the Tsuchihashi procedure is very similar to the spectrum of the protein prepared entirely by chromatographic procedures. Bannister et al. (176) described a well resolved band at 322 nm in the absorption spectrum. Calabrese et al. (177) showed that the band persisted in the apoprotein and suggested the presence of persulphide (RSSH) as a possible explanation for the observation. However, Briggs and Fee (178) claimed that this absorption band is due to sul-phydryl groups reacting with a variety of sulphur compounds including zero-valent sulphur and considered that the absorption is an artefact of the purification procedures employing organic solvents. Although a physiological reason cannot be easily found for the presence of labile sulphur in human erythrocuprein it is unlikely to be an artefact of the preparation as Hartz and Deutsch (173) also found a similar absorption band using erythrocuprein prepared without organic solvents. It is quite likely that the presence of the 322 nm band depends on the state of the starting material. Human erythrocuprein is usually prepared from out-dated red cells. The age of these cells is never taken into account. It is therefore not unreasonable to suggest that the labile sulphur present is a consequence of the ageing of the red cells and that it is probably arising as a result of the degradation of glutathione.

Despite the various misgivings about the use of organic solvents, the Tsuchihashi procedure is still widely used in the preparation of erythrocuprein or as it should preferably be called copper/zinc superoxide dismutase. The enzyme has also been purified from *Neurospora crassa* (118), green peas (121), yeast (116,117), wheat germ (122), spinach (123), chicken liver (146), horse liver (177), and swordfish liver (145) to mention a few sources of purified superoxide dismutase. Puget and Michelson (66) and Vignais et al. (67) purified the only two known bacterial copper/zinc superoxide dismutases by conventional procedures. The need to employ organic solvents to purify copper/zinc superoxide dismutase from non-hemoglobin containing sources does not arise.

(ii) <u>Manganese and iron superoxide dismutase</u>. The manganese and iron enzymes were first purified from *Escherichia coli* B (17,18). Both enzymes were purified by conventional protein purification procedures. In both cases ammonium sulphate precipitation was used as the major initial purification step. The two activities could be separated by anion-exchange cellulose. The manganese enzyme was found to bind to carboxymethyl-cellulose equilibrated with 2 mM acetate buffer, pH 5.5, while no binding to diethylaminoethyl-cellulose took place in 5 mM phosphate buffer, pH 7.8. The opposite was found to be the case with the iron enzyme. Ion-exchange chromatography has been applied in the purification of the manganese and iron enzymes from various sources. The manganese enzyme has been purified from *Streptococcus mutans* (95), *Paracoccus dentitrificans* (103), *Saccharomuces cerevisiase* (114), *Thermus thermophilus* (101), *Mycobacterium lepraemium* (98), *Mycobacterium phlei* (96), *Mycobacterium* sp. (91), *Bacillus stearothermophilus Thermus aquatics* (100), and *Pleurotus olearius* (115).

An iron enzyme has been purified from *Bacillus megaterium* (93), *Desulfovibrio desulfuricans* (Norway 4) (75), *Chlorobium thiosulfatophilum* (79), *Thiobacillus denitrificans* (180), *Photobacterium* species (94), *Mycobacterium tuberculosis* (90), *Anacystis nidulans* (110), *Propionibacterium shermanii* (81), and *Pseudomonas ovalis* (92). The iron enzyme was also purified from the algal species *Spirulina platensis* (181) and *Plectonema boryanum* (62,109).

In higher species the iron and manganese enzymes have been purified from plant sources while in vertebrates the presence of a second form of superoxide dismutase with a molecular weight higher than the copper/zinc enzyme was first noted by Marklund in bovine liver extracts (182). However, the first complete purification was carried out by Weisiger and Fridovich (146) using chicken liver mitochondria. The enzyme was found to be inhibited by organic solvents as was also the pig heart enzyme. However, Michelson et al. (183) have claimed that the purification of the manganese superoxide dismutase from human liver can be achieved using organic solvents. McCord et al. (158) described the isolation of the human liver manganese enzyme following essentially the same procedures utilized by Weisiger and Fridovich (146) for the preparation of the chicken liver mitochondrial manganese enzyme. A similar procedure was sued by Salin et al. (184) to purify the enzyme from rat liver. A preparation of the manganese enzyme from bovine heart was found to be highly heterogeneous (185).

Physicochemical studies on the copper/zinc superoxide dismutases

(i) Introduction. Physicochemical studies on the superoxide dismutases have included (a) spectroscopic investigations of the metal binding sites and their reactions: these investigations date back much earlier than the discovery of the superoxide dismutase activity of erythrocuprein; (b) kinetic studies on the mechanism of enzyme action: these studies were initiated following the suggestion that the superoxide radical could be the physiological substrate for the enzyme; and finally (c) X-ray diffraction analysis of the crystallized protein which proved invaluable to interpretative trends outlined by the other lines of research.

Erythrocuprein or its equivalent protein from other tissues, was actually an early candidate for spectroscopic investigations in the frame of the nascent field of copper protein spectroscopy. Since the pioneering work of Malmstrom and Vanngard (186) utilizing epr spectroscopy as a probe for specific copper binding sites, erythrocuprein has had its distinctive place. In this work, erythrocuprein was introduced as a typical example of a copper protein with a "normal" hyperfine splitting value, as compared to the small value characteristic of "blue" copper proteins. As a matter of fact the value reported by Malmstrom and Vanngard ($A_{||} = 0.016$ cm^{-1}) was not confirmed by further work and is rather similar to that of more regular square-planar geometries as found in low-molecular weight copper chelates and less distorted copper-protein complexes. The actual $A_{||}$ value is significantly lower and reflects an intermediate degree of distortion between square planar and tetrahedral as demonstrated from experimental and theoretical studied on other copper proteins (187,188). This large $A_{||}$ value remained uncorrected in the literature for more than a decade. It was reported by Carrico and Deutsch in 1969 (7) who, on the other hand, displayed the first detailed epr spectrum of the protein (cytocuprein) showing the typical broadness of the $g_{\perp}$ absorption which was later interpreted as indicative of rhombic distortion.

In the decade between 1960 and 1970, Malmstrom and coworkers were developing a concept that the extinction coefficient of copper proteins between 600 and 700 nm was strictly related to the degree of deviation of the epr spectrum, in particular the $A_{||}$ value from the parameters that are typical of low-molecular weight complexes. In this context it was noted (189) that the optical spectrum of erythrocuprein was characterized by a broad absorption band with a maximum between 650 and 700 nm and an extinction coefficient, per copper atom, of approximately 150 M^{-1} cm^{-1} (172). It was pointed out that such a value was one order of magnitude less than that of "blue" copper proteins but still significantly higher than values for low-molecular weight complexes and other non-blue copper proteins. This feature also reflected a specifically distorted geometry of the erythrocuprein copper.

It was also in the same decade that another fundamental spectroscopic property of the protein was taken into consideration, namely, the ultraviolet spectrum. In the case of the bovine copper/zinc superoxide dismutase this is characterized by a higher extinction coefficient at 260 nm than at 280 nm with a clear fine structure due to phenylalanine residues (Fig. 2a). The human copper/zinc enzyme also (sometimes) exhibits a unique band in the 330 nm region (Fig. 2b). While the higher extinction at 260 nm can be related to the lack of tryptophan and low tyrosine content in the bovine enzyme, the additional band present in the human enzyme was the subject of controversial interpretations until it was assigned to an unusual sulphur-containing residue. It was shown that the band does not depend on protein-bound copper. It was, however, abolished by cyanide, by reducing agents and by denaturing agents such as quanidine and sodium lauryl sulphate. A persulphide group, R-S-SH such as that described for xanthine oxidase and rhodanese appears to be the most likely structure for this chromophore (177). It is not associated with the catalytic function of the enzyme and may be related to the peculiar

162

accessibility to external reagents, including thiols and disulphides which as
already suggested could arise in the degradation of glutathione, of the fourth
cysteine residue also unique to the human copper/zinc superoxide dismutase (190).

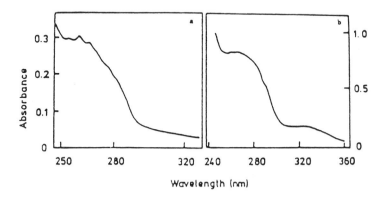

Fig. 2. Ultraviolet spectrum of (a) bovine and (b) human copper/zinc superoxide
dismutases.

(ii) <u>Spectroscopic studies on the copper-binding site.</u> Two companion papers
by Bannister and co-workers were the first to define the optical and circular
dichroism spectra of bovine erythrocyte copper/zinc superoxide dismutase (175,
197). The typical ultraviolet spectrum was found to be preserved after metal
removal. However, both metals and the copper in particular were found to have a
strong hyperchromic effect on the absorption. The ultraviolet circular dichroism
spectrum was also profoundly modified by removal of the metals (Fig. 3). These
results were the first demonstration of the conformational role of the metals in
copper/zinc superoxide dismutase. The first detailed spectroscopic investigations
of the copper-binding site were published by Rotilio et al. (192). Reversible
epr changes were observed following titration of the bovine enzyme as a function
of pH in the alkaline range and with cyanide (Fig. 4). In both cases the epr
line shaped reverted from an apparently rhombic to a more axial one. The $A_{\parallel}$
established to be 0.014 cm^{-1} in the native protein increased from approximately
130 to approximately 150 gauss at pH 11 and to 190 gauss with cyanide. An evident superhyperfine structure was apparent in the $g_{\perp}$. The latter was interpreted

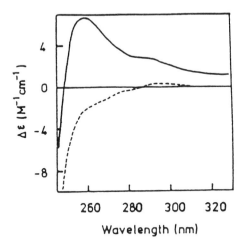

Fig. 3. Ultraviolet cicular dichroism spectrum of bovine copper/zinc superoxide dismutase. Holoprotein (———), apoprotein (-----).

as indicative of the presence of 3 to 4 nitrogens as planar ligands. Since both changes were fully reversible to native spectrum on dialysis these results marked the first observation of hyperfine structure due to endogenous ligands for a copper-binding site of a protein in the native state. Coordination of at least one water molecule was also suggested in view of the specific and reversible exchange of exogenous molecules. The electronic and circular dichroism spectra in the different conditions were also recorded; in particular the broad absorption at 680 nm was shown to be due to the overlapping of two bands, most likely being d-d transitions of a distorted copper geometry. Circular dichroism spectra in the ultraviolet region were carried out by Wester et al. (193) and suggested a very low helical content in the protein.

The copper binding site was also exhaustively characterized by epr by Rotilio et al. (219). The two copper atoms in the dimer were shown to be equivalent and rhombic (g_z = 2.26_5, g_y = 2.10_8 and g_x = 2.02_3). The symmetry changes into axial on binding of singly charged anions such as cyanide, fluoride and azide. Cyanide apparently binds in the ratio 1:1 via its carbon end and gives rise to a novel spectrum with a nitrogen hyperfine structure on the copper hyperfine line at lowest field. By means of ^{63}Cu and ^{13}C substitutions this hyperfine pattern was interpreted as due to three equivalent nitrogen nuclei coordinated as in plane ligand and a water molecule was suggested to be present as a fourth weaker

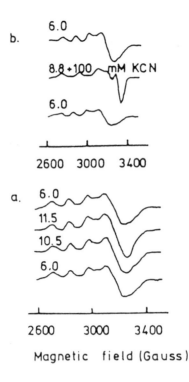

b.

6.0

8.8 + 100 mM KCN

6.0

2600 3000 3400

a. 6.0

11.5

10.5

6.0

2600   3000   3400

Magnetic field (Gauss)

Fig. 4. Epr spectra of bovine copper/zinc superoxide dismutase as (a) function of pH and (b) effect of KCN.

in plane ligand ready for substitution by anionic exogeneous molecules, including the superoxide substrate or for deprotonation to give a stronger OH^- complex.

Water coordination and the pattern of anion binding was confirmed by Fee and Gaber (212) using nuclear magnetic relaxation of water protons by the protein bound copper as a specific probe of the effects occurring on direct binding of the copper ion. The results obtained with cyanide, cyanate and thiocyanate, were taken to suggest binding to the zinc site and to affect the copper epr spectrum "indirectly." This interpretation proved to be wrong and was later corrected (194) but the rationalization made in terms of a close vicinity of the two metals to explain the "indirect" effects of zinc ligands on the copper epr spectrum were substantially shown to be true following detailed spectroscopic studies and eventually from the X-ray structure of the protein. Measurements at varying magnetic field refined the nuclear magnetic resonance data on water coordination (220). The exchange time for the copper-bound water was estimated to be in the range of 4×10^{-6}

to 10^{-8}s and the copper-water distance of approximately 2.0 Å. These values
are relevant to the possible role of the metal-bound water in the mechanism of
the dismutation reaction.

(iii) <u>Metal-removal and substitution of the copper/zinc superoxide dismutase.</u>
McCord and Fridovich (8) while assigning a function to erythrocuprein also
established that copper was essential for its superoxide dismutase activity. It
was also shown that no other metal could replace the copper in restoring the
activity to the apoprotein. The procedure used for making the apoprotein--
extensive dialysis against EDTA at pH 3.8--resulted in the loss of all the metals.
The preparation of a stable and reconstitutable apoprotein by a much faster procedure than dialysis against chelating agent was reported by Weser et al. (208).
Apoprotein was prepared by gel filtration at room temperature through a Sephadex
G-25 column previously equilibrated with 10 mM EDTA at pH 3.8 (Fig. 5). This method
of preparation leaves small amounts of EDTA bound to the protein. It can be
removed by dialysis against high concentrations of sodium perchlorate (194).

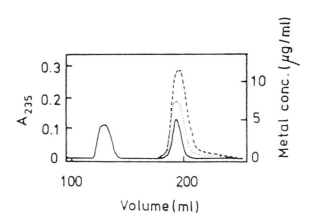

Fig. 5. Preparation of apo-superoxide dismutase on Sephadex G-25. Copper
content (---), zinc content (••••).

Carrico and Deutsch (9) reported that the metals could be removed by dialysis
against potassium cyanide at pH 8.0. The use of cyanide in the preparation of
apoprotein was extensively investigated by Rotilio et al. (195). By selecting
the pH of the dialysis buffer, copper could be reversibly removed without affecting the zinc content of the enzyme. This method allowed the characterization of

The copper-free protein and the role of zinc in stabilizing the native protein
conformation was established. No spectroscopic contribution by the zinc could
be observed, while copper was shown to contribute entirely to the increase of
the ultraviolet absorption occurring on reconstitution of the holoprotein. This
behavior is now well explained in a recent report in charge-transfer ultraviolet
absorption of copper(II) imidazolate chromophores (196). This spectroscopic
property was the first evidence for coordination of the copper to histidine
residues although its relevance was overlooked. Rotilio et al. (195) also observed the reduction of copper by hydrogen peroxide. This reaction turned out
to be of particular relevance in studies on the mechanism of enzyme action, as
hydrogen peroxide is a product of the dismutation reaction. The inertness of the
reduced enzyme toward reoxidation by molecular oxygen was also established in this
work confirming the earlier observation of Mann and Keilin (1). This property
is not usual with reduced copper proteins and complexes and is related to the
catalytic action of the enzyme.

In 1972, Weser et al. (197) established the extinction coefficient of the apoprotein to be only one-third that of the holoprotein. In the same publication the
role of copper in determining the conformation of the protein was supported by
the fact that only addition of copper reversed the electrophoretic mobility of the
apoprotein to that typical of the holoprotein, while the zinc-apoprotein complex
had the same mobility as the apoprotein. The role of zinc was again shown to be
important for proper binding of the copper by monitoring the position of the
visible optical absorption maximum. Additional information on the metals was
provided by an X-ray photoelectron study of the protein (198). This technique
which is unfortunately of little use for the study of protein-bound metal centres
because of the drastic conditions to which the sample has to be subjected, was
nevertheless valuable in this case suggesting that the cupric ion was likely to
be located on the surface of the protein, while the zinc was more buried inside
the protein.

The structural role of zinc was confirmed by Forman and Fridovich (199) who
also reported the effect of metals on the stability of the copper/zinc protein.
The activity of the enzyme was shown to be unaffected in the presence of 10 M urea
and 4% sodium lauryl sulphate. This information proved to be relevant for the
study of the subunits of the enzyme. Guanidine hydrochloride was, however,
reported to inhibit the enzyme activity without causing any structural perturbations. This inhibition was later reported to be related to ionic strength effects
(200).

Four articles by Fee and co-workers (200-203) dealt extensively with the
problem of reconstitution of the metal-free protein with cobalt, copper and
zinc. Cobalt was first introduced in the protein by Calabrese et al. (204) who
used dialysis of the holoprotein against cobalt and showed that (a) cobalt

substitution occurs at the zinc site; (b) cobalt does not affect the activity; (c) according to the optical spectrum the cobalt is in a tetrahedral site; (d) not more than 1 cobalt per dimer can be introduced by exchange dialysis; and finally (e) cobalt and by analogy zinc, is close to the copper, as the epr spectrum of the cobalt substituted enzyme indicated magnetic coupling between the two paramagnetic metal centers. The fact that only one cobalt per dimer could be introduced in the protein indicated possible conformational constraints on the protein structure arising from subunit interaction. The results obtained by Fee and coworkers (200-203) can be summarized as follows: (a) a zinc-free protein containing copper bound at its native binding site could be obtained. This form of the protein displayed an epr spectrum that was distinctly more axial than when zinc was present confirming that the properties of the active site require both metal ions; (b) binding of excess copper to the zinc-free protein gave an epr spectrum indicative of dipolar coupling between neighbor copper ions suggesting that copper can bind to the zinc-binding site. This result indicates that the metal-binding sites are very close in the protein confirming the result obtained by Calabrese et al. (204) on the cobalt substituted protein.

The binuclear copper-copper complex obtained by addition of four copper atoms to the apoprotein was further characterized by epr spectroscopy between 50 and 100°K (Ref. 205). A coupling constant of approximately 52 cm^{-1} for the antiferromagnetic interaction between the two copper ions could then be calculated. The zinc-free copper-containing protein was prepared by slow infusion of a 15 mM cuprous chloride into a 0.3 mM apoprotein solution at pH 5.5. A similar reconstitution procedure had earlier been reported by Beem et al. (205). These workers prepared the zinc-free protein and also other metallo-derivatives when zinc was replaced by either cadmium or mercury. Epr and absorption spectroscopy confirmed the results of other investigators (195) that full recovery of the properties of the copper-binding site can only be achieved in the presence of zinc in an equivalent metal binding at the zinc site. Variable specific activities (20 to 80% of normal activity) were reported for the protein reconstituted with copper only. The apoprotein reconstituted with two coppers displayed only half the activity of the native enzyme (205). This result was recently explained by Valentine et al. (207) who demonstrated that copper binds preferentially at its native site at pH values lower than neutral, but migrates to the vacant sites at more alkaline pH values, thus disproportionating the fully active copper binding site into a half of fully active copper-copper pairs and a half of metal depleted sites. This condition is also likely to occur during the enzyme assay carried out at alkaline pH values.

The properties of the metal binding sites were refined following a series of investigations using cobalt substituted protein. A magnetic circular dichroism

study of the d-d transitions of the cobalt chromophore (209) showed that the
cobalt coordination environment in superoxide dismutase was almost identical to
that of cobalt in the carbonic anhydrase-cyanide adduct (four coordinated, nearly
regular tetrahedron). It was also shown that the cobalt was able to specifically
sense changes in the valence of the copper. A pulsed-NMR investigation showed
that the copper loses its ability to relax water in the copper/cobalt enzyme,
indicating that the cobalt was magnetically coupled to the copper very strongly
(210). These results were confirmed by epr spectroscopy carried out at liquid
helium temperatures (Fig. 6) (211). The epr spectra definitely demonstrated that
the two metal centers were coupled by an exchange interaction. This is only
possible if they are bridged by a common ligand. X-ray data were to prove later
that the copper and zinc share a common imidazole ligand. The epr parameters of
the cobalt obtained after reduction of the copper to release the magnetic coupling were obtained in this investigation. The parameters obtained were found to
indicate a tetrahedral coordination with some degree of distortion from the zero
field splitting constant $Z = 23 \text{ cm}^{-1}$. The zinc site was also shown not to be
accessible to external ligands such as cyanide and azide, thus ruling out that
the precocious effects observed by Fee and Gaber (212) in the epr spectrum of
copper following binding of azide were due to coordination to the zinc.

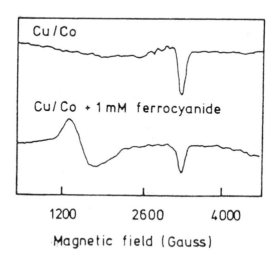

Fig. 6. Epr spectra of bovine copper/cobalt superoxide dismutase.

Cobalt has also recently been shown to bind to the copper site (213). Nuclear magnetic resonance spectral changes obtained on addition of zinc to the apoprotein had indicated that the zinc can bind to the copper-binding site (214,215). In the cobalt/zinc protein, the cobalt chromophore was found to exhibit similar pseudo-tetrahedral spectral features as compared to the cobalt resident in the zinc site, although the two situations can be clearly discriminated either spectro-scopically or by the response to external perturbations. In particular the cobalt in the copper site is sensitive to phosphate and to pH in the range 7.0 to 8.0 (216). It can also bind cyanide stoichiometrically forming a stable adduct (217). The cobalt in the zinc site is affected by alkaline pH and by cyanide only when the copper is removed (218). The reaction of cyanide and OH$^-$ with the copper/cobalt protein does not lead to uncoupling of the antiferromagnetic interaction between the two metals.

The value of the coupling constant between copper and cobalt is relevant to whether the copper and the cobalt share a common ligand. Preliminary magnetic susceptibility measurements by Moss and Fee (221) in the temperature range 1.4 to 5°K were extended by Desideri et al. (22) who established by exploring the temperature range 30-200°K a lower limit for the coupling constant ($J \geq 600$ cm^{-1}). This indicates that the system is still coupled at room temperature and the mag-nitude of the value indicates that a chemical bond links the two metal centers. Recent investigations on binuclear imidazole-bridged copper(II) complexes of copper-copper distance comparable to that established by X-ray analysis for the copper and the zinc in the protein has substantially confirmed that these model compounds reproduce the properties of the bimetal cluster of the enzyme (223). The only difference is that OH$^-$ is capable of breaking the bimetal bridge of the model complexes in alkaline solution while this is apparently not the case with the enzyme. However, the models and the enzyme have the same behavior in acidic solutions. At low pH the bridge is broken in the complexes and in the enzyme (223,224). Recent work (225,226) has indicated that at pH 3.4 any metal occupying the zinc site is released from the protein while the copper is still bound to the protein. On the basis of these results a scheme (Fig. 7) has been proposed incorporating previous data by Morpurgo et al. (227) showing that copper, if released from the zinc at low pH, is not reduced by ferrocyanide and forms a typical complex with this ligand. According to the scheme (228) the bimetal is broken above pH 5.0, only by reduction of the copper, through the protonation of the copper-facing imidazole nitrogen, while at more acidic pH values the copper(II) redox potential is significantly lowered and the bridge is broken by protonation of the zinc, facing imidazole nitrogen.

The mechanism of action of copper/zinc superoxide dismutase

The first studies on the dismutation reaction were carried out using pulse radiolysis (45,46). The substrate, O$_2^-$, was produced by water radiolysis under

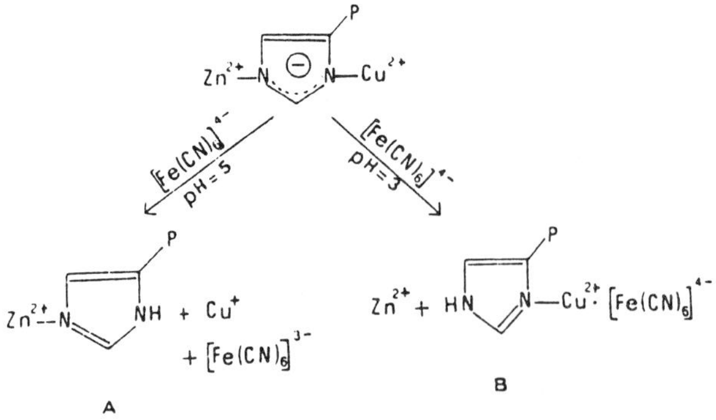

Fig. 7. Proposed structure for the zinc-copper bridge of bovine superoxide dismutase when copper is reduced (A) and at acid pH (B).

high energy electrons and its decay in the presence of catalytic amounts of the enzyme was studied by fast-recording photometry in steady state conditions. A second order rate constant of 2×10^9 $M^{-1}s^{-1}$ was determined for the enzyme-O_2^- reaction (Fig. 8). This rate constant is almost independent of pH in the range 5-10. This result is relevant to the biological role of the enzyme as the spontaneous and metal-catalyzed dismutations are strongly pH-dependent. The decrease of activity below pH 5 supports O_2^- rather than HO_2 (pK = 4.8) being the active form of the substrate which is in turn in line with the inhibitory effect of cyanide (45) and other singly charged anions. However, while cyanide inhibition could be quantitated by pulse radiolysis, inhibition by other anions could not be investigated because of the limiting experimental conditions (e.g., too high azide concentration in a pulse radiolysis experiment interfered with the absorption of the high energy electrons).

The oxidation state of the copper turned out to be one of the main features of the catalytic reaction of the enzyme. Fee and Di Corleto (229) and Rotilio et al. (230) carried out the first extensive investigation of the redox properties of the copper/zinc enzyme. An Eo value of approximately 0.40 V was calculated from the reaction with ferrocyanide. It was also shown that anions such as azide and cyanide (230) stabilized the oxidized state and that reoxidation of the reduced protein by oxygen is very slow. These redox properties are probably related to the unusual symmetry of the native copper-binding site. This is

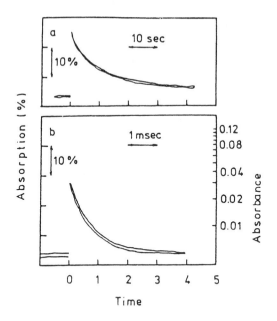

Fig. 8. Decay of superoxide radicals in the absence (a) and presence (b) of bovine copper/zinc superoxide dismutase. (Reproduced from Klug et al. (1972) J. Biol. Chem., 247, 4839-4842).

supported by evidence that at low pH, when the copper epr spectrum becomes axial, ferrocyanide is unable to reduce the metal, but rather binds to it in a binuclear complex with an unusual epr spectrum (227). The pH-dependence of the mid-point potential of the copper between pH 5 and 8.7 indicated that one proton binds on reduction (221). It was suggested that this proton is bound by a ligand which is released from the reduced copper. The results obtained from redox studies on the enzyme contributed significantly to the understanding of the mechanism of the enzyme. Klug-Roth et al. (231) and Fielden et al. (232) demonstrated by pulse radiolysis that the enzymatic reaction consists of two redox steps of equal rate involving first reduction and then reoxidation of the copper by superoxide. The rate constant for the reaction was found to be independent of the initial state of the enzyme--oxidized or reduced. A very important point that emerged from these investigations was that the steady-state level of oxidized copper in the enzyme, which must be 50% in view of the equal rate of the reduction and re-oxidation reactions, is approximately 75%. Klug-Roth et al. (231) explained this result by assuming that the copper ions in the active dimeric molecule are not initially equivalent but have different molar absorptivities at 680 nm.

Fielden et al. (232) however showed the spectroscopic equivalence of the two
copper ions in the resting enzyme and alternatively proposed that only half of
the active sites participate in the turnover of the substrate. Further investigations by Cockle and Bray (233), however, showed that 50% steady state levels
of oxidized copper could be approached with higher superoxide concentrations. A
possible explanation for these results is an anticooperative interaction between
the subunits. Evidence for interactions between subunits in the dimer has been
presented (234). Using ^{19}F nuclear magnetic resonance relaxation Viglino et al.
(235) have shown that the steady state level of the oxidized is actually 50% but
can change to 75% in previously lyophilized samples without a concomitant change
of activity. These results, though difficult to interpret in molecular terms,
show that the previous investigations are in some way reproducible and reflect
possible intrinsic properties of the protein.

The study of the dismutation of superoxide by the copper/zinc superoxide dismutase has led to investigations being carried out on the interaction between the
enzyme and the major product of the reaction, hydrogen peroxide. Bray et al.
(236) carried out a kinetic study of the reduction of the copper with hydrogen
peroxide and showed that after reduction of the copper(II) to copper(I) the reduced enzyme further reacts with hydrogen peroxide in a slow reaction leading to
destruction of histidine residues probably adjacent to the metal with consequent
inactivation of the enzyme. The reaction was reinvestigated by Hodgson and
Fridovich (237,28) who pointed out additional interesting features. Superoxide
dismutase was found to catalyze the peroxidation of a variety of compounds. This
point is of relevance to the frequent misinterpretation in the literature of
apparently paradoxical effects of superoxide dismutase. It should be pointed out,
however, that in an ideal system producing hydrogen peroxide from superoxide and
containing no peroxide removing enzymes, superoxide dismutase will behave as a
catalyst of oxidative reactions rather than a beneficial system against oxidative
injury (239). The same workers (237,238) also found that cyanide protected
the enzyme against hydrogen peroxide inactivation while azide did not. This
result was later shown to be due to the very different inhibition constant
for the two inhibitors (50,65). The result obtained by Hodgson and Fridovich
(237,238), however, led to the suggestion that azide could bind at a second
binding site for anions, and in particular could replace a histidine ligand of
the enzyme. This suggestion however gives a different interpretation of the
active site of the copper/zinc superoxide dismutase. Hodgson and Fridovich
(237,238) presented interesting speculations concerning the mechanisms of the
enzyme. They observed the absence of an isotope effect when the dismutation
reaction is carried out in deuterium oxide and the requirement of an efficient
proton carrier for the protonation of the peroxide anion produced in the reoxidation step of the dismutation process. A possible source of this proton

was suggested to be an imidazolate bridging the copper and the zinc which would release the copper and become protonated in the reduction step. This bridging imidazolate later identified from X-ray investigations to be His-63 is one of the major issues in the mechanism of enzyme activity. Spectral changes recorded during a study of the dismutation reaction by the copper/cobalt enzyme by pulse radiolysis (240) unequivocally demonstrated that rapid protonation and deprotonation by His-63 nitrogen is a concurrent act of catalysis. The rapidity of the event permits the possibility that the same imidazole could be the proton donor in the formation of the peroxide product.

Interaction of the copper and the zinc through a bridging imidazole ligand has recently been challenged following investigations carried out using the cadmium substituted enzyme. Cadmium substitution in place of the zinc is an analog of cobalt substitution of the zinc and was previously reported by Beem et al. (206). While cobalt is paramagnetic and strongly chromophoric (113), cadmium(II) allows direct observation of the cadmium nuclear spin by nuclear magnetic resonance (NMR) and of its nuclear quadrupole interaction by perturbed angular correlation of X-rays (PAC). Two investigations using ^{113}Cd NMR have been carried out. Armitage et al. (241) found different chemical shifts in the copper-free and in the copper(I) enzyme while Bailey et al. (242) observed almost identical chemical shifts in both derivatives thereby confirming the assumptions made on the basis of the changes observed in the spectrum of the cobalt enzyme during dismutation. The PAC study (243) was not able to detect any influence on the cadmium spectrum by the valence state of the copper and concluded that a bridging imidazole is not coordinated to both copper and zinc. The conclusions drawn from ^{113}Cd NMR and PAC data point to the difficulties usually encountered by spectroscopists working with protein derivatives that need manipulation likely to affect the conformation of the whole molecule. The copper/zinc superoxide dismutase used in these investigations were reconstituted with ^{113}Cd by different procedures. Different reconstitution procedures were used in three investigations and in none of the investigations was explicit evidence of reconstitution, such as epr spectra, provided. We have reproduced the experimental procedures reported (see Fig. 9) and it appears that while the method of Bailey et al. (242) results in an epr spectrum similar to that of the native enzyme, the method described by Bauer et al. (243) leads to binding of copper at sites which are not typical of those occupied in the native enzyme. It is therefore reasonable to conclude that the cadmium investigations result in substantial agreement with previous data obtained with the cobalt enzyme and represent a typical case of how crucial is the preparation of the protein sample. The imidazole bridge was also investigated using X-ray absorption near edge spectroscopy (XANES) (Ref. 244). The results showed that reduction of the copper does not affect the XANES spectrum of zinc, thus demonstrating that its ligands with

174

the protein remain intact when the copper is reduced and no charge-transfer occurs from the copper to the zinc. A XANES analysis of the cobalt derivatives showed that the structure of the cobalt site is identical in the copper-free and copper(I) derivatives. Although it was found to be significantly different in the copper(II) derivative it still maintained the same tetrahedral coordination to the same ligands (245). This study provides the definitive evidence that the conclusion reached by McAdam et al. (240) is correct.

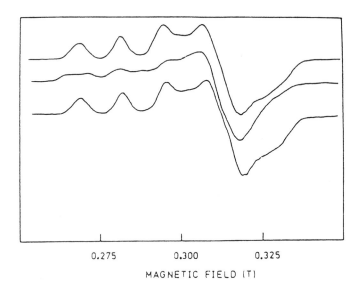

0.275   0.300   0.325

MAGNETIC FIELD (T)

Fig. 9. Epr spectra of cadmium-reconstituted bovine copper/zinc superoxide dismutase at 77°K. From top: native protein; protein reconstituted according to Bauer et al. (243) and protein reconstituted by addition of the two metals together and incubating for several hours at room temperature.

Another major line of investigation concerning the mechanism of action of the copper/zinc superoxide dismutase concerns the mode of interaction of the superoxide radical with the copper. This line of research can be defined as dealing with the anion binding site of the enzyme as the superoxide radical is a singly charged anion and therefore halides and pseudohalides are to be considered as substrate analogs and potential inhibitors. In spite of many contradictory reports, a great deal of spectroscopic and catalytic evidence indicates that there is a single anion binding site.

In fact single charged anions change the epr spectrum of the protein from rhombic to axial (219) and this conversion produces a change of the redox

potential of the copper, which is revealed by the hastened reoxidation of the
reduced enzyme (230). This result is in line with the established lack of reduction of the axial forms of the enzyme by mild reducing agents that are effective with the native enzyme (227). Other changes observed as a result of anion
binding are decrease of the water proton relaxation rate and catalytic inhibition
(246). The change of enzyme activity, epr spectra and water nuclear magnetic
relaxation rate that are observed between pH 10 and 12 are reasonably accounted
for by OH$^-$ ligation to the copper (247) and therefore may be included in the
general pattern of anion effects. The report that the azide adduct is active and
could be reduced by hydrogen peroxide (237,238) suggests that azide could bind
in place of one of the histidine copper ligands. Although these results were
due to an incomplete determination of the azide inhibition constant (50,65,246)
they are still used to corroborate evidence that would support the presence of
a second anion-binding site in the copper coordination sphere, besides that provided by the displacement of the copper bound water. This second site could
arise either from the displacement of the imidazole nucleus of the bridging
histidine (248) or from an in plane histidine (249). However, the former conclusion does not take into account that neither cyanide nor OH$^-$ break the antiferromagnetic coupling between the copper and cobalt in the cobalt-substituted
enzyme (218). On the other hand Bertini et al. (249) report that thiocyanate
binds to the copper in a concentration range where the enzyme activity and the
water relaxation rate are not affected whereas the epr spectra show that the
copper is converted to an axial form. However, while the water relaxation rate
and enzyme activity are tested in the liquid state, the epr spectra reported
were taken on frozen solutions. It can be easily appreciated that most anions,
even those that do not strongly bind to the copper, convert the epr spectrum to
an axial line shape *only on freezing* (see Fig. 10). It is clear that just a
single approach cannot lead to any conclusive evidence. More reliable conclusions
can be drawn from a comparative study which should include: (a) demonstration
that all the effects observed are reversible, as displacement of protein ligands
is hardly compatible with reversibility, (b) determination of the enzyme activity
to prove that binding of anions may occur without enzyme inhibition, and (c)
rigorous control of specificity, especially regarding charge effects which become
predominant at very high anion concentrations, such as those used by Bertini
et al. (249). Such a comprehensive approach has shown that all single charged
anions, including OH$^-$ are competitive between each other and with superoxide
(246) strongly suggesting that binding of all anionic species of a single site,
the water coordination site, is responsible for the observed changes in the
spectral and functional properties of the copper in the presence of anions.
Evidence for a complex between superoxide and the enzyme copper (250) has been
obtained from the saturation effects at high superoxide concentration with an

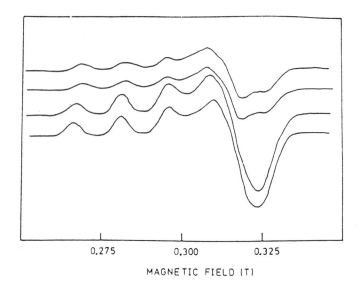

MAGNETIC FIELD (T)

Fig. 10. Epr spectra of bovine copper/zinc superoxide dismutase in the presence of different anions. From top: native enzyme at room temperature; enzyme plus 0.1 M NCS⁻ or ClO_4^- at room temperature; enzyme plus 0.1 M NCS⁻ at 77°K. The spectrum of the native enzyme at 77°K is reported in Fig. 9.

estimated Michaelis constant of 3.6×10^{-4} M and from the inhibition of the enzyme activity at high ionic strength (200). From the slope of the linear plot of log k versus $\sqrt{\mu}$ the formation of inner sphere complexes of superoxide with both copper(II) and copper(I) at the active site is inferred. Direct anion binding to copper(I) is supported by ^{35}Cl NMR investigations (251) and by observed perturbations of the histidine resonances liganding the copper(I) from NMR investigations (252).

All the evidence obtained has been incorporated in a mechanistic scheme which involves reversible protonation of the bridging histidine and the displacement of the bound water by superoxide prior to electron transfer from both the reduced and oxidized copper (253). This mechanism clearly implies a double displacement of the water molecule bound to the copper by superoxide (Fig. 11). Cass and Hill (252) point out that the rate of exchange of water is too low to allow such a mechanism, and therefore propose outer sphere electron transfer from superoxide to copper and vice versa. However, ^{19}F NMR relaxation measurements (55) have shown that anionic ligands can be exchanged very fast at the copper center of the enzyme ($T_M = 4 \times 10^{-8}$ s for ^{19}F) and this supports the contention that superoxide has actually the time for water replacement and electron donation within the turnover limits of the enzyme.

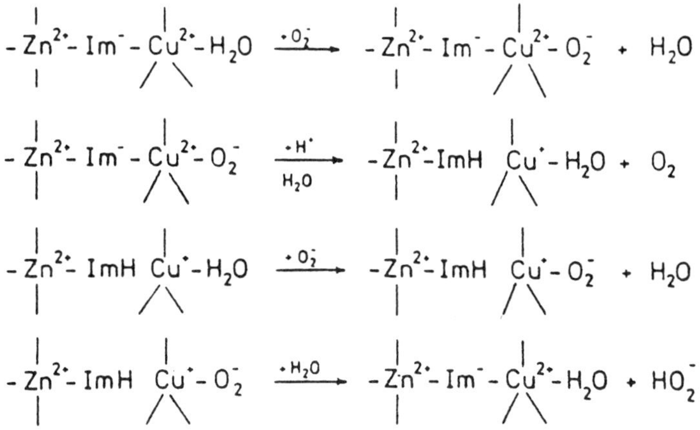

$$-\overset{|}{\underset{|}{Zn}}{}^{2+}-Im^- - \overset{|}{Cu}{}^{2+}-H_2O \xrightarrow{\cdot O_2^-} -\overset{|}{\underset{|}{Zn}}{}^{2+}-Im^- - \overset{|}{Cu}{}^{2+}-O_2^- \ + \ H_2O$$

$$-\overset{|}{\underset{|}{Zn}}{}^{2+}-Im^- - \overset{|}{Cu}{}^{2+}-O_2^- \xrightarrow[H_2O]{\cdot H^\cdot} -\overset{|}{\underset{|}{Zn}}{}^{2+}-ImH \ \overset{|}{Cu}{}^\cdot-H_2O \ + \ O_2$$

$$-\overset{|}{\underset{|}{Zn}}{}^{2+}-ImH \ \overset{|}{Cu}{}^\cdot-H_2O \xrightarrow{\cdot O_2^-} -\overset{|}{\underset{|}{Zn}}{}^{2+}-ImH \ \overset{|}{Cu}{}^\cdot-O_2^- \ + \ H_2O$$

$$-\overset{|}{\underset{|}{Zn}}{}^{2+}-ImH \ \overset{|}{Cu}{}^\cdot-O_2^- \xrightarrow{\cdot H_2O} -\overset{|}{\underset{|}{Zn}}{}^{2+}-Im^- - \overset{|}{Cu}{}^{2+}-H_2O \ + \ HO_2^-$$

Fig. 11. Scheme for copper/zinc superoxide dismutase incorporating the bridging histidine.

In the mechanism outlined in Fig. 11, the protonation-deprotonation of the imidazole nucleus of the bridging histidine is important in two respects. First, the alternate change of the copper coordination number between 5 and 4 would kinetically favor change by providing appropriate geometries to copper(II) and copper(I) without rearrangement of the surrounding nuclei. Second, the deprotonation occurring in the reoxidation step could be the source of a proton for the developing peroxide anion, and this may explain the pH-independence of the enzyme activity. These properties prove that the active site of the enzyme is specifically adapted to the molecular function of superoxide dismutation, in contrast to the rather indiscriminate reactivity (towards H^+, O_2^- and H_2O_2) of low molecular weight complexes of copper with amino acids that may even dismute superoxide faster than the enzyme under the same conditions.

Further evidence regarding the specificity of the protein structure around the copper site comes from the fact that Arg-143 is essential for enzyme activity (254). This residue is located within 6 Å of the active site and may provide electrostatic attractions for the incoming superoxide. The importance of positively charged amino acid residues in determining the rate of electron exchange of proteins with superoxide has been pointed out by Koppernol (255) for cytochrome c and can apply for the copper/zinc superoxide dismutase as well. This effect is in line with the established inhibition of the enzyme with high ionic strength (200). Arginine-143 has also been proposed as a possible proton source during the second half of the catalytic cycle (254). However, this proposed function is in conflict with the established absence of an isotope (D_2O) effect on the enzyme activity as the exchange of an acid-base proton of ionic groups should be heavily affected by deuteration (237,238). General acid catalysis by amino acid side chain is also excluded because catalysis is not pH-dependent (45). Deprotonation of Arg-143 may however be involved, together with deprotonation of copper-bound water (247) in the reversible decrease of the enzyme activity at alkaline pH (200,256).

Physical properties of the noncopper superoxide dismutases

Investigations on the manganese and iron superoxide dismutases have been rather scanty compared with the numerous investigations carried out on the copper/zinc enzyme. Important catalytic differences between this class of enzyme and the copper/zinc enzyme were first pointed out by Forman and Fridovich (42) who in a careful study redetermined the rate constants for the dismutation reaction by kinetic competition with reagents of known kinetics with superoxide. Identical rate constants as those obtained by pulse radiolysis can be measured at very low steady state level of superoxide radicals (10^{-8} to 10^{-13}M) and it was shown that the constants for the manganese and iron enzyme drop sharply between pH 7 and 10. A detailed mechanistic study of the manganese superoxide dismutase from *Escherichia coli* indicated a complex reaction mechanism which included a fast rate (1.5×10^9 $M^{-1}s^{-1}$ at pH 7.9) for slight excesses of superoxide radicals and a much slower rate (2×10^7 $M^{-1}s^{-1}$) for an additional reaction which removes higher superoxide excesses (49). The nature of the enzyme form involved in such a reaction was not clarified, but at least four valence states of the manganese (I to IV) were proposed to be present in the catalytic cycle. The valence of the metal in the resting protein was established to be manganese(III) by a variety of spectroscopic techniques (257-259). A much simpler catalytic mechanism was proposed by McAdam et al. (260) using the manganese enzyme prepared from the thermophile *Bacillus stearothermophilus*. This mechanism involves a fast redox cycle similar to that observed with the copper/zinc enzyme and likely to involve conversion between manganese(III) and manganese(II). In the presence of excess superoxide a rather stable complex appears to form with the enzyme species originated by the fast reaction with low superoxide (possibly manganese(II)) and this species slowly decreases back to the native enzyme in a slower first order reaction. In fact appearance of the manganese(II) epr spectrum occurs after treatment of the manganese superoxide dismutase with hydrogen peroxide which also bleaches the optical absorption spectrum (258). However, in the short time scale hydrogen peroxide does not affect the activity of the enzyme (260). External ligands such as azide and even cyanide have little or no effect on the enzyme activity. This activity is strongly pH-dependent (44,260).

Nuclear magnetic resonance investigations suggest that a water molecule is bound to the manganese(III) in the native enzyme (257). This exchange rate for this water molecule was found to be too low to allow an inner sphere mechanism. Also the lack of an effect by azide and cyanide suggests an outer sphere electron transfer between manganese and superoxide. Similar conclusions are reported for the iron superoxide dismutase following proton relaxation rate (T_1) measurements and by the absence of any effect by cyanide on the T_1 rates and on enzyme activity.

The mechanism of action of the iron superoxide dismutase was found to be similar to the copper/zinc superoxide dismutase (261). A similar redox cycling between iron(III) and iron(II) with rates equal to the overall turnover rate ($k = 5.5 \times 10^8$ $M^{-1}s^{-1}$ at pH 8.0) has been demonstrated. Also the sensitivity to hydrogen peroxide inactivation is higher for the iron enzyme than for the manganese enzyme. Furthermore, azide and fluoride, at variance with cyanide, change the optical absorption and epr spectrum although no clear conclusions have been reached concerning the inhibition of the enzyme activity. A possible suggestion is that two fluoride or azide atoms per iron atom have to bind to affect catalysis (262). The activity of the iron superoxide dismutase is also pH-dependent and also its epr spectrum changes with pH (262).

The major problem in the study of the physical properties of both the iron and manganese superoxide dismutase has been the variability of the metal to protein stoichiometry in the various preparations. Another problem is that it is difficult to obtain reconstitutable apoproteins. The preparation of manganese-free superoxide dismutase involves the use of chaotropic agents at acidic pH (263,264). Reconstitution of the apoprotein with manganese chloride was carried out (262). The reconstituted protein was found to be fully active. However, no spectral properties were reported for the reconstituted protein. Other metals were found to compete with the manganese during reconstitution. Some of these metals--cobalt(II), zinc(II), nickel(II) and iron(III)--were shown to bind to the enzyme. None of these derivatives were, however, catalytically active. Milder conditions were used for the preparation of apoprotein for iron superoxide dismutase (265). A reconstitutable apoprotein was obtained following treatment with urea, EDTA and dithiothreitol in 3-(N-morpholino)propanesulfonic acid buffer, pH 7.0 under anerobic conditions.

Chemical characterization of superoxide dismutases

(i) Molecular weight. The copper/zinc superoxide dismutase is a homodimer of about 32,000 daltons. The molecular weights determined for the enzyme from a variety of sources are all substantially in agreement. By contrast the manganese and iron forms of the enzyme have a slightly higher molecular weight of about 40,000 daltons. While all the copper/zinc and the iron superoxide dismutases have been shown to be dimeric, the manganese enzyme has been found to form tetramers. The extent of polymerization does not apparently depend on the

source of the enzyme. Manganese superoxide dismutase from *E. coli* is a dimer
(17) while the enzyme from chicken liver (146), *Thermus aquaticus* (100) and
yeast mitochondria (114) is a tetramer.

(ii) Metal content. The copper/zinc superoxide dismutase is assumed to contain
up to 2 atoms of copper and 2 atoms of zinc calculated on the basis of a molecular weight of 32,000 dalton. The values reported in the literature are 1.8
atoms of copper and 1.8 atoms of zinc. Puget and Michelson (66) reported the
presence of 1 atom of copper in the enzyme from *Photobacterium leiognathi*. This
may however be due to loss of copper during the purification procedure.

The metal content of the iron and manganese enzymes varies between 1.0 and
2.0 atoms per dimer. Whether this variation is due to loss of manganese
content can only be determined once the number of metal binding sites is determined from the X-ray structure.

(iii) Subunits. All the various forms of superoxide dismutase are composed of
identical subunits. In earlier investigations (17) bovine copper/zinc superoxide dismutase was considered to have covalently bound subunits because dissociation could only be obtained in the presence of β-mercaptoethanol, however,
the primary sequence determination (266) has shown that the subunits are non-
covalently bound. Hartz and Deutsch (267) proposed that the human copper/zinc
superoxide dismutase has nonidentical subunits, again the primary sequence
determination (268,269) has shown the subunits to be identical.

Dissociation of the copper/zinc enzyme into subunits has been reported in the
presence of 8 M urea (270). However, these results were obtained solely from
gel chromatography. Sedimentation equilibrium analysis showed that a single
species was present when bovine copper/zinc superoxide dismutase was dissolved
in 8 M urea. Malinowski and Fridovich (272) reported an apparent molecular
weight of 32,000 daltons under these conditions. However in a similar experiment, Bannister and Bannister (unpublished observations) obtained a molecular
weight of 19,000 daltons.

Monomerization into subunits does, however, occur in the presence of 1 to 4%
sodium lauryl sulphate. This has been demonstrated in the yeast (116), fungal
(118) and wheat germ variant I (122,273) but not for the bovine (17), human (267)
or wheat germ variant II (122,273) copper/zinc superoxide dismutases. Succinyla-
tion has recently been shown to lead to dissociation of the bovine copper/zinc
enzyme forming nondenatured subunits (274). The succinylated protein had,
however, only 10% activity of the native enzyme. This was interpreted to be
possibly due to charge effects on the protein-substrate interaction

(iv) Primary structure. The complete amino acid sequence has been determined
for seven superoxide dismutases. The copper/zinc superoxide dismutases sequenced
were obtained from bovine and human erythrocytes (266,268,269), horse liver (275)
and yeast (276,277). The amino acid sequences obtained are compared in Fig. 12.

A great deal of homology is found in the sequences which are characterized by a
hypervariable region between residues 20 and 33.   The copper/zinc proteins have
a number of unusual features.   Tryptophan is absent in the bovine and yeast
enzymes while tyrosine is absent from the human enzyme.   Both residues are
absent in the horse enzyme.   The human enzyme is also characterized by the
presence of a unique cysteine in position III.

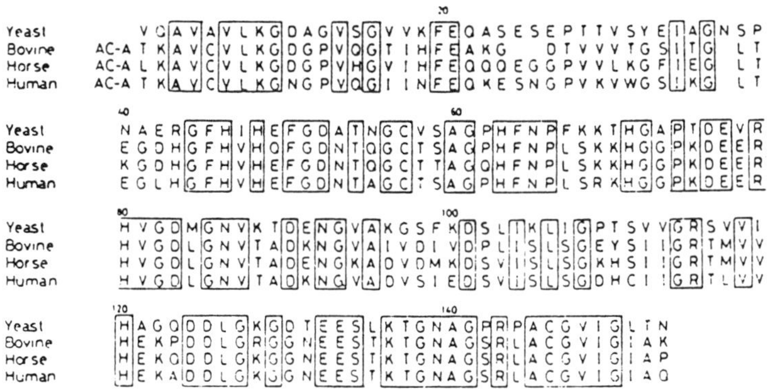

Fig. 12.   Amino acid sequence of yeast, bovine, horse and human copper/zinc
superoxide dismutase.

The manganese superoxide dismutases sequenced have been obtained from E. coli
(278), B. Stearothermophilus (279) and yeast mitochondria (280).   They exhibit
a significant degree of homology.   No complete amino acid sequence has as yet
been obtained for an iron superoxide dismutase.   However, the N-terminal sequence
of a variety of iron and manganese superoxide dismutases has been determined.
A high degree of homology has been obtained between the two metalloproteins (281).
(v)   Crystal structure.   Bovine copper/zinc erythrocyte superoxide dismutase is
the only form of the enzyme to have its crystal structure determined.   Two
crystalline forms have been obtained (282).   A monoclinic and orthorhombic
form were crystallized.   Structural determinations at 5, 3 and 2 Å resolution
maps were obtained for the monoclinic form (283-285).   Crystals were found to
contain four subunits per asymmetric unit, i.e., the protein exists as a dimer
with each monomeric form containing dimeric subunits.   The dimeric subunits are

identical in the crystal form and the area of contact between the subunits is due to Van der Waals contact between approximately 14 sidechains. Each single subunit appears as a slightly flattened cylindrical barrel of β-pleated sheet made up of 8 antiparallel chains from which two long loops extend. The upper loop consisting of residues 119 to 141 is highly hydrophilic and is not involved in each subunit contact or metal binding. The lower loop consisting of residues 48 to 79. This loop has two regions. One region is attached to the strand of the β-barrel that contains two of copper ligands, histine 46 and 48 (Fig. 11). The other region has three of the histidine zinc ligands; histidine 63, 71 and 80 (Fig. 11). Histidine 63 is a common ligand while the fourth zinc ligand, aspartate 83 is in the β-barrel. The fourth copper ligand is histidine 120.

The crystal structure of the enzyme has been found to have a striking resemblance to the three-dimensional structure of immunoglobin despite the fact that there are no sequence homologies between the two proteins (286). A further analysis (287) speculated that the present protein evolved initially as a copper protein and that gene duplication occurred very early. Only preliminary data has appeared on the manganese and iron superoxide dismutase (288-291).

Acknowledgments: J. V. Bannister thanks the Wellcome Trust for a Senior Research Fellowship. We thank our friends and colleagues at the Universities of Rome, Camerino and Venice for many stimulating discussion.

References

1. Mann, T. and Keilin, D. (1939) Proc. Roy. Soc. B., 126, 303-315.
2. Mohamed, M.S. and Greenberg, D. (1954) J. Gen. Physiol., 37, 433-439.
3. Porter, H. and Folch, J. (1957) J. Neurochem., 1, 260-271.
4. Porter, H. and Ainsworth, S. (1959) J. Neurochem., 5, 91-98.
5. Markowitz, H., Cartwright, G.E., and Wintrobe, M.M. (1959) J. Biol. Chem., 24, 40-45.
6. Kimmel, J.R., Markowitz, H., and Brown, D.M. (1959) J. Biol. Chem., 234, 46-50.
7. Carrico, R.J. and Deutsch, H.F. (1969) J. Biol. Chem., 244, 6087-6093.
8. McCord, J. and Fridovich, I. (1969) J. Biol. Chem., 244, 6049-6055.
9. Carrico, R.J. and Deutsch, H.F. (1970) J. Biol. Chem., 245, 723-727.
10. McCord, J. and Fridovich, I. (1977) in Superoxide and Superoxide Dismutase Michelson, A.M., McCord, J.M., and Fridovich, I., eds., New York and London: Academic Press, pp. 1-10.
11. Fridovich, I. and Handler, P. (1962) J. Biol. Chem., 237, 916-921.
12. Fridovich, I. (1962) J. Biol. Chem., 237, 584-586.
13. Michelson, A.M., McCord, J.M., and Fridovich, I., eds. (1977) Superoxide and Superoxide Dismutases, New York and London: Academic Press, 569 pp.
14. Bannister, J.V. and Hill, H.A.O., eds. (1980) Chemical and Biochemical Aspects of Superoxide and Superoxide Dismutase, New York: Elsevier/North Holland, 411 pp.
15. Bannister, W.H. and Bannister, J.V., eds. (1980) Biological and Clinical Aspects of Superoxide and Superoxide Dismutase, New York: Elsevier/North Holland, 433 pp.
16. Hayaishi, O. and Asada, K., eds. (1977) Biochemical and Medical Aspects of Active Oxygen, Tolyo: Japan Scientific Societies Press, 200 pp.

17. Keele, B.B., McCord, J.M., and Fridovich, I. (1970) J. Biol. Chem., 245, 6176-6181.
18. Yost, F.J. and Fridovich, I. (1973) J. Biol. Chem., 248, 4905-4908.
19. Fridovich, I. (1974) Adv. in Enzymol., 40, 35-97.
20. Azzi, A., Montecucco, C. and Richter, C. (1975) Biochem. Biophys. Res. Commun., 65, 579-603.
21. Buchanan, A.G. and Lees, H. (1976) Can. J. Microbiol., 22, 1643-1646.
22. Beauchamp, C. and Fridovich, I. (1971) Anal. Biochem., 44, 276-287.
23. Rajagopalan, K.V. and Handler, P.J. (1964) J. Biol. Chem., 239, 2022-2026.
24. Miller, R.W. (1970) Can. J. Biochem., 48, 935-941.
25. Auclair, C., Torres, M., and Hakim, J. (1978) FEBS Letts., 89, 26-28.
26. Rapp, U., Adams, W.C., and Miller, R.W. (1973) Can. J. Biochem., 51, 158-171.
27. Massey, V., Strickland, S., Mayhew, S.G., Howell, L.G., Engel, P.C., Matthews, R.G., Schuman, M., and Sullivand, P.A. (1969) Biochem. Biophys. Res. Commun., 36, 891-897.
28. Misra, H.P. and Fridovich, I. (1972) J. Biol. Chem., 247, 3170-3175.
29. Sun, M. and Zigman, S. (1978) Anal. Biochem., 90, 81-89.
30. Green, S., Maxur, A., and Shorr, J. (1956) J. Biol. Chem., 220, 237-255.
31. Ball, E.G. and Chen, T.T. (1933) J. Biol. Chem., 102, 691-719.
32. Elstner, E.F., Stoffer, C., and Heupel, A. (1975) Z. Naturforsch., 30c, 53-56.
33. Elstner, E.F. and Heupel, A. (1976) Anal. Biochem., 70, 616-620.
34. Kono, Y. (1978) Arch. Biochem. Biophys., 186, 189-195.
35. Nishikimi, M. (1975) Arch. Biochem. Biophys., 166, 273-279.
36. Heikkila, R.E. and Cabbat, F. (1976) Anal. Biochem., 75, 356-362.
37. Marklund, S. and Marklund, G. (1974) Euro. J. Biochem., 47, 469-474.
38. McCord, J.M. and Fridovich, I. (1969) J. Biol. Chem., 244, 6056-6063.
39. Tyler, D.D. (1975) Biochem. J., 147, 493-504.
40. Misra, H.P. and Fridovich, I. (1977) Arch. Biochem. Biophys., 181, 308-312.
41. Misra, H.P. and Fridovich, I. (1977) Arch. Biochem. Biophys., 183, 511-515.
42. Forman, H.J. and Fridovich, I. (1973) Arch. Biochem. Biophys., 158, 396-400.
43. Sawada, Y. and Yamazaki, I. (1973) Biochim. Biophys. Acta, 327, 257-265.
44. Ballou, D., Palmer, G., and Massey, V. (1969) Biochem. Biophys. Res. Commun., 36, 898-904.
45. Rotilio, G., Bray, R.C., and Fielden, E.M. (1972) Biochim. Biophys. Acta, 268, 605-609.
46. Klug, D., Rabani, J., and Fridovich, I. (1972) J. Biol. Chem., 247, 4839-4482.
47. Bannister, J.V., Bannister, W.H., Bray, R.C., Fielden, E.M., Roberts, P.B. and Rotilio, G. (1973) FEBS Letts., 32, 303-306.
48. Klug, D., Fridovich, I., and Rabani, J. (1973) J. Amer. Chem. Soc., 95, 2786-2790.
49. Pick, M., Rabani, J., Yost, F., and Fridovich, I. (1974) J. Amer. Chem. Soc., 96, 7329-7333.
50. Rigo, A., Viglino, P., and Rotilio, G. (1975) Anal. Biochem., 68, 1-9.
51. McClune, G.J. and Fee, J.A. (1976) FEBS Letts., 67, 294-298.
52. Marklund, S. (1976) J. Biol. Chem., 251, 7504-7507.
53. Viglino, P., Rigo, A., Argese, E., Calabrese, L., Cocco, V., and Rotilio, G. (1981) Biochem. Biophys. Res. Commun., 100, 125-130.
54. Rigo, A., Viglino, P., Argeses, E., Terenzi, M., and Rotilio, G. (1979) J. Biol. Chem., 254, 1759-1760.
55. Viglino, P., Rigo, A., Stevenato, R., Ranieri, G.A., Rotilio, G., and Calabrese, L. (1979) J. Magnet. Res., 34, 265-274.
56. Kelly, K., Barefoot, C., Sehan, A., and Petkau, A. (1978) Arch. Biochem. Biophys., 190, 531-538.
57. Del Villano, B.C. and Tischfield, J.A. (1979) J. Immunol., Meths., 29, 253-262.
58. Holme, E., Bunkel, L., Lundberg, P.A., and Waldenstrom, J. (1980) in Ref. 15, pp. 262-270
59. Baret, A., Schinvi, P. and Michelson, A.M. (1980) in Ref. 15, pp. 252-261.
60. Baret, A., Schiavi, P., Michel, P., Michelson, A.M., and Puget, K. (1980) FEBS Letts., 112, 25-29.
61. Baret, A., Bacterman, M.A., Mattei, J.F., Michel, P., Broussole, B., and Giraud, F. (1981) Biochem. Biophys. Res. Commun., 98, 1035-1043.

62. Asada, K., Moshikawa, K., Takahashi, N., Maeda, Y., and Enmangi, K. (1975) J. Biol. Chem., 250, 2801-2807.
63. Britton, L., Malinowski, D.P., and Fridovich, I. (1978) J. Bacteriol., 134, 229-236.
64. McEuen, A.R., Hill, H.A.O., Dring, G.J., and Ingram, G.S. (1980) in Ref. 14, pp. 284-289.
65. Misra, H. and Fridovich, I. (1978) Arch. Biochem. Biophys., 189, 317-322.
66. Puget, K. and Michelson, A.M. (1974) Biochem. Biophys. Res. Commun., 58, 830-838.
67. Vignais, P.M., Henry, M-F., Terech, A., and Chabert, J. (1980) in Ref. 14, pp. 154-159.
68. Salin, M.L. and Bridges, S.M. (1980) in Ref. 14, pp. 176-184.
69. Grigoryan, N.A. and Nalbandyan, R.M. (1980) in Ref. 14, pp. 196-200.
70. Hewitt, J. and Morris, J.E. (1975) FEBS Letts., 50, 315-318.
71. McCord, J.M., Keele, B.B., and Fridovich, I. (1971) Proc. Natl. Acad. Sci., 68, 1024-1027.
72. Lumsden, J. and Hall, D.O. (1975) Nature, 257, 670-672.
73. Carlsson, J., Werthau, C., and Beckman, G. (1977) J. Clin. Microbiol., 6, 280-284.
74. Gregory, E.M., Kowalski, J.B., Holdeman, L.V. (1977) J. Bact., 129, 1298-1302.
75. Hatchikan, E.C. and Henry, Y.A. (1977) Biochimie, 59, 153-161.
76. Tally, F.P., Golden, B.R., Jacobus, N.V., and Gorbach, S.L. (1977) Infec. Immunity, 16, 20-25.
77. Kanematsu, S. and Asada, K. (1978) FEBS Letts., 91, 94-98.
78. Gregory, E.M., Moore, W.E.C., Holdeman, L.V. (1978) Appl. Environ. Microbiol., 35, 988-991.
79. Kanematsu, S. and Asada, K. (1978) Arch. Biochem. Biophys., 185, 473-482.
80. Yano, K. and Nishie, H. (1978) J. Gen. Appl. Microbiol., 24, 333-339.
81. Meier, B. and Schwartz, A.C. (1980) in Ref. 14, pp. 160-167.
82. Martin, J.P. and Fridovich, I. (1981) J. Biol. Chem., 256, 6080-6089.
83. Asada, K., Kanematsu, S., Okaka, S., and Hayakawa, T. (1980) in Ref. 14, pp. 136-153.
84. Dougherty, H.W., Sadowski, S.J., Baker, E.E. (1978) J. Biol. Chem., 253, 5220-5223.
85. Hassan, H.M. and Fridovich, I. (1979) J. Bacteriol., 129, 1574-1583.
86. Hassan, H.M. and Fridovich, I. (1977) J. Biol. Chem., 252, 7667-7672.
87. Kanematsu, S. and Asada, K. (1977) Proc. Agr. Chem. Soc. Jap., 266.
88. Nishie, H. and Yano, K. (1977) Proc. Agr. Chem. Soc. Jap., 266.
89. Slykhouse, T.O. and Fee, J.A. (1976) J. Biol. Chem., 251, 5472-5477.
90. Kusunose, E., Ichihara, K., Noda, Y., and Kusunose, M. (1976) J. Biochem., 80, 1343-1352.
91. Kusunose, M., Noda, Y., Ichihara, K., and Kusunose, E. (1976) Arch. Microbiol., 108, 65-73.
92. Yamakura, F. (1976) Biochim. Biophys. Acta, 422, 280-294.
93. Anastasi, A., Bannister, J.V., and Bannister, W.H. (1976) Int. J. Biochem., 7, 541-546.
94. Puget, K., Lavelle, F., and Michelson, A.M. (1977) in Ref. 13, pp. 139-150.
95. Vance, P.G., Keele, B.B., and Rajagopolan, K.V. (1972) J. Biol. Chem., 247, 4782-4786.
96. Chikata, Y., Kusunose, E., Ichihara, K., and Kusunose, M. (1975) Osaka City Med. J., 21, 127-136.
97. Lumsden, J., Cammack, R., and Hall, D.O. (1976) Biochim. Biophys., Acta, 438, 380-392.
98. Ichihara, K., Kusunose, E., Kusunose, M., and Mori, T. (1977) J. Biochem., 81, 1427-1433.
99. Harris, J.I. (1977) in Ref. 13, pp. 151-158.
100. Sato, S. and Harris, J.I. (1977) Eur. J. Biochem., 73, 373-381.
101. Sato, S. and Nakazowa, K. (1978) J. Biochem., 83, 1165-1171.
102. Kirby, T., Blum, J., Kahami, I. and Fridovich, I. (1980) Arch. Biochem. Biophys., 201, 551-555.

103. Terech, A. and Vignais, P.M. (1981) Biochim. Biophys. Acta, 657, 411-424.
104. Asada, K., Kanematsu, S., Takahashi, M., and Knon, Y. (1976) in Iron and Copper Proteins, Yasunobu, K.T., Mower, H.F., and Hayaishi, O., eds., New York: Plenum Press, pp. 551-564.
105. Asada, K. and Kanematsu, S. (1978) in Evolution of Protein Molecules, Matsubara, H. and Yamanaka, T., eds., Tokyo: Jap. Sci. Soc. Press, pp. 361-372.
106. Asada, K., Kanematsu, S., and Uchida, K. (1977) Arch. Biochem. Biophys., 179, 243-251.
107. Henry, L.E.A. and Hall, D.O. (1977) in Photosynthetic Organelles, Miyachi, S., Fugita, Y., and Shibata, K., eds., Kyoto: Jap. Soc. Plant Physiol., pp. 377-382.
108. Misra, H.P. and Fridovich, I. (1977) J. Biol. Chem., 252, 6421-6423.
109. Misra, H.P. and Keele, B.B. (1975) Biochim. Biophys. Acta, 379, 418-425.
110. Cseke, C., Horvath, L.I., Simon, P., Borbely, G., Keszthelyi, L., and Farkas, G.L. (1979) J. Biochem., 85, 1397-1404.
111. Kanematsu, S. and Asada, K. (1979) Arch. Biochem. Biophys., 115, 535-545.
112. Kanematsu, S. and Asada, K. (unpublished).
113. Lindmark, D.G. and Muller, M. (1974) J. Biol. Chem., 249, 4634-4637.
114. Ravindranath, S.V. and Fridovich, I. (1975) J. Biol. Chem., 250, 6107-6112.
115. Lavelle, F. and Michelson, A.M. (1975) Biochimie, 57, 375-381.
116. Gossin, S.A. and Fridovich, I. (1972) Biochim. Biophys. Acta, 289, 276-283.
117. Weser, U., Fretzdorff, A., and Prinz, R. (1972) FEBS Letts., 27, 267-269.
118. Misra, H.P. and Fridovich, I. (1972) J. Biol. Chem., 247, 3410-3414.
119. Shatzman, A.R. and Kosman, D.J. (1979) J. Bacteriol., 137, 313-320.
120. Bridges, S.M. and Salin, M.L. (1981) Plant Physiol., 68, 275-278.
121. Sawada, Y., Ohyama, T., and Yamazaki, I. (1972) Biochim. Biophys. Acta, 268, 305-312.
122. Beauchamp, C. and Fridovich, I. (1973) Biochim. Biophys. Acta, 317, 50-64.
123. Asada, K., Urano, M., and Takahashi, M. (1973) Eur. J. Biochem., 36, 257-266.
124. Kono, Y., Takahashi, M., and Asada, K. (1979) Plant Cell Physiol., 20, 1229-1235.
125. Baker, J.E. (1976) Plant Physiol., 58, 644-657.
126. Giannopolitis, C.N. and Ries, S.K. (1977) Plant Physiol., 59, 309-314.
127. Giannopolitis, C.N. and Ries, S.K. (1977) Plant Physiol., 59, 315-318.
128. Del Rio, L.A., Sevilla, F., Gomez, M., Yanez, J., and Lopez, J. (1978) Planta, 140, 221-225.
129. Arron, G.P., Henry, L., Palmer, J.M., and Hall, D.O. (1976) Biochem. Soc. Trans., 4, 618-620.
130. Hakamada, F., Kanematsu, S., and Asada, K. (1978) Study of Tea, 54, 6-10.
131. Sevilla, F., Lopez Gorge, J., and Del Rio, L. (1980) in Ref. 14, pp. 185-195.
132. Baum, J.A. and Scandalius, J.G. (1981) Arch. Biochem. Biophys., 206, 249-264.
133. Manwell, C. (1977) Comp. Biochem. Physiol., 58B, 331-338.
134. Lin, A.L. (1979) Comp. Biochem. Physiol., 62B, 425-431.
135. Bannister, J.V. (unpublished observations).
136. Albergoni, V., Cassini, A., and Tallandini, L. (personal communication).
137. Wolf, G.H., Heyneman, R., and Decleir, W. (1981) Comp. Biochem. Physiol., 69B, 865-867.
138. Fernandez-Sousa, J.M., and Michelson, A.M. (1976) Biochem. Biophys. Res. Commun., 73, 217-223.
139. Massie, H.R., Aiello, U.R., and Williams, T.R. (1980) Mech. Age Dev., 12, 279-286.
140. Massie, H.R., Williams, T.R., and Aiello, V.R. (1981) Gerontol., 27, 205-208.
141. Lee, Y.M., Ayala, F.J., and Misra, H.P. (1981) J. Biol. Chem., 256, 8506-8507.
142. Maral, J., Puget, K., and Michelson, A.M. (1977) Biochem. Biophys. Res. Commun., 77, 1525-1535.
143. Mazeud, F., Maral, J., and Michelson, A.M. (1979) Biochem. Biophys. Res. Commun., 86, 1161-1168.
144. Morris, S.M. and Albright, J.T. (1981) Cell. Tissue Res., 220, 739-752.
145. Bannister, J.V., Anastasi, A., and Bannister, W.H. (1977) Comp. Biochem., Physiol., 56B, 235-238.
146. Weisiger, R.A. and Fridovich, I. (1973) J. Biol. Chem., 248, 3582-3592.
147. Salin, M.L. and Wilson, W.W. (1981) Mol. Cell. Biochem., 36, 157-161.

148. Bhuyan, K.C. and Bhuyan, D.K. (1978) Biochim. Biophys. Acta, 542, 28-38.
149. Hicks, C.L., Korycka-Dahl, M. and Richardson, T. (1975) J. Dairy Sci., 58, 796.
150. Hill, R.D. (1975) Aust. J. Dairy Technol., 30, 26.
151. Asada, K. (1976) Agr. Biol. Chem., 40, 1659.
152. Keen, C.L., Lonnendal, B., Stein, T.N., and Hurley, L.S. (1980) Biol. Trace Elements Research, 2, 221-227.
153. Froman, D.P. and Thurston, R.J. (1981) Biology of Reproduction, 24, 193-200.
154. Rotilio, G., Calabrese, L., Finazzi-Agro, A., Argento-Ceru, M.P., Autuori, F., and Mondovi, B. (1973) Biochim. Biophys. Acta, 321, 98-102.
155. Weisiger, R.A. and Fridovich, I. (1973) J. Biol. Chem., 248, 4793-4796.
156. Peeters-Joris, C., Vandervoorde, A-M., and Baudhuin, P. (1975) Biochem. J., 150, 31-39.
157. Panchenko, L.F., Brusov, O.S., Gerasimov, A.M., Loktaeva, T.D. (1975) FEBS Letts., 55, 84-87.
158. Rest, R.F. and Spitznagel, J.K. (1977) Biochem. J., 166, 145-153.
159. McCord, J.M., Boyle, J.A., Day, Jr., Ed., Rizzolo, L.J., and Salim, M.L. (1977) in Ref. 13, pp. 129-138.
160. Gregory, E.M., Yost, F.J., and Fridovich, I. (1973) J. Bact., 115, 987-991.
161. Britton, L. and Fridovich, I. (1977) J. Bact., 131, 815-820.
162. Okada, S., Kanematsu, S., and Asada, K. (1979) FEBS Letts., 103, 106-110.
163. Lumsden, J. and Hall, D.P. (1974) Biochim. Biophys. Res. Commun., 58, 35-41.
164. Elstner, E.F. and Heupel, A. (1975) Planta, 123, 145-154.
165. Jackson, C., Dench, J., Moore, A.L., Halliwell, B., Foyer, C.H., and Hall, D.O. (1978) Eur. J. Biochem., 91, 339-344.
166. Salin, M.L. and Bridges, S.M. (1980) Z. Pflan. Physiol., 99, 37-45.
167. Salin, M.L. and Bridges, S.M. (1981) Biochem. J., 195, 229-233.
168. Nyman, P.O. (1960) Biochim. Biophys. Acta, 45, 387-389.
169. Porter, H., Sweeney, M., and Porter, E.M. (1964) Arch. Biochem. Biophys., 105, 319-325.
170. Shields, G.S., Markowitz, H., Klassen, W.H., Cartwright, G.E., and Wintrobe, M.M. (1961) J. Clin. Invest., 40, 2007-2015.
171. Stansell, M.J. and Deutsch, H.F. (1965) J. Biol. Chem., 240, 4299-4305.
172. Stansell, M.J. and Deutsch, H.F. (1965) J. Biol. Chem., 240, 4306-4311.
173. Hartz, J.W. and Deutsch, H.F. (1969) J. Biol. Chem., 244, 4565-4572.
174. Bannister, W.H. and Wood, E.J. (1970) Life Sci., 9, 229-233.
175. Bannister, J.V., Bannister, W.H., and Wood, E.J. (1971) Eur. J. Biochem., 18, 178-186.
176. Bannister, W.H., Dalgleish, D.G., Bannister, J.V., and Wood, E.J. (1972) Int. J. Biochem., 3, 560-568.
177. Calabrese, L., Federici, G., Bannister, W.H., Bannister, J.V., Rotilio, G., and Finazzi-Agro, A. (1975) Eur. J. Biochem., 56, 305-309.
178. Briggs, R.G. and Fee, J.A. (1978) Biochim. Biophys. Acta, 400, 86-89 and 100-109.
179. Albergoni, V. and Cassini, A. (1974) Comp. Biochem. Physiol., 47B, 767-777.
180. Baldensperger, J.B. (1978) Arch. Microbiol., 119, 237-244.
181. Lumsden, J., Cammack, R. and Hall, D.O. (1976) Biochim. Biophys. Acta, 438, 380-392.
182. Marklund, S. (1973) Acta Chem. Scand., 27, 1458-1460.
183. Michelson, A.M., Puget, K., Durosay, A., and Rousselet, A. (1981) in Ref. 15, pp. 348-366.
184. Salin, M.L., Day, E.D., Crapo, J.D. (1978) Arch. Biochem. Biophys., 187, 223-228.
185. Marklund, S. (1978) Int. J. Biochem., 9, 299-306.
186. Malmstrom, B. and Vanngard, T. (1960) J. Mol. Biol., 2, 118-134.
187. Desideri, A., Morpurgo, L., Rotilio, G., and Mondovi, B. (1979) FEBS Letts., 98, 339-341.
188. Morpurgo, L., Calabrese, L., Desideri, A., and Rotilio, G. (1981) Biochem. J., 193, 639-643.
189. Malkin, R. and Malmstrom, B. (1970) Adv. Enzymol., 33, 177-244.

190. Barra, D., Martini, F., Bossa, F., Rotilio, G., Bannister, J.V., and Bannister, W.H. (1978) Biochem. Biophys. Res. Commun., 81, 1195-2000.
191. Wood, E., Dalgleish, D., and Bannister, W. (1971) Eur. J. Biochem., 18, 187-193.
192. Rotilio, G., Finazzi-Agro, A., Calabrese, L., Bossa, F., Guerrieri, P., and Mondovi, B. (1971) Biochemistry, 10, 616-621.
193. Weser, U., Bunnerberg, E., Cammack, R., Djerassi, C., Flohé, L., Thomas, G., and Voelter, W. (1971) Biochim. Biophys. Acta, 243, 203-213.
194. Fee, J.A. (1973) J. Biol. Chem., 248, 4229-4234.
195. Rotilio, G., Calabrese, L., Bossa, F., Barra, D., Finazzi-Agro, A., and Mondovi, B. (1972) Biochemistry, 11, 2182-2186.
196. Fawcett, T.G., Bernaducci, E.E., Krogh-Jesperson, K., and Shuyan, H.J. (1980) J. Amer. Chem. Soc., 102, 2598-2604.
197. Weser, U., Barth, G., Djerassi, C., Hartmann, H.-J., Krauss, P., Voelcker, G., Voelter, W., and Voetsch, W. (1972) Biochim. Biophys. Acta, 278, 28-44.
198. Jung, G., Otand, M., Bohnenkamp, W., and Weser, U. (1972) FEBS Letts., 25, 346-349.
199. Forman, H.J. and Fridovich, I. (1973) J. Biol. Chem., 248, 2645-2649.
200. Rigo, A., Viglino, P., Rotilio, G., and Tomata, R. (1975) FEBS Letts., 50, 86-88.
201. Fee, J.A. (1973) Biochim. Biophys. Acta., 295, 87-95.
202. Fee, J.A., Natter, R., and Baker, G.S.T. (1973) Biochim. Biophys. Acta, 295, 96-106.
203. Fee, J.A. (1973) Biochim. Biophys. Acta, 295, 107-116.
204. Calabrese, L., Rotilio, G., and Mondovi, B. (1972) Biochim. Biophys. Acta, 263, 827-829.
205. Fee, J.A. and Briggs, R.G. (1975) Biochim. Biophys. Acta, 400, 439-450.
206. Beem, K.M., Rich, W.E., and Rajagopolan, K.V. (1974) J. Biol. Chem., 249, 7298-7305.
207. Valentine, J.S., Pantoliano, M.W., McDonnell, P.J., Burger, A.R., and Lippard, S.J. (1979) Proc. Natl. Acad. Sci. USA, 76, 4245-4249.
208. Weser, U. and Hartmann, H.J. (1971) FEBS Letts., 17, 78-80.
209. Rotilio, G., Calabrese, L., and Coleman, J. (1973) J. Biol. Chem., 248, 3855-3859.
210. Rigo, A., Terenzi, M., Franconi, C., Mondovi, B., Calabrese, L., and Rotilio, G. (1974) FEBS Letts., 39, 154-156.
211. Rotilio, G., Calabrese, L., Mondovi, B., and Blumberg, B. (1974) J. Biol. Chem., 249, 3157-2160.
212. Fee, J.A. and Gaber, B.P. (1972) J. Biol. Chem., 247, 60-65.
213. Calabrese, L., Cocco, D., and Desideri, S. (1979) FEBS Letts., 106, 142-144.
214. Lippard, S.J., Burger, A.R., Ugurbil, K., Pantoliano, M.W., and Valentine, J.S. (1977) Biochemistry, 16, 1136-1141.
215. Cass, A.E.G., Hill, H.A.O., Bannister, J.V., and Bannister, W.H. (1979) Biochem. J., 177, 477-486.
216. Calabrese, L., Cocco, D., Desideri, A., and Rotilio, G. (1979) in Metallo-proteins, Weser, U., ed., Stuttgart: G. Thieme Verlag, pp. 36-42.
217. Desideri, S., Calabrese, L., Cocco, D. and Rotilio, G. (1980) Abs. IX Int. Conf. Mag. Res. Biol., France, p. 17.
218. Calabrese, L., Cocco, D., Morpurgo, L., Mondovi, B., and Rotilio, G. (1976) Eur. J. Biochem., 64, 465-470.
219. Rotilio, G., Morpurgo, L., Giovangnoli, C., Calabrese, L., and Mondovi, B. (1972) Biochemistry, 11, 2187-2192.
220. Gaber, B.P., Brown, R.D., Koenig, S.H., and Fee, J.A. (1972) Biochim. Biophys. Acta, 271, 1-5.
221. Moss, T.H. and Fee, J.A. (1975) Biochem. Biophys. Res. Commun., 66, 799-808.
222. Desideri, A., Cerdonio, M., Mogno, F., Vitale, S., Calabrese, L., Cocco, D., and Rotilio, G. (1978) FEBS Letts., 89, 83-85.
223. O'Young, C.C., Dewen, J.C., Lilienthal, H.R., and Lippard, S. (1978) J. Amer. Chem. Soc., 100, 7291-7300.
224. Calabrese, L., Cocco, D., Morpurgo, L., Mondovi, B., and Rotilio, G. (1975) FEBS Letts., 59, 29-31.

225. Pantoliano, M.W., McDonald, P.J., and Valentine, J.S. (1979) J. Amer. Chem. Soc., 101, 6454-6456.
226. Hirose, J., Iwatzuka, K., and Kidani, Y. (1981) Biochem. Biophys. Res. Commun., 98, 58-65.
227. Morpurgo, L., Mavelli, I., Calabrese, L., Finazzi-Agro, A., and Rotilio, G. (1976) Biochem. Biophys. Res. Commun., 70, 607-614.
228. Rotilio, G., Morpurgo, L., Calabrese, L., Finazzi-Agro, A., and Mondovi, B. (1977) in Metal-Ligand Interactions in Organic Chemistry and Biochemistry, p. 243-253.
229. Fee, J.A. and DiCorletto, P.E. (1973) Biochemistry, 13, 4893-4899.
230. Rotilio, G., Morpurgo, L., Calabrese, L., and Mondovi, B. (1973) Biochim. Biophys. Acta, 302, 229-235.
231. Klug-Roth, D., Fridovich, I., and Rabani, J. (1973) J. Amer. Chem. Soc., 95, 2786-2790.
232. Fielden, E.M., Roberts, P.B., Bray, R.C., Loewe, D.J., Mautner, G.H., Rotilio, G., and Calabrese, L. (1974) Biochem. J., 139, 49-60.
233. Cockle, S. and Bray, R.C. (1977) in Ref. 13, pp. 215-216.
234. Rotilio, G., Rigo, A., Viglino, P., and Calabrese, L. (1977) in Ref. 13, pp. 207-214.
235. Viglino, P., Rigo, A., Argese, E., Calabrese, L., Cocco, D., and Rotilio, G. (1981) Biochem. Biophys. Res. Commun., 100, 125-130.
236. Bray, R.C., Cockle, S.A., Fielden, E.M., Roberts, P.B., Rotilio, G., and Calabrese, L. (1974) Biochem. J., 139, 43-48.
237. Hodgson, E. and Fridovich, I. (1975) Biochemistry, 14, 5294-5298.
238. Hodgson, E. and Fridovich, I. (1975) Biochemistry, 14, 5299-5303.
239. Rigo, A. and Rotilio, G. (1981) in Ref. 14, pp. 56-64.
240. McAdam, M.E., Fielden, E.M., Lavelle, F., Calabrese, L., Cocco, D., and Rotilio, G. (1977) Biochem. J., 167, 271-274.
241. Armitage, I.M., Schoot-Uiterkamp, A.J.M., Chlebowski, J.F., and Coleman, J.E. (1978) J. Mag. Res., 29, 375-392.
242. Bailey, D.B., Ellis, P.D., and Fee, J.A. (1980) Biochemistry, 19, 591-596.
243. Bauer, R., Demeter, I., Haseman, V., and Johansen, J.T. (1980) Biochem. Biophys. Res. Commun., 94, 1296-1302.
244. Blumberg, W.E., Peisach, J., Eisenberger, P., and Fee, J.A. (1976) Biochemistry, 17, 1842-1846.
245. Desideri, A., Comin, F., Morpurgo, L., Cocco, D., Calabrese, L., Mondovi, B., Maret, W., and Rotilio, G. (1981) Biochim. Biophys. Acta, 661, 312-315.
246. Rigo, A., Stevanto, R., Viglino, P., and Rotilio, G. (1977) Biochem. Biophys. Res. Commun., 79, 776-783.
247. Terenzi, M., Rigo, A., Franconi, C., Mondovi, B., Calabrese, L., and Rotilio, G. (1974) Biochim. Biophys. Acta, 351, 230-236.
248. Boden, N., Homes, M.C., and Knowles, P.F. (1979) Biochem. J., 177, 303-309.
249. Bertini, I., Luchinat, C., Scozzafava, A. (1980) J. Amer. Che. Soc., 102, 7349-7353.
250. Rigo, A., Viglino, P., and Rotilio, G. (1975) Biochem. Biophys. Res. Commun., 63, 1013-1018.
251. Fee, J.A. and Ward, R.L. (1976) Biochem. Biophys. Res. Commun., 71, 427-437.
252. Cass, A.E.G. and Hill, H.A.O. (1981) in Ref. 14, pp. 290-298.
253. Rotilio, G., Rigo, A., and Calabrese, L. (1978) in Frontiers in Physico-chemical Biology, Pullman, B., ed.
254. Malinowski, D. and Fridovich, I. (1979) Biochemistry, 18, 5909-5917.
255. Koppenol, W.H. (1981) Bull. Europ. Physiopath. Resp., 17 (suppl), 85-89.
256. Roberts, P.B., Fielden, E.M., Rotilio, G., Calabrese, L., Bannister, J.V., and Bannister, W.H. (1974) Rad. Res., 60, 441-452.
257. Villafranca, J.J., Yost, F.J., and Fridovich, I. (1974) J. Biol. Chem., 249, 3532-3536.
258. McAdam, M.E., Fox, R.A., Lavelle, F., and Fielden, E.M. (1977) Biochem. J., 165, 71-79.
259. Fee, J.A., Shapiro, E.R., and Moss, T.H. (1976) J. Biol. Chem., 251, 6157-6159.

260. McAdam, M.E., Fox, R.A., Lavelle, F., and Fielden, E.M. (1977) Biochem. J., 165, 81-87.
261. Lavelle, F., McAdam, M.E., Fielden, E.M., Roberts, P.B., Puget, K., and Michelson, A.M. (1977) Biochem. J., 161, 3-11.
262. Slykhouse, T.O. and Fee, J.A. (1976) J. Biol. Chem., 251, 5472-5477.
263. Brock, C.J., Harris, J.I., and Sato, S. (1976) J. Mol. Biol., 107, 175-178.
264. Ose, D. and Fridovich, I. (1979) Arch. Biochem. Biophys., 194, 360-364.
265. Yamakura, F. (1978) J. Biochem., 83, 849-857.
266. Steinman, H.M., Naik, V.R., Abernethy, J.L., and Hill, R.L. (1974) J. Biol. Chem., 249, 7376-7338.
267. Hartz, J.W. and Deutsch, H.F. (1972) J. Biol. Chem., 247, 7043-7050.
268. Barra, D., Martini, F., Bannister, J.V., Schinan, M.E., Rotilio, G., Bannister, W.H., and Bossa, F. (1980) FEBS Letts., 120, 53-56.
269. Jabusch, J.R., Farb, D.L., Kerschesteinen, D.A., and Deutsch, H.F. (1980) Biochemistry, 19, 2310-2316.
270. Bannister, J.V., Anastasi, A., and Bannister, W.H. (1978) Biochem. Biophys. Res. Commun., 81, 469-472.
271. Marmocchi, F., Venardi, G., Bossa, F., Rigo, A., and Rotilio, G. (1978) FEBS Letts., 94, 109-111.
272. Malinowski, D.P. and Fridovich, I. (1979) Biochemistry, 18, 237-244.
273. Rigo, A., Marmocchi, F., Cocco, D., Viglino, P., and Rotilio, G. (1978) Biochemistry, 17, 534-537.
274. Marmocchi, F., Mavelli, I., Rigo, A., Stevenato, R., Boss, F., and Rotilio, G. (1982) Biochemistry, 21, 2853-2858.
275. Lerch, K. and Ammer, D. (1981) J. Biol. Chem., 256, 11545-11551.
276. Johansen, J.T., Overballe-Petersen, C., Martin, B., Haseman, V., and Svensen, F. (1979) Carlsberg Res. Commun., 44, 201-207.
277. Steinman, H.M. (1980) J. Biol. Chem., 255, 6758-6765.
278. Steinman, H.M. (1978) J. Biol. Chem., 253, 8707-8720.
279. Brock, C.J. and Walker, J.E. (1980) Biochemistry, 19, 2873-2882.
280. Ditlow, C., Johansen, J.T., Martin, B.M., and Ivendsen, I.B. (1982) Carlsberg Res. Commun., 47, 81-91.
281. Harris, J.I., Auffret, A.D., Northrop, F.D., and Walker, J.E. (1980) Eur. J. Biochem., 106, 297-303.
282. Richardson, D.C., Bier, C.J., and Richardson, J.S. (1972) J. Biol. Chem., 247, 6368-6369.
283. Thomas, K.A., Rubin, B.H., Bier, C.J., Richardson, J.S., and Richardson, D.C. (1974) J. Biol. Chem., 249, 5677-5683.
284. Richardson, J.S., Thomas, K.A., and Richardson, D.C. (1975) Biochem. Biophys. Res. Commun., 63, 986-992.
285. Richardson, J.S., Thomas, K.A., Rubin, B.H., and Richardson, D.C. (1975) Proc. Natl. Acad. Sci. USA, 72, 1349-1353.
286. Richardson, J.S., Richardson, D.C., Thomas, K.A., Silverton, E.W., and Davis, D.R. (1976) J. Mol. Biol., 102, 221-235.
287. McLachlan, A.D. (1980) Nature, 285, 267-268.
288. Smit, J.D.G., Pulver-Sladek, J., and Jansonius, J.N. (1977) J. Mol. Biol., 112, 491-494.
289. Stallings, W.C., Partridge, K.A., Powers, T.B., Fee, J.A., and Ludwig, M.L. (1981) J. Biol. Chem., 256, 5857-5859.
290. Yamakura, F., Suzuki, K., and Mitsui, Y. (1976) J. Biol. Chem., 251, 4792-4793.
291. Powers, T.B. Slykhouse, T.O., Fee, J.A., and Ludwig, M.L. (1978) J. Mol. Biol., 123, 689-690.

CHAPTER 9 SUPEROXIDE AND OXIDATIVE KILLING BY PHAGOCYTES

BERNARD M. BABIOR
Blood Research Laboratory and Department of Medicine,
Tufts-New England Medical Center, Boston, MA 02111, USA

The killing of pathogens by phagocytes is a critical element of host defense. The ability of these cells to destroy invading bacteria, fungi, and parasites is indispensible for life, and when this function fails the organism rapidly succumbs to overwhelming infection. In part because of their physiological importance but also because of their availability, phagocytes have been the object of intensive study, the level of which has been increasing rapidly over the past few years.

A major objective of the investigations of phagocyte function has been to understand the mechanisms by which these cells kill their targets. These investigations have revealed that these mechanisms can be divided into two classes: those which require oxygen, and those which do not. With regard to the oxygen-dependent microbcidial mechanisms of phagocytes, it is now clear that superoxide is the key. This article will discuss how superoxide is produced by phagocytes, and how it is used to kill invading pathogens.

Neutrophils

The phagocytes responsible for the destruction of pathogens can be subdivided in three cell types: neutrophils, eosinophils, and mononuclear phagocytes (monocytes a macrophages). These three types differ in their morphology and their physiological role, but all are capable of generating O_2^- in large quantities in response to appropriate stimuli.

The cell first shown to manufacture O_2^- was the human neutrophil (Ref. 1). This is an end cell, incapable of dividing, which is produced in the bone marrow, then released into the blood stream from which it rapidly migrates into the tissue (Ref. It appears to be the first line of defense against bacteria which have established themselves in tissue (as opposed to bacteria circulating in the blood stream, which appear to be cleared primarily by the mononuclear phagocyte system).

The neutrophil is shown in Fig. 1. Its main structural features are its vestiga nucleus, which is segmented generally into 3 or 4 lobes, and its granules. The cel contains two types of granules: the azurophil (primary) granules, containing hydrolytic enzymes (Refs. 3,4) and myeloperoxidase (Ref. 4), and the specific (secondary granules, containing the iron-binding protein apolactoferrin (Ref. 5), a cobalamin-binding protein (Ref. 6), lysozyme (Ref. 4) and a collagenase (Ref. 7). As will be seen below, myeloperoxidase is an essential component of one of the oxygen-dependen microbicidal systems of this cell.

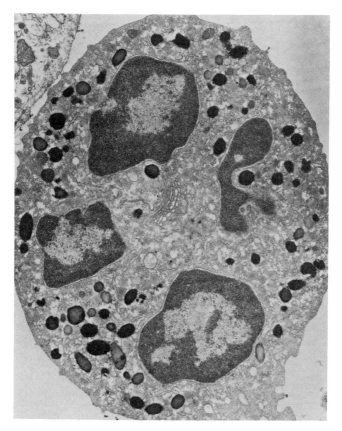

Fig. 1. The neutrophil. (Figure by courtesy of D. F. Bainton.)

The neutrophil finds its target by chemotaxis (Ref. 8), attracted by substances released by the interaction of tissue fluids with the microorganism at the site of infection. Interaction with tissue fluids also results in the opsonization of the microorganism (Ref. 9), a term which refers to the deposition on the invading organism of certain plasma-derived proteins which serve to mark the organism as a target for ingestion by phagocytes. Having encountered an opsonized organism, the neutrophil ingests it by phagocytosis, a process in which the organism together with a small amount of extracellular fluid is incorporated into the neutrophil within a vesicle (the phagocytic vesicle) which is lined with what was originally a portion of the plasma membrane (Fig. 2). Granules then fuse with the internalized plasma membrane,

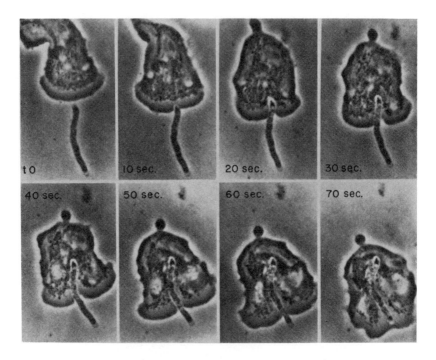

Fig. 2. Phagocytosis. (Reproduced from Hirsch, J.G. (1962) J. Exp. Med., 116, 827-834.)

their contents into the phagocytic vesicle (Fig. 3) (Ref. 10). At the same time, an oxidase in the plasma membrane is activated, initiating the series of metabolic events known as the "respiratory burst" on which all oxygen-dependent killing depends (Ref. 11).

The respiratory burst

The term "respiratory burst" refers to the simultaneous increases in oxygen uptake O_2^- and H_2O_2 production, and oxidation of glucose *via* the hexosemonophosphate shunt which are observed when neutrophils and other phagocytes are exposed to appropriate stimuli. These changes in oxygen metabolism are not inhibited by CN^- or other heme enzyme inhibitors, a property which distinguishes them from metabolic changes due to alterations in mitochondrial activity (Ref. 11). The respiratory burst begins 30-60 seconds after the exciting stimulus (Ref. 12) and lasts 20-30 minutes (Fig. 4). It antedated by changes in the transmembrane potential whose connection with the onset of the burst remain to be elucidated (Ref. 13). Activation of the respiratory burst requires neither phagocytosis nor degranulation (Ref. 14), is reversible under some circumstances (Ref. 14), and can be accomplished by a remarkably wide variety of stimulating agents (Table 1). The mechanism responsible for the activation of the

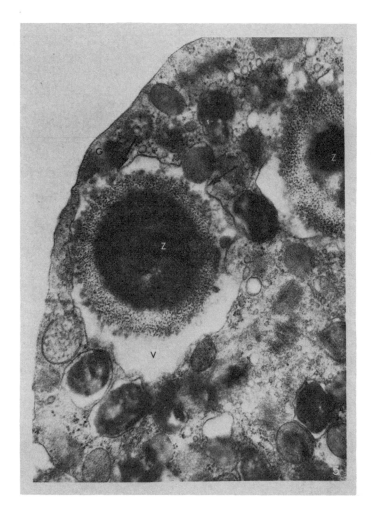

Fig. 3. Degranulation. (Reproduced from Ref. 10).

burst in unknown, except that it appears to be an energy-requiring process.

TABLE 1

Examples of agents capable of activating the respiratory burst in neutrophils

Particulate.	Soluble
Latex beads	F-met-leu-phe
Opsonized bacteria	Phorbol myristate acetate
Opsonized zymosan	A23187 (a calcium ionophore)
	Concanavalin A
	Digitonin
	Fluoride ion

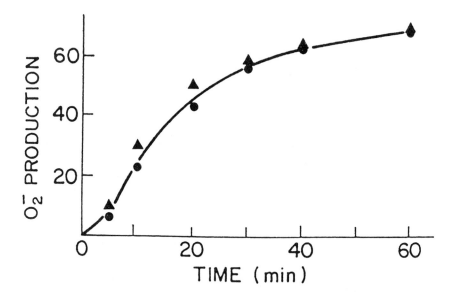

Fig. 4. Time course of O_2^- production by neutrophils. (Adapted from Curnutte, J.T. and Babior, B.M. (1974) J. Clin. Invest., 53, 1662-1672.

It is universally agreed that the biochemical basis for the respiratory burst is the activation of an enzyme, dormant in resting cells, which catalyzes the one-electron reduction of oxygen to O_2^- at the expense of a reduced pyridine nucleotide (Ref. 15):

$$2 O_2 + NAD(P)H \longrightarrow 2 O_2^- + NAD(P)^+$$

Most, but not all, of this O_2^- reacts with itself either spontaneously or under catalysis by superoxide dismutase to generate hydrogen peroxide (Ref. 16):

$$2 O_2^- + 2 H^+ \longrightarrow H_2O_2 + O_2$$

All the hydrogen peroxide produced during the respiratory burst has been shown to arise by the dismutation of O_2^-. During the course of the respiratory burst, $NADP^+$ is generated as a result of the reduction of a portion of the H_2O_2 by the gluta-thione-dependent peroxide detoxifying system (Ref. 17):

$$2 \text{ GSH} + H_2O_2 \xrightarrow{\text{glutathione peroxidase}} \text{GSSG} + 2 \text{ H}_2O$$

$$\text{GSSG} + \text{NADPH} \xrightarrow{\text{glutathione reductase}} 2 \text{ GSH} + NADP^+$$

Most workers hold that $NADP^+$ is also generated through the action of the O_2^- forming oxidase, which is widely believed to use NADPH as the physiological substrate; this view, however, is not unanimous, as will be discussed. The $NADP^+$ is reconverted to NADPH through the first two reactions of the hexosemonophosphate shunt (Refs. 7,18):

$$\text{Glucose-6-phosphate} + NADP^+ \longrightarrow \text{6-Phosphogluconate} + \text{NADPH}$$

$$\text{6-Phosphogluconate} + NADP^+ \longrightarrow \text{Ribulose-5-phosphate} + \text{NADPH} + CO_2$$

Oxygen uptake and O_2^- production thus result from the activity of the primary oxidase, H_2O_2 is produced as a consequence of the dismutation of O_2^-, and glucose is oxidized *via* the hexosemonophosphate shunt in order to re-reduce the $NADP^+$ generated during the course of the respiratory burst.

The primary oxidase

The first report of an enzyme from neutrophils capable of catalyzing the uptake of oxygen at the expense of a reduced pyridine nucleotide was published by Iyer and Quastel (Ref. 19), who proposed this enzyme as a candidate primary oxidase. Since that report a great deal of study has been devoted to the question of the identity of the primary oxidase, with conflicting findings from various laboratories generating confusion and controversy. At the present time a consensus seems to be forming as to the identity of the oxidase, but the controversy is not yet fully settled. In dis-cussing this question I will first describe the enzyme most widely considered to be the primary oxidase. I will then discuss in briefer terms other candidate oxidases.

Prior to a discussion of the oxidases themselves, it is useful to consider the criteria by which a choice can be made as to which enzyme is the "real" oxidase. A thoughtful discussion of these criteria has been presented by Karnovsky and his associates (Ref. 20). In my view, the two most important of these, representing the *sine qua non* for the primary oxidase, are as follows:

1. Activity is present in cell-free preparations from stimulated but not resting neutrophils;

2. There is no activity in cell-free preparations from stimulated neutrophils

obtained from patients with chronic granulomatous disease (CGD), an inherited condition in which neutrophils are unable to express a respiratory burst.

The only candidate oxidase described to date that fulfills these criteria is the particulate NADPH oxidase first described by Rossi and his co-workers (Ref. 21), and it is for this reason that this enzyme is now regarded by most investigators as the primary oxidase. For awhile it was thought that this oxidase required manganese. Recently, though, it was discovered that his apparent metal requirement was an artifact which introduced complications into early studies (Ref. 22). Work done subsequent to this discovery has shown that the particulate NADPH oxidase is a membrane-bound flavoprotein which catalyzes the one-electron reduction of oxygen to O_2^- at the expense of a reduced pyridine nucleotide according to the following stoichiometry (Refs. 23-25):

$$2 \ O_2 \ + \ NAD(P)H \ \longrightarrow \ 2 \ O_2^- \ + \ NAD(P)^+$$

The enzyme is insensitive to N_3^- (Ref. 24). Either pyridine nucleotide can serve as substrate, but kinetic data indicate that the enzyme prefers NADPH (K_m 33 μM) over NADH (K_m 930 μM). Little oxidase activity can be obtained from normal resting neutrophils or (with the human enzyme) from stimulated CGD cells. The enzyme from human neutrophils has been solubilized by detergents, but has not yet been purified (Ref. 26).

A number of alternative enzymes and activities have been proposed as the primary oxidase. These include the following:

1. Myeloperoxidase. Myeloperoxidase is able to catalyze the oxidation of reduced pyridine nucleotides, particularly at low pH and most particularly in the presence of Mn^{++} (Ref. 27). This catalytic property, a manifestation of the well-known peroxidase -oxidase activity displayed by a large number of heme peroxidases, has been a source of confusion in studies on the respiratory burst of neutrophils, and has led to proposals that myeloperoxidase is the primary oxidase. The normal respiratory burst seen in cells from patients with inherited myeloperoxidase deficiency and the presence of myeloperoxidase in CGD cells rule this possibility out for all practical purposes (Refs. 28,29). Parenthetically, it should be noted that the activity of the particulate NADPH oxidase is normal in neutrophils from myeloperoxidase-deficient patients

2. D-amino oxidase. The fact that D-amino acids are constituents of bacterial cell walls led to the proposal that D-amino acid oxidase might be the primary oxidase, its action on D-amino acids released from the surface of an ingested microorganism leading to oxygen uptake and H_2O_2 production. The presence of normal D-amino acid oxidase levels in CGD neutrophils suggests that this enzyme is unlikely to be the primary oxidase (Ref. 30).

3. NADH oxidase. A soluble flavoprotein oxidase showing absolute specificity for

NADH was described in homogenates of human and guinea pig neutrophils (Refs. 31,32). The guinea pig enzyme has been purified to homogeneity and characterized rather extensively. From the finding that levels of this oxidase are diminished to 30% of normal in CGD cells, this enzyme was proposed as the primary oxidase. The contrast between the rather modest reduction in the activity of this enzyme and the total absence of the respiratory burst in CGD cells suggests that this enzyme is not as attractive a candidate for primary oxidase as the particulate NADPH oxidase, an enzyme which cannot be detected in preparations from CGD cells. In addition, other laboratories have found normal levels of soluble NADH oxidase in CGD cells (Refs. 33,34), a finding which remains to be reconciled with the reduced levels initially reported.

4. Cytochrome b. A heme protein with the spectral properties of a b-type cytochrome has been shown by several groups to be present in neutrophil membranes (Refs. 35,36). This cytochrome appears to be absent from some, but not all, cases of chronic granulomatous disease (Refs. 36,37). The proposal that this cytochrome represents the primary oxidase is unlikely in view of the fact that CN^-, an inhibitor of every terminal heme oxidase described to date, does not inhibit the respiratory burst. On the other hand, its absence from patients with CGD suggests that it is closely connected with the respiratory burst, perhaps as a component of the oxidase activating system.

On the basis of the foregoing, it seems likely that the particulate NADPH oxidase is the enzyme responsible for the respiratory burst, and that the alternative candidates are not. Conclusive evidence as to this point, however, must await the purification and characterization of the particulate oxidase. Studies of the purified enzyme could reveal hitherto unsuspected roles for some of the alternative enzymes in the production of reactive oxidants by neutrophils.

Oxygen-dependent killing mechanisms

The products of the respiratory burst are used as microbicidal agents. To date, two microbicidal systems are known which employ these products. One system depends on myeloperoxidase; the other does not.

Myeloperoxidase. Myeloperoxidase is a heme enzyme that catalyzes a number of H_2O_2-mediated oxidations, the most important of which is probably the oxidation of chloride to hypochlorite (Ref. 38):

$$Cl^- + H_2O_2 \longrightarrow OCl^- + H_2O$$

In the human neutrophil, it is a green protein of MW 150,000 which is present in high concentrations in the azurophil granules (Ref. 39).

A role for myeloperoxidase in bacterial killing by neutrophils was first proposed by Klebanoff, who showed that the combination of myeloperoxidase, H_2O_2 and a halide ion constituted a remarkably effective microbicidal system (Ref. 40). This system operates in vivo as well as in vitro, as indicated by the finding that neutrophils from patients with inherited myeloperoxidase deficiency show a pronounced delay in the killing of S. *aureus* as compared with normal neutrophils (Ref. 41). The peroxidase-halide-myeloperoxidase system is thus an important component of the microbicidal capacity of the neutrophils.

Of the halides which could be used by this system (F^- was not active), Cl^- was t least effective, in that the concentration of Cl^- required for microbicidal activit was greater than that for any of the other halides (Br^-, I^- and the pseudohalide SC Nevertheless, Cl^- is probably the halide employed by this system under physiologica conditions. This is supported by the fact that the concentration of Cl^- within the neutrophil is adequate to support bacterial killing by the isolated system (Ref. 42 as well as by studies showing that neutrophils undergoing the respiratory burst car out the myeloperoxidase-dependent oxidation of ambient Cl^- with the production of C and the incorporation of chlorine into trichloroacetic acid-precipitable material (Ref. 38,43). The probable site of OCl^- production is the phagocytic vesicle, sinc myeloperoxidase and H_2O_2 are delivered into the vesicle in phagocytosing neutrophil and Cl^-, as mentioned above, is abundant both inside and outside the cell.

Present evidence suggests that the proximate microbicidal agent generated by the peroxide-halide-myeloperoxidase system is OCl^- itself. This compound is known to b a potent antiseptic, and is used commercially for the purification of water. It ox dizes amines to chloroamines, and reacts with peptides to produce N-terminal chloro amines which subsequently cleave, leading to degradation of the halogenated polypep tide (Ref. 44). Sulfhydryl groups are also oxidized by OCl^- as well as by N-chloro amines, and there is some evidence to suggest that sulfhydryl oxidation may be related to bacterial killing, because when microorganisms are exposed to a source c OCl^-, death and sulfhydryl oxidation occur *pari passu* (Ref. 45). The biochemical basis for killing, however, has not been established for this or any other lethal mechanism of phagocytes.

The other candidate microbicidal agent which has been proposed in the context of the peroxide-halide-myeloperoxidase system is singlet oxygen. There are several reactions by which singlet oxygen might be produced in stimulated neutrophils. One is the reaction of hypochlorite with H_2O_2, well-documented to produce singlet oxyge (Ref. 46):

$$H_2O_2 + OCl^- \longrightarrow {}^1O_2 + H_2O + Cl^-$$

Another is the spontaneous dismutation of O_2^-, during which singlet oxygen has been said to arise (Ref. 47):

$$2O_2^- + 2H^+ \longrightarrow {}^1O_2 + H_2O_2$$

Finally, evidence has been presented that singlet oxygen is produced when O_2^- reacts with H_2O_2 (Ref. 48):

$$2O_2^- + 2H^+ \longrightarrow {}^1O_2 + OH^{\bullet} + OH^-$$

Its production is therefore feasible *a priori* on chemical grounds. Whether it is actually formed by neutrophils, however, has been a controversial topic for a number of years.

The first piece of evidence cited in support of singlet oxygen production by neutrophils was the finding that during phagocytosis, these cells emit light by a process that is dependent on the respiratory burst (Ref. 49). Singlet oxygen was proposed as the source of this light because its production in this system is chemically feasible, as discussed above, and because it is known to participate in light-emitting chemical reactions. Experiments with singlet oxygen scavengers and traps provided further support for this idea (Ref. 50), as did experiments showing that bacteria deficient in singlet oxygen-scavenging carotenoids were unusually susceptible to killing by neutrophils (Ref. 51). These studies were all consistent with the idea that singlet oxygen is produced by neutrophils, but they did not represent conclusive proof.

Meanwhile, evidence against singlet oxygen production began to appear. The spectrum of the light emitted by phagocytosing neutrophils was shown to be different from that produced by the relaxation of singlet oxygen to triplet (ground-state) oxygen (Ref. 52). This plus other characteristics of the emitted light suggested that it arose concomitant with the oxidation of unspecified compounds by the oxidizing agents generated by stimulated neutrophils. Most of the traps and scavengers were found not to be specific for singlet oxygen, reacting (interestingly) with HOCl to yield the same products obtained with $^1O_2$ (Ref. 53). Studies with carotenoid-deficient organisms are ambiguous insofar as the scavenging ability of carotenoids has not been shown to be confined to singlet oxygen. Finally, studies with the only specific $^1O_2$ trap so far employed--namely, cholesterol, which reacts with $^1O_2$ to yield the 5α-hydroperoxide--revealed little if any $^1O_2$ production by phagocytosing neutrophils.

It appears from the data available at present that $^1O_2$ is not a major product of the respiratory burst of neutrophils. It is likely that all the results provisionally interpreted to support its formation can be explained in terms of HOCl or other securely established products of the respiratory burst.

Oxidizing radicals. As discussed above, there are microbicidal mechanisms which require the products of the respiratory burst but do not use myeloperoxidase. These mechanisms appear to employ reactive oxidizing radicals as the microbicidal agents.

The production of reactive oxidizing radicals by phagocytes was first postulated on the basis that both O_2^- and H_2O_2 are produced during the respiratory burst, and that these can react in the presence of Fe^{++} to form $OH^{\cdot}$ (Ref. 54). Neither O_2^- not H_2O_2 is especially potent as a microbicidal agent, yet myeloperoxidase-deficient neutrophils express an efficient respiratory burst-dependent microbicidal capacity that must be explained in terms of a killing agent generated in a myeloperoxidase-independent reaction from O_2^-, H_2O_2, or both. The highly reactive $OH^{\cdot}$ radical provides such an explanation, at least in principle.

Evidence that such reactive oxidizing radicals are produced by neutrophils was first obtained through the study of the oxidation of methional by activated cells (Ref. 55). Methional reacts with $OH^{\cdot}$ and oxidizing radicals of similar reactivity, but not with O_2^- or H_2O_2, to yield ethylene according to the following reaction:

$$CH_3-S-CH_2-CH_2-CHO + OH^{\cdot} \longrightarrow 1/2(CH_3-S)_2 + HCOOH + CH_2=CH_2$$

Neutrophils were found to release ethylene from methional, but only when they were undergoing the respiratory burst. No ethylene was produced by resting neutrophils or by "activated" neutrophils from patients with chronic granulomatous disease. Similar observations were made with monocytes (see below) (Ref. 56). Ethylene is also released from 2-keto-4-methylthiobutyric acid by neutrophils and monocytes undergoing the respiratory burst (Ref. 57), while stimulated neutrophils are able to generate methane from dimethylsulfoxide (Ref. 58). Both these reactions represent oxidations mediated by $OH^{\cdot}$ or radicals with similar properties. These results indicate that during the respiratory burst, phagocytes are able to manufacture highly reactive oxidizing radicals.

It has been consistently demonstrated that O_2^- is essential for the production of these oxidizing radicals by phagocytes. H_2O_2, however, seems to be involved in the production of only a portion of these radicals, since oxidizing radical production is inhibited only partially by catalase (Ref. 56). This raises the question as to how much of the total oxidizing radical output is represented by $OH^{\cdot}$ which has been generated by the reaction between O_2^- and H_2O_2, as well as questions concerning the identities of radical species produced by H_2O_2-independent processes. Spin trapping experiments have shown that at least part of the output of oxidizing radicals is in the form of $OH^{\cdot}$ (Refs. 59,60), but quantitation has not been possible as yet, nor has it been possible to identify other radical species--for example, alkoxy radicals, alkyl radicals or acyl radicals--that might in principle be expected to be generated in this system.

Regardless of the radicals' identity, there is good evidence that they participate in killing by neutrophils. A superoxide-generating system consisting of acetaldehyde and xanthine oxidase is able to kill bacteria by means of an agent which is neutralized by oxidizing radical scavengers and whose production is blocked by either superoxide dismutase or catalase (Ref. 61). From these observations, this agent is probably $OH^{\cdot}$, produced by the reaction between O_2^- and H_2O_2. It is of interest that bacterial killing by this system followed a time course similar to that seen with myeloperoxidase-deficient neutrophils, and that the addition of myeloperoxidase both increased the potency of the system and altered the time course of bacterial killing to one very similar to that of normal neutrophils. The killing of bacteria by neutrophils themselves can also be prevented by either superoxide dismutase or catalase,

provided the enzyme is introduced directly into the microorganism-containing phagocytic vesicle, accomplished in these experiments by means of enzyme-coated latex
particles which were taken up into the same phagocytic vesicle as the microorganism
(Ref. 62). These results, like the results obtained with the acetaldehyde-xanthine
oxidase system, implicate OH* in the microbicidal activity of neutrophils. Finally,
activated neutrophils can also kill nearby endothelial and other cells by a process
mediated at least in part by OH* (Ref. 63).

Thus, neutrophils produce powerful oxidizing radicals during the respiratory burst
and use these radicals for the destruction of microorganisms and (probably inadvert-
ently) nearby cells. What radicals (other than OH*) are produced by these cells
remains to be determined, as does the biochemical basis for the radicals' microbicidal activity.

Eosinophils

Like neutrophils, eosinophils express a respiratory burst when appropriately stimulated (Ref. 64). The burst appears to result from the activation of an enzyme similar
if not identical, to the neutrophil oxidase (Ref. 65). As with neutrophils, the
respiratory burst in eosinophils is manifested by the production of O_2^- and H_2O_2 and
an increase in the oxidation of glucose via the hexosemonophosphate shunt. Initial
rates of oxygen uptake and O_2^- production are similar in the two types of cells. However, the burst in eosinophils lasts much longer than it does in neutrophils, possibly
because the mechanisms for terminating the respiratory burst are less efficient in the
former than the latter.

Recent work has indicated that eosinophils, like neutrophils, are involved in the
destruction of invading organisms, the eosinophils specializing in metazoan pathogens
such as the larval forms of trichinella (Refs. 66,67) and schistosomes (Refs. 68,69).
The fact that eosinophils express a respiratory burst which is even more vigorous than
that of neutrophils implies that the products of the burst are likely to participate
in the mechanisms by which these pathogens are killed. Data concerning this point,
however, are incomplete and to a certain extent conflicting. The killing of trichinella larvae by eosinophils has been demonstrated to involve the respiratory burst,
H_2O_2 being the parasiticidal agent in this case (Ref. 67). Killing of schistosomulae,
however, is said not to involve the respiratory burst, but rather to be mediated by
"major basic protein," the main constituent of the eosinophil granule (Ref. 70). Much
more work needs to be done to define the role of the respiratory burst in eosinophil-
mediated host defense mechanisms.

A further puzzle related to the role of the respiratory burst in eosinophil
function has to do with eosinophil peroxidase. Eosinophil granules contain large
amounts of a peroxidase which appears to be unique to this type of phagocytes; it is
clearly different from myeloperoxidase (Ref. 71), most significantly in its inability
to catalyze the oxidation of Cl^- by H_2O_2 (Ref. 72). What little evidence is available

202

suggests that the eosinophil peroxidase does not participate in the destruction
of pathogens (Ref. 72). Beyond this, nothing is known about its function.

Mononuclear phagocytes

Mononuclear phagocytes include the monocytes, which circulate in the blood, and the
tissue macrophages, which are present in all tissues but are particularly abundant in
the spleen, lymph nodes, liver (Kupffer cells) and lung (alveolar macrophages). The
tissue macrophages constitute a population of cells whose function is the removal of
particulate impurities (e.g., bacteria, foreign bodies, effete cells) from the blood
circulating through the organ. Their origin has been under dispute for many years,
but most now believe that they are derived from circulating monocytes which enter the
tissue from the blood and mature into full-fledged macrophages (Ref. 73).

Like the neutrophil, the circulating monocyte can kill bacteria with great
efficiency. Indeed, monocytes can replace neutrophils in vivo, as shown by the degree
of resistance to bacterial infections seen in patients with benign congenital neutro-
penia, an inherited condition in which virtually all the circulating phagocytes are
monocytes (normally, neutrophils represent over 80% of the circulating phagocytes)
(Ref. 74). Monocytes express a respiratory burst which is similar to that of neutrophils (Ref. 75), manufacturing O_2^- (Refs. 76-78) by an enzyme which has not as yet
been characterized but is likely to be the same as the neutrophil oxidase, and
liberating H_2O_2 and oxidizing radicals (Ref. 56). A comparison of the burst in
neutrophils and monocytes is given in Table 2. Monocytes also contain myeloperoxidase
which they presumably employ for the destruction of invading bacteria (Ref. 79). The
similarities between the oxygen-dependent microbicidal mechanisms of neutrophils and
monocytes are evident.

TABLE 2

A Comparison of the Respiratory Burst in Neutrophils and Monocytes[a]

	O_2^- production	
	Neutrophils (nmoles/min/10^6 cells)	Monocytes
Resting	0	0
Stimulated	1.3	0.8

[a]Adapted from Ref. 78.

Studies of O_2^- production by macrophages yielded variable results, and on the basis
of some of these it was thought for awhile that the respiratory burst may have little
to do with macrophage function. Further studies, however, disclosed that the variability was largely related to the source of the cells and particularly to their state

of activation at the time of testing (Ref. 76).

The term "activation" is used in a special sense when applied to macrophages (Refs. 80,81). It refers to a group of changes in macrophage properties which take place when the cells are stimulated by certain agents, usually immunological in nature. Activation can be induced by prior infection of the animals from which the macrophages are to be obtained with BCG or *Listeria monocytogenes*. In the case of peritoneal macrophages, cells which have been at least partially activated can be obtained by elicitation with intraperitoneally administered inflammatory substances such as endotoxin or casein. Some activation also takes place during monocyte culture. The mechanism of activation in vivo is thought to involve a cooperative interaction between T lymphocytes and resident macrophages whereby the lymphocytes, stimulated by the infection or the inflammatory substance, secrete soluble effectors (lymphokines) which stimulate the macrophage to undergo activation.

The alterations that take place during activation greatly augment the power of the macrophage as an effector cell. The size of the cell, its motility and its ability to spread on a surface all increase. There is a rise in the content of lysosomal enzymes, and an increase in the rate at which secreted proteins such as plasminogen activator and lysozyme are released into the medium. Rates of phagocytosis and pinocytosis increase. The cell acquires the ability to kill organisms which it was previously unable to handle. In Mackaness' term, the cell turns into an "angry macrophage."

Among the functions altered by activation is the ability of the macrophage to express a respiratory burst (Refs. 76,82,83). In studies of peritoneal macrophages, resident cells (i.e., macrophages obtained by rinsing the peritoneal cavity with saline) produced relatively little O_2^- when stimulated with phorbol myristate acetate, whereas activated cells generated large quantities of this radical under the same conditions (Fig. 5)(Ref. 76). Unstimulated macrophages produced little O_2^- regardless of their state of activation. It is of interest that when opsonized zymosan was used as stimulus, resident peritoneal macrophages produced nearly as much O_2^- as activated macrophages, in sharp contrast to the wide disparity in O_2^- production seen with phorbol myristate acetate (Ref. 76). It is clear that the nature of the stimulus is as important a factor in determining respiratory burst activity as is the state of activation of the cell.

Alveolar macrophages have also been examined from the point of view of the respiratory burst. These cells differ from peritoneal macrophages in that they consume large amounts of oxygen in the resting state, a property reflecting their unusual (for phagocytes) degree of reliance on mitochondrial metabolism for energy production (Ref. 84). A further difference is that, as isolated, alveolar macrophages appear to be activated, a finding that is not surprising in view of their location at the interface between the organism and the environment. Because of their high baseline oxygen uptake, the respiratory burst as expressed in terms of an increase in oxygen consump-

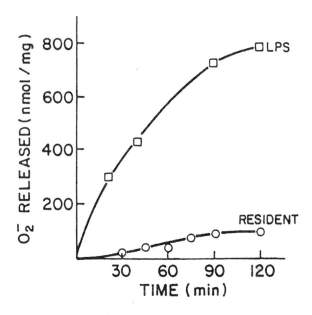

Fig. 5. Superoxide production by resident and lipopolysaccharide-activated macrophages in response to phorbol myristate acetate. (Adapted from Ref. 76.)

tion over baseline levels seems relatively modest. As measured by O_2^- production, however, it is substantial (Ref. 85). H_2O_2 production and hexosemonophosphate shun activation also takes place in stimulated alveolar macrophages (Ref. 86). The respiratory burst in these cells is therefore similar to that in other phagocytes.

One of the reasons why peritoneal and alveolar macrophages have been studied so extensively is that they are wandering cells which can be isolated easily in large numbers from their respective locations. Fixed tissue macrophages such as Kupffer cells are much less readily obtained, and consequently have been studied to a much smaller extent. Though it is likely that these cells, too, express a respiratory burst, conclusive studies regarding this point remain to be carried out.

In the macrophage, as in the monocyte and the neutrophil, the function of the respiratory burst is to supply oxidizing agents for use in microbicidal processes. There are however, differences between macrophages on one hand and monocytes and neutrophils on the other in the way in which these microbicidal oxidants are used. These differences relate largely to differences in the amounts of myeloperoxidase i the different types of cells. As macrophages undergo maturation, they appear to lo myeloperoxidase (as measured cytochemically), and fully mature macrophages appear t be devoid of this enzyme (Refs. 88,89). Oxygen-dependent microbicidal mechanisms are likely to operate in all cells expressing a respiratory burst, including fully activated macrophages. Cells with low to absent myeloperoxidase, however, will employ oxidizing radicals as the major or exclusive oxygen-derived microbicidal agents.

The presence of potent microbicidal systems in mononuclear phagocytes, their demonstrated capacity to kill bacteria in vitro and their ability to assume the functions of neutrophils in benign congenital neutrophenia all indicate an important role for these cells in host defense against bacteria. Over and above this important function, recent evidence has shown that mononuclear phagocytes play an important role in defense against protozoan parasites. Moreover, oxygen-dependent killing mechanisms are central to the antiprotozoal action of these phagocytes. Recent studies have disclosed that *Trypanosoma cruzi* are readily killed by activated peritoneal macrophages, though not by resident cells, and that the anti-trypanosomal activity of these cells is mediated by the H_2O_2 generated in the respiratory burst (Ref. 90). Macrophages also kill *Toxoplasma gondii* by oxygen-dependent mechanisms, but with this organism $OH^{\cdot}$ appears to be the anti-protozoal agent (Ref. 91). It seems reasonable to speculate that other protozoan pathogens will also be shown to be destroyed by the oxygen-requiring microbicidal mechanisms of mononuclear phagocytes.

ACKNOWLEDGMENT

1. Babior, B.M., Kipnes, R.S., and Curnutte, J.T. (1973) J. Clin. Invest., 52, 741-744.
2. Dancey, J.T., Deubelbeiss, K.A., Harker, L.A., and Finch, C.A. (1976) J. Clin. Invest., 58, 705-715.
3. Avila, J.L. and Convit, J. (1973) Biochim. Biophys. Acta, 293, 397-408.
4. Bretz, U. and Baggiolini, M. (1974) J. Cell. Biol., 63, 251-269.
5. Leffell, M.S. and Spitznagel, J.K. (1972) Infect. Immun., 6, 761-765.
6. Kane, S.P. and Peters, T.J. (1975) Clin. Sci. Mol. Med., 49, 171-182.
7. Murphy, G., Reynolds, J.J., Bretz, U., and Baggiolini, M. (1977) Biochem. J., 162, 195-197.
8. Keller, H.U., Hess, M.W., and Cottier, H. (1975) Semin. Hematol., 12, 47-57.
9. Stossel, T.P. (1975) Semin. Hematol., 12, 83-116.
10. Zucker-Franklin, D. and Hirsch, J.G. (1964) J. Exp. Med., 120, 569-576.
11. Sbarra, A.J. and Karnovsky, M.L. (1959) J. Biol. Chem., 234, 1355-1362.
12. Newburger, P.E., Chovaniec, M.E., and Cohen, H.J. (1980) Blood 55, 85-92.
13. Korchak, H.M. and Weissmann, G. (1978) Proc. Natl. Acad. Sci. USA, 75, 3818-3822.
14. Curnutte, J.T., Babior, B.M., and Karnovsky, M.L. (1979) J. Clin. Invest., 63, 785-792.
15. Babior, B.M. (1978) N. Engl. J. Med., 298, 659-668.
16. Root, R.K. and Metcalf, J.A. (1977) J. Clin. Invest., 60, 1266-1279.
17. Reed, P.W. (1969) J. Biol. Chem., 244, 2459-2464.
18. Iyer, G.Y.N., Islam, M.F., and Quastel, J.H. (1961) Nature, 192, 535-541.
19. Iyer, G.Y.N. and Quastel, J.H. (1963) Canad. J. Biochem., 41, 427-434.
20. Badwey, J.A., Curnutte, J.T., and Karnovsky, M.L. (1979) N. Engl. J. Med., 300, 1157-1160.

21. Patriarca, P., Cramer, R., Moncalvo, S., Rossi, F., and Romeo, D. (1971) Arch. Biochem. Biophys., 145, 255-262.
22. Curnutte, J.T., Karnovsky, M.L., and Babior, B.M. (1976) J. Clin. Invest., 57, 1059-1067.
23. Babior, B.M., Curnutte, J.T., and McMurrich, B.J. (1976) J. Clin. Invest., 58, 989-996.
24. Babior, B.M. and Kipnes, R.S. (1977) Blood, 50, 517-524.
25. Dewald, B., Baggiolini, M., Curnutte, J.T., and Babior, B.M. (1979) J. Clin. Invest., 63, 21-29.
26. Gabig, T.G. and Babior, B.M. (1979) J. Biol. Chem., 254, 9070-9074.
27. Roberts, J. and Quastel, J.H. (1964) Nature, 202, 85-86.
28. Rosen, H.S. and Klebanoff, S.J. (1976) J. Clin. Invest., 58, 50-60.
29. Baehner, R.L., Karnovsky, M.T., and Karnovsky, M.L. (1969) J. Clin. Invest., 48, 187-192.
30. Eckstein, M.R., Baehner, R.L., and Nathan, D.G. (1971) J. Clin. Invest., 50, 1985-1991.
31. Cagan, R.H. and Karnovsky, M.L. (1964) Nature, 204, 255-257.
32. Baehner, R.L. and Karnovsky, M.L. (1968) Science, 162, 1277-1279.
33. Holmes, B., Page, A.R., and Good, R.A. (1967) J. Clin. Invest., 46, 1422-1432.
34. Iverson, D., DeChatelet, L.R., Spitznagel, J.K., and Wang, P. (1977) J. Clin. Invest., 59, 282-290.
35. Shinagawa, Y., Tanaka, C., Teraoka, A., and Shinagawa, Y. (1966) J. Biochem., 59, 622-624.
36. Segal, A.W., Jones, O.T.G., Webster, D., and Allison, A.C. (1978) Lancet, 2, 446-449.
37. Borregaard, N., Johansen, K.S., Taudorff, E., and Wandall, J.H. (1979) Lancet, 1, 949-951.
38. Harrison, J.E. and Schultz, J. (1976) J. Biol. Chem., 251, 1371-1374.
39. Ehrenberg, A. and Anner, K. (1958) Acta Chem. Scand., 12, 95-100.
40. Klebanoff, S.J. (1968) J. Bacteriol., 95, 2131-2138.
41. Klebanoff, S.J. (1970) Science, 169, 1095-1097.
42. Klebanoff, S.J. and Hamon, C.F. (1972) J. Reticuloendothel. Soc., 12, 170-196.
43. Zgliczynski, J.M. and Stelmaszynska, T. (1975) Eur. J. Biochem., 56, 157-162.
44. Stelmaszynska, T. and Zgliczynski, J.M. (1978) Eur. J. Biochem., 92, 301-308.
45. Thomas, E.L. (1979) Infect. Immun., 23, 522-531.
46. Seliger, H.H. (1960) Anal. Biochem., 1, 60-65.
47. Khan, A.U. (1970) Science, 168, 476-477.
48. Kellogg, E.W., III and Fridovich, I. (1975) J. Biol. Chem., 250, 8812-8817.
49. Allen, R.C., Stjernholm, R.L., and Steele, R.H. (1972) Biochem. Biophys. Res. Commun., 47, 679-684.
50. Rosen, H. and Klebanoff, S.J. (1977) J. Biol. Chem., 252, 4803-4810.
51. Krinsky, N.I. (1974) Science 186, 363-365.
52. Cheson, B.D., Christensen, R.L., Sperling, R., Kohler, B.E., and Babior, B.M. (1976) J. Clin. Invest., 58, 789-796.
53. Held, A.M. and Hurst, J.K. (1978) Biochem. Biophys. Res. Commun., 81, 878-885.
54. McCord, J.M. and Day, E.D. (1978) FEBS Lett., 92, 321-326.
55. Tauber, A.I. and Babior, B.M. (1977) J. Clin. Invest., 60, 374-379.
56. Weiss, S.J., King, G.W., and LoBuglio, A.F. (1977) J. Clin. Invest., 60, 370-373.
57. Weiss, S.J., Rustagi, P.K., and LoBuglio, A.F. (1978) J. Exp. Med., 147, 316-323.
58. Repine, J.E., Eaton, J.W., Anders, M.W., Hoidal, J.R., and Fox, R.B. (1979) J. Clin. Invest., 64, 1642-1651.
59. Green, M.R., Hill, H.A.O., Okolow-Zubkowska, M.J., and Segal, A.W. (1979) FEBS Lett., 100, 23-26.
60. Rosen, H. and Klebanoff, S.J. (1979) J. Clin. Invest., 64, 1725-1729.
61. Rosen, H. and Klebanoff, S.J. (1979) J. Exp. Med., 149, 27-39.
62. Johnston, R.B., Keele, B.B., Misra, H.P., Lehmeyer, J.E., Webb, L.S., Baehner, R.L., and Rajagopalan, R.V. (1975) J. Clin. Invest., 55, 1357-1373.

63. Sacks, T., Moldow, C.F., Craddock, P.R., Bowers, T.K., and Jacob, H.S. (1978) J. Clin. Invest., 61, 1161-1167.
64. Baehner, R.L. and Johnston, R.B. (1971) Brit. J. Haematol., 20, 277-285.
65. Tauber, A.I., Goetzl, E.A., and Babior, B.M. (1979) Inflammation, 3, 261-272.
66. Grove, D.I., Mahmoud, A.A.F., and Warren, K.S. (1977) J. Exp. Med., 145, 755-759.
67. Bass, D.A. and Szejda, P. (1979) J. Clin. Invest., 64, 1558-1564.
68. David, J.R. and Butterworth, A.E. (1977) Fed. Proc., 36, 2176-2180.
69. Grove, D.I., Mahmoud, A.A.F., and Warren, K.S. (1977) J. Exp. Med., 145, 755-759.
70. Butterworth, A.E., Wassom, D.L., Gleich, G.J., Loegering, D.A., and David, J.R. (1979) J. Immunol., 122, 221-229.
71. Salmon, S.E., Cline, M.J., Schultz, J., and Lehrer, R.I. (1970) N. Engl. J. Med., 282, 250-253.
72. Migler, R., DeChatelet, L.R., and Bass, D.A. (1978) Blood, 51, 445-456.
73. Van Furth, R., Cohn, Z.A., Hirsch, J.G., Humphry, J.H., Spector, W.G., and Langevoort, H.L. (1972) Bull. World Health Org., 46, 845-852.
74. Cutting, H.O. and Lang, J.E. (1964) Ann. Int. Med., 61, 876-887.
75. Oren, R., Farnham, A.E., Saito, K., Milofsky, E., and Karnovsky, M.L. (1963) J. Cell. Biol., 17, 487-501.
76. Johnston, R.B. (1978) Fed. Proc., 37, 2759-2764.
77. Sagone, A.L., King, G.W., and Metz, E.N. (1976) J. Clin. Invest., 57, 1352-1358.
78. Reiss, M. and Roos, D. (1978) J. Clin. Invest., 61, 480-488.
79. Bos, A., Wever, R., and Roos, D. (1978) Biochim. Biophys. Acta, 525, 37-44.
80. Karnovsky, M.L. and Lazdins, J.K. (1978) J. Immunol., 121, 809-813.
81. Cohn, Z.A. (1978) J. Immunol., 121, 813-816.
82. Nathan, C.F. and Root, R.K. (1978) J. Exp. Med., 146, 1648-1662.
83. Pabst, M.J. and Johnston, R.B. (1980) J. Exp. Med., 151, 101-114.
84. Simon, L.M., Robin, E.D., Phillips, J.R., Acevedo, J., Axline, S.G., and Theodore, J. (1977) J. Clin. Invest., 59, 443-448.
85. Holian, A. and Danielle, R.P. (1979) FEBS Lett., 108, 47-50.
86. Rister, M. and Baehner, R.L. (1977) Brit. J. Haematol., 36, 241-248.
87. Hoidal, J.R., Repine, J.E., Beall, G.D., Rasp, F.L., and White, J.G. (1978) Am. J. Pathol., 91, 469-476.
88. Bainton, D.F. and Golde, D.W. (1978) J. Clin. Invest., 61, 1555-1569.
89. Van der Meer, J.W.M., Reelen, R.H.J., Fluitsma, D.M., and van Furth, R. (1979) J. Exp. Med., 149, 17-26.
90. Nathan, C., Nogueira, N., Juangbhanich, C., Ellis, J., and Cohn, Z.A. (1979) J. Exp. Med., 149, 1056-1068.
91. Murray, H.W. and Cohn, Z.A. (1979) J. Exp. Med., 150, 938-949.

CHAPTER 10   SUPEROXIDE DISMUTASE AND DISEASE

W. H. BANNISTER
Nuffield Department of Clinical Biochemistry, University of Oxford,
Radcliffe Infirmary, Oxford OX2 6HE, U.K.

INTRODUCTION

    The discovery of the enzyme superoxide dismutase (SOD) is an interesting example
of convergence of a number of lines of research. In 1939, Mann and Keilin (Ref. 1)
isolated from bovine erythrocytes a copper protein, which they called hemocuprein.
Later renamed erythrocuprein (Ref. 2), the protein was shown to be identical with
other tissue proteins, notably hepatocuprein and cerebrocuprein (Ref. 3), and to
contain zinc as well as copper (Ref. 4). In 1969, McCord and Fridovich (Ref. 5)
reported the far-reaching discovery that erythrocuprein was a superoxide dismutase
(superoxide:superoxide oxidoreductase, EC 1.15.1.1) with remarkable catalytic
activity. Fridovich and collaborators went on to show the existence of other
superoxide dismutases containing manganese or iron, instead of copper, at the
active site besides differing in the protein moiety (Ref. 6). Generally speaking
copper-zinc uperoxide dismutase (CuZn-SOD) is found in the cytoplasm of eukaryotic
cells, while manganese superoxide dismutase (Mn-SOD) is found in the mitochondria
(Ref. 7). These forms of the enzyme appear to be evolutionarily unrelated (Ref. 8).
In man both CuZn-SOD and Mn-SOD are present in liver cytosol, a finding confirmed
in another primate, the baboon (Ref. 9). SOD is an intracellular enzyme with only
traces in the extracellular fluids (Ref. 10). At the time of the pioneering work
of McCord and Fridovich (Ref. 5), CuZn-SOD had been under study as indophenol
oxidase (Ref. 11), tetrazolium oxidase (Ref. 12), tetrazolium reductase inhibitor
(Ref. 13) and orgotein (Ref. 14), without knowledge of its true enzymatic activity.
    Biological production of superoxide is a potentially dangerous crossroad of
oxygen metabolism. The question of whether superoxide can be an initiating or
contributing factor in disease is part of the more general problem of the nature
and pathogenicity of toxic oxygen (in the widest sense of this term), whose elucidation and reduction to coherent order are the ultimate goal of studies on active
oxygen. Aetiological factors in disease admit of a wide variety of antecedent
causes. Michelson et al. (Ref. 15) put forward a concept of superoxide-related
disease according to which both high and low levels of SOD can be pathogenic. Their
arguments imply that SOD strikes a balance between any utilization (which is poorly
understood) and elimination of superoxide. This is a useful way of looking at
SOD under physiological and pathological circumstances. As in other aetiological
studies, three sets of evidence are required to substantiate Michelson's concept of

Superoxide-related disease (Refs. 15,16), namely, evidence of association of high
and low levels of SOD with disease, evidence of mechanisms by which such associations
could be causally linked, and experimental data to support the cause-and-effect
interpretation. The purpose of this article is to give a coherent description,
where possible, of the state of the problem of superoxide-related disease. The
article does not set out to represent SOD as an enzyme in search of a disease.

POPULATION GENETICS OF SUPEROXIDE DISMUTASE

Studies on the population genetics of SOD began before its true nature was discovered. Brewer (Ref. 11) observed a constant achromatic band after electrophoresis
of hemolysates on starch gel and tetrazolium staining. One subject out of several
thousands from different parts of the world had three achromatic bands. Pedigree
study suggested an electrophoretic variant of an enzyme with autosomal inheritance,
which behaved as an indophenol oxidase. With tissue extracts Brewer (Ref. 11)
noticed two achromatic bands, one (A) identical to that in hemolysates and another
(B) with lower anodic mobility. The isozymes appeared to have separate genetic
loci, since the observed deviation of the phenotype of isozyme A was not reflected
in isozyme B. Beauchamp and Fridovich (Ref. 17) and Lippitt and Fridovich (Ref. 18)
confirmed the identity of SOD and indophenol oxidase. In fact isozyme A of Brewer
(Ref. 11) corresponded to CuZn-SOD and isozyme B corresponded to Mn-SOD (Ref. 19).

Electrophoretic polymorphism of CuZn-SOD (SOD A) has been widely investigated
in relation to population genetics following the initial work of Brewer (Ref. 11).
After further observations of a deviating phenotype from Finland (Ref. 20), Southern
Germany (Ref. 21) and the Westray Island of the Orkneys (Ref. 22), Beckman (Ref. 23)
reported the first of a series of studies from Northern Sweden and Northern Finland
which formalized the genetics of SOD A. Beckman (Ref. 23) proposed the existence
of two genes, SOD^1 and SOD^2, with associated phenotypes, SOD 1, SOD 2-1 and SOD 2.
In starch gel electrophoresis, at pH 8.6, the rare phenotype SOD 2 shows a slower
anodic mobility than the common phenotype SOD 1. The phenotype SOD 2-1 shows, in
addition to SOD 1 and SOD 2 bands, a hybrid enzyme with intermediate electrophoretic
mobility (Refs. 19,23,24). The SOD^2 variant allele has a relatively high frequency
(1% to 3%) only in Northern Sweden (Ref. 25), Northern Finland (Refs. 25,26), the
Westray Island of the Orkneys (Ref. 22) and the West Coast of Newfoundland (Ref. 27).
This concentration supports a hypothesis of successive population migrations and
gene flow from a single Scandinavian, probably Northern Finnish, source, where
genetic drift, rather than any selective advantage, may have played an important
role in establishing the SOD^2 gene (Ref. 25). In other populations the gene appears
to be very rare and overwhelmingly Caucasian (Refs. 25-33).

Visual study of the electrophoretic phenotype SOD 2-1 indicates weaker staining
of the SOD 2 band in comparison with the SOD 1 band, suggesting that the SOD^2 gene
might be associated with lower enzymatic activity (Ref. 25). The fact that the

incidence of SOD 1, SOD 2-1 and SOD 2 individuals in the Tornedalen area of Northern Sweden, where the frequency of the SOD^2 allele is about 3%, appears to conform to the Hardy-Weinberg principle, and the observation that SOD 2-1 and SOD 2 individuals from families in which the gene segregates show no accumulation of any particular disease imply that the SOD^2 gene causes no selective disadvantage for SOD 2-1 heterozygotes and SOD 2 homozygotes (Ref. 34).

The CuZn-SOD variant SOD A2 has been isolated from the erythrocytes of an SOD 2 homozygote by Marklund et al. (Ref. 35) and compared with SOD A1. In isoelectric focusing, carried out as a preparative step, the variant had a pI of 4.85 compared with a pI of 4.7 for the common SOD. The variant showed small changes in amino acid composition, but no definite amino acid substitution could be pinpointed. Subunit molecular weight and the ultraviolet spectrum showed no change. Specific activity and sensitivity to inhibition by cyanide and hydrogen peroxide were virtually the same as for the common SOD. The variant SOD was quantitated on the assumption of normal copper content (and molecular weight). On this basis the measured zinc content was normal. The variant enzyme was significantly less stable than common SOD to heat (70°C) and pH extremes of 4.1 and 11.0. The physiological significance, if any, of this instability is difficult to interpret. The variant was as stable as common SOD when kept for more than three weeks in 50 mM phosphate buffer, pH 7.0, at 37°C. However, some relative instability or ageing effect in the erythrocyte may still explain a weaker SOD 2 band compared to the SOD 1 band in electrophoresis of hemolysates from SOD 2-1 heterozygotes, since a weaker SOD 2 band is not seen with placenta extracts (Refs. 24,35).

Polymorphism of Mn-SOD (SOD B) has been reported from Japan and Malaysia (Refs. 36,37). In an examination of 98 Japanese autopsy liver specimens, Shinoda et al. (Ref. 36) found two with a deviating phenotype for SOD B in starch gel electrophoresis. The normal pattern for SOD B was one intense and one weaker band. The two variant specimens showed three bands, one correspondingly to the normal (intense) band, one intense variant band migrating anodally behind the normal band, and another weaker variant band migrating the slowest of all three bands. This was considered the phenotypic expression of heterozygosity at the SOD B locus. Tan and Teng (Ref. 37) in a study of SOD zymograms of saliva specimens from racial groups in Malaysia found polymorphism for SOD B among the Senoi aborigines. The variant phenotype SOD B 2-1 showed two intense bands for SOD B, one with the mobility of the normal band and another with slightly slower anodal migration than the normal band. The estimate of the frequency of the $SOD B^2$ gene was 1.2%. Genetic variation of SOD A was not found. Identity of the SOD B variant in the Senoi and Japanese is considered likely by Tan and Teng (Ref. 37) although the phenotyping evidence needs a firmer basis.

The balance of evidence suggests that the variant allele is harmless in populations with polymorphism for SOD A or SOD B and its physiological effects, if any, are small enough to escape observation. Considering the crucial role of SOD in the metabolism of active oxygen, it is possible that only variants not significantly affecting the enzymatic activity can be tolerated (Ref. 35).

SUPEROXIDE DISMUTASE IN TRISOMY 21

By means of a human-mouse somatic cell hybridization technique that causes preferential loss of human chromosomes, the gene for CuZn-SOD has been assigned to chromosome 21 in man (Ref. 38). The gene is on chromosome 16 of the mouse (Refs. 39,40). The gene for Mn-SOD has been assigned to chromosome 6 in man (Ref. 41,42).

Chromosome 21 in man is of special interest because trisomy 21 is the factor responsible for Down's syndrome. This is a common syndrome of developmental defects and mental retardation with an incidence of about 1 in 600 live births. The genes responsible for this syndrome when present in the trisomic state are localized on the distal part of the long arm of chromosomes 21 (Ref. 43). Consistent with triplication of the gene for CuZn-SOD an increase of 50% in erythrocyte SOD activity can be demonstrated (Refs. 44-48). The increase in activity is due to increase in the level of enzyme protein as shown by immunoassay (Ref. 49). A similar increase in CuZn-SOD activity has been demonstrated in platelets (Ref. 50) and in leukocytes and fibroblasts (Ref. 51). In platelets, the 50% increase in the activity of CuZn-SOD is associated with a 33% decrease in the activity of Mn-SOD. Sinet et al. (Ref. 50), who made this observation, suggested that the level of Mn-SOD might be regulated by that of CuZn-SOD. Their data show an interesting inverse proportion between CuZn-SOD and Mn-SOD activities in platelets. Thus the product (CuZn-SOD activity) x (Mn-SOD activity) is 260 units/mg protein for normal and 271 units/mg protein, i.e., very similar, for trisomy 21 platelets. This supports the idea of an inverse decrease in synthesis of Mn-SOD with increase in synthesis of CuZn-SOD, other things being equal, but it is not possible to go into any regulatory process.

The gene for CuZn-SOD is probably located in the region of sub-band 21q22.1 of chromosome 21. This is indicated by the correlation between the erythrocyte SOD level and the chromosome abnormality in cases of monosomy and trisomy 21 (Refs. 52-55). Thus partial monosomy or trisomy for the segment 21pter →21q21 is associated with an erythrocyte level in the normal range, and partial trisomy for the segment 21q21 → 21q22.1 is associated with an erythrocyte SOD level in the range observed for full trisomy 21 (Ref. 52). The gene-dosage effect for erythrocyte SOD in trisomy 21 by centromeric D/G or G/G translocation was the same as in free trisomy 21 in six cases of unbalanced translocation studied by Garber et al. (Ref. 56) but was problematically absent in three cases studied by Kedziora et al. (Ref. 57).

Aula et al. (Ref. 43) considered that 21q22 trisomy is sufficient to explain the pathology of Down's syndrome. This is generally accepted (Refs. 53.58) but the genes implicated in the syndrome have not been specifically identified. The role of the CuZn-SOD gene is difficult to evaluate. Speculation is possible (Ref. 15). A high level of SOD may impair the utilization of superoxide as a free-radical chain terminator (Refs. 15,16), but it is doubtful whether a 50% increase in CuZn-SOD by itself is pathological (see discussion of erythrocyte SOD levels, next section).

The mitochondrial electron transport chain is a significant source of superoxide production in respiring cells (Refs. 59,60). Superoxide so produced may diffuse preferentially into the mitochondrial matrix. Decrease in mitochondrial Mn-SOD activity, as observed in platelets (Ref. 50), might therefore expose the mitochondria to oxygen free-radical damage in trisomy 21. It has been suggested that mitochondria where over 90% of the oxygen consumed by mammals is utilized, may serve as a biological clock, and that maximum life-span may be a reflection of the rate of mitochondrial degradation (Ref. 61). Some features of trisomy 21 are broadly consistent with rapid ageing. The central nervous system seems to be particularly sensitive, as indicated by rapid deterioration of the low IQ of the patients and the frequent occurrence of presenile dementia of the Alzheimer type (Ref. 62) with senile plaques and ganglion-cell degeneration (Ref. 63). Cultured fibroblasts show phenomena of early senescence (Refs. 64,65), reminiscent of those seen in fibroblasts taken from patients with accelerated ageing syndromes (Ref. 66). According to Orgel's error catastrophe hypothesis, ageing of post-mitotic cells is by cumulation of transcription and translation errors in protein synthesis that leads to a cascading process whereby, as the cell ages, altered proteins appear and the synthesis of altered proteins accelerates the ageing process (Ref. 67). Although lately put in doubt in fibroblasts (Ref. 68), this hypothesis is particularly attractive to explain degenerative changes in neurons in which there is no possibility of selection by mitosis in postnatal life. Anyway it would be of interest in trisomy 21 to explore the reason and implications of decrease in mitochondrial Mn-SOD activity within this conceptual framework in accessible cells.

An acceleration of oxidative processes in trisomy 21 has been postulated largely from observations on erythrocytes (Ref. 69). The erythrocyte can be considered to be at increased risk of damage by active oxygen species because of oxygen (and carbon dioxide) transport and the autoxidizability of hemoglobin. Carrell et al. (Ref. 70) have postulated that oxidation of oxyhemoglobin and reduction of methemoglobin constitute a cycle producing a continuous flux of superoxide in the erythrocyte. According to this hypothesis, any factor that increases the production or diminishes the elimination of superoxide (and hydrogen peroxide) is a potential threat to the erythrocyte leading to oxidative hemolysis. Glutathione peroxidase (GSH-Px) may be the primary enzyme which eliminates hydrogen peroxide in the erythrocyte (Ref. 71), although a more cautious view can be taken (Refs. 72,73). At any rate it is of interest to find an approximately 50% increase in the GSH-Px activity of trisomy 21 erythrocytes (Ref. 74), which has been confirmed in fibroblasts (Ref. 69). Catalase activity is unchanged (Ref. 74,75). The erythrocytes also show increased activity of the hexose monophosphate shunt which generates NADPH for reduction of oxidized glutathione by glutathione reductase (Ref. 69). The significance to be placed on these observations is not sufficiently clear at the present time. It is generally considered that trisomy 21 patients have essentially normal red cell indices and maturity (Refs. 76,77). Whether or not the erythrocytes (and other cells) are exposed to increased oxidative stress as a result of the trisomy 21 genotype but are adequately protected by the increased levels of CuZn-SOD and GSH-Px is not known. It is to be noted that GSH-Px reduced not only hydrogen peroxide but also (and more preferentially) lipid peroxides, which are more toxic (Ref. 73). The gene for GSH-Px has been assigned to chromosome 3 in man (Ref. 78). It is a matter for speculation whether its activity is influenced by that of the CuZn-SOD gene or by accelerated peroxidative processes in trisomy 21.

It is of interest to note that reduction of nitroblue tetrazolium (NBT) by resting leukocytes is significantly higher in trisomy 21 patients than in normal subjects, as observed in three to nineteen-year olds (Ref. 79). This difference is not seen after stimulation of phagocytosis. Apart from patients with bacterial infections (Ref. 80), spontaneous NBT activation is found regularly in newborn infants (Ref. 81) in patients with osteogenesis imperfecta and their relatives without manifest disease (Ref. 80), and in hemophiliacs (Ref. 80). Superoxide released by neutrophils (Ref. 82) can be considered to promote reduction of the dye in the NBT test (Ref. 83). In osteogenesis imperfecta spontaneous NBT reduction is associated with increased leuko-cyte respiration and hexose monophosphate shunt activity (Ref. 84), which are not unlikely also in trisomy 21 as a manifestation of a generalized increase in cellu-lar oxidative metabolism.

THE VARIATION OF SUPEROXIDE DISMUTASE

Erythrocytes have provided convenient access to the levels of CuZn-SOD under various conditions. Michelson et al. (Ref. 15) have presented extensive data on erythrocyte SOD levels in normal subjects and patients suffering from various diseases. Erythrocyte SOD is best expressed per unit mass of hemoglobin. This index necessarily varies with hemoglobin concentration. From the data for 200 white French rural subjects of Michelson et al. (see Table III, in Ref. 15) the variation is given by the regression: μg SOD/g Hb = [727.7 − 20.8 x (g Hb/100 ml)] ± 4.7. Observed SOD levels are compared with expected levels, given by this regression, in Table 1 which gives the data of Michelson et al. (Ref. 15) in condensed form. The mean SOD level in the normal population studied by Michelson et al. (Ref. 15) agrees with the estimated (500 μg SOD/g Hb) given by Winterbourn et al. (Ref. 85). There was no significant variation with respect to sex or age. Furthermore it appeared that SOD level does not vary within the life span of the mature erythrocyte. The ratio SOD_{obs}/SOD_{exp} in trisomy 21 needs no further comment. Of some interest is the increase in the value of the ratio for psychiatric cases,

TABLE 1

Variation of erythrocyte superoxide dismutase[a]

Cases	Number	Hb (g/100 ml)	SOD_{obs} (µg/g Hb)	$\dfrac{SOD_{obs}}{SOD_{exp}}$
Normal rural whites	200	12.67+1.3	461.4+ 45.8	0.99
Hemodialysis	24	8.01+1.1	540.3+ 38.3	0.96
Hemochromatosis	5	11.72+0.9	468.0+ 28.4	0.96
Splenomegaly (myeloid)	4	11.09+3.06	480.0+ 91.7	0.97
Alcoholic cirrhosis	8	12.06+1.41	439.0+ 29.3	0.94
Porphyria	2		433.0	
Polycythaemia rubra vera	2		609.5	
Trisomy 18	1	7.1	691.0	1.19
Mothers (after parturition)	6	11.2 +1.18	504.2+ 44.1	1.02
Newborns	6	11.95+1.74	501.2+ 18.9	1.05
Trisomy 21 (6-48 years)	41	12.55+1.13	679.4+ 62.8	1.46
Psychiatric cases	30	12.54+0.85	587.0+ 66.4	1.26
Old age (70-99 years)	23	11.81+1.57	463.3+ 44.3	0.96
Geriatric cases	34	12.08+1.45	460.9+113.4	0.97
Touaregs	7	10.46+1.86	506.7+ 67.8	0.99
Hb matched rural whites	39	10.83+0.58	506.6+ 45.6	1.01
Negroids (Paris)	40	14.26+1.85	672.5+ 81.9	1.56
Hb matched rural whites	46	14.37+0.88	431.2+ 44.6	1.01
Whites (Paris)	20	15.57+1.40	593.6+ 43.1	1.47

[a] Values are mean $\pm$ SD. SOD_{obs} is the measured SOD level. SOD_{exp} is the SOD level given by the regression of SOD_{obs} on Hb in the normal rural whites. Data from Ref. 15.

which included paranoid psychosis (one case), schizophrenia (six cases), and other psychoses. The value of the ratio in geriatric cases showed wide dispersion perhaps due to the variety of ailments. The hemoglobin concentration in these cases varied within a narrow range. Quite interesting are two cases of hyperlipidaemia (of unspecified type), one with arterial hypertension and an SOD level of 702 µg/g Hb and one with hemiplegia and an SOD level of 232 µg/g HB. On the basis of the mean hemoglobin concentration for the group of geriatric cases, these patients had an SOD_{obs}/SOD_{exp} ratio of 1.47 and 0.49, respectively. This range of variation (of unclear origin) suggests that study of erythrocyte SOD in the various types of hyperlipidaemia might be rewarding.

Autor et al. (Ref. 86) found significantly greater SOD activity in blood in adults compared to normal term infants. SOD activity was measured after ethanol-chloroform treatment of clotted whole blood. Values were 93 $\pm$ 3 (SE) and 60 $\pm$ 5 (SE) units/µmole

heme in the two groups, respectively. According to Legge et al. (Ref. 87), the
adult erythrocyte SOD level is reached about three months after birth. Augmented
erythrocyte SOD can occur in normal adults, as found by Michelson et al. (Ref. 15)
for Parisian negroids and whites (see Table 1), possibly as a response to increased
environmental or nutritional oxidative stress or both. An augmentation which
appears to reflect a specific metabolic response has been found in black alcoholics
(Refs. 88,89). In the rat the activity of CuZn-SOD is significantly elevated in
fetal liver after administration of ethanol to dams during pregnancy (Ref. 90). The
activity of the enzyme in maternal liver is not appreciably elevated. Normally
maternal liver has considerably higher CuZn-SOD activity than fetal liver (Refs. 90,
91). Increase in activity occurs during postpartum development in parallel with
decrease in lipid peroxidation (Ref. 91).

Ueda and Ogata (Ref. 92) have claimed a significant decrease in erythrocyte SOD
in the old age group of a sample of Japanese, but their data are difficult to interpret because hemoglobin levels (and age range) are not given. They refer to the
old age group (60-69 years) in the normal sample of Michelson et al. (see Table I in
Ref. 15). For this group the ratio SOD_{obs}/SOD_{exp} is 0.91 and can hardly be taken
as evidence of decreased erythrocyte SOD in old age. Furthermore, the value of the
ratio is 0.96 for still older individuals (70-99 years; see Table 1) studied by
Michelson et al. (Ref. 15). In an earlier study of erythrocyte SOD activity
Stevens et al. (Ref. 93) found that this remained constant well into the eighth
decade of life, and more recently Joenje et al. (Ref. 94) also reported that human
erythrocyte SOD does not decline with donor age. The transcriptional and trans-
lational processes for CuZn-SOD synthesis in human erythrocyte precursor cells may
remain intact throughout life, as suggested by Stevens et al. (Ref. 93).

The competence of the entire protein-synthesizing mechanism may generally be
quite high for SOD. In human fibroblasts in tissue culture SOD activity, measured
according to Misra and Fridovich (Ref. 95), shows a tendency to increase with
population doubling in the initial life span of the cultures and then to remain
elevated. The activity attained by the fibroblasts appears to increase with donor
age when fetal, newborn and adult cells are compared (Ref. 96). Preliminary work
on WI-38 fibroblasts has shown a slight increase in cytoplasmic and mitochondrial
SOD with ageing of the cells. A partial inactivation of cytoplasmic SOD was
observed in old cells, apparently due to loss of a stabilizing factor (Ref. 97).

Observations on a transient tissue--the placenta--have shown that SOD activity,
determined according to Misra and Fridovich (Ref. 95), increases with the age of
the organ (Ref. 98). The SOD activity increases rapidly in the first ten weeks of
gestation (by a factor of about 4.0 between the 4th and the 11th week) and then
more slowly (by a factor of about 1.4) to term. A similar report for placental SOD,
measured according to Beauchamp and Fridovich (Ref. 17), has confirmed the increase
in activity and indicated a two-to-three-fold increase between early gestation and

term (Ref. 99). This may be related quite generally to homeostasis in the feto-maternal unit, one aspect of which may be the control of lipid peroxidation as the data of Sekiba and Yoshioka (Ref. 99) would appear to suggest.

Placental SOD activities are systematically lower than normal in cases of spontaneous abortion and stillbirth, and peroxide-decomposing enzymes show similar behavior (Ref. 100). The reported data (Ref. 100) show approximately 50% decrease in placental SOD for cases of abortion around the 15th week of gestation. At this time Holme et al. (Ref. 10) found a significantly higher concentration of CuZn-SOD in amniotic fluid than in serum in pregnant women over the age of thirty-five, screened for absence of fetal chromosomal aberrations. It is of interest to note that about half of all miscarriages, irrespective of aetiology occur during the 10th to 13th week of gestation, but comment in relation to placental SOD activity is not possible without further study because this peak incidence (of abortion) is partially correlated with the fact that most abnormal ova abort at this time.

Michelson et al. (Ref. 15) found no difference in erythrocyte SOD level between maternal and cord blood. The ratio SOD_{obs}/SOD_{exp} was around unity in both cases (see Table 1). Kobayashi et al. (Ref. 101) and Yoshioka et al. (Ref. 102 have reported similar observations. According to Autor et al. (Ref. 86), SOD activities (determined on clotted whole blood and expressed in units/μmole heme) in the blood of normal premature and normal full-term infants do not differ significantly. These workers also found no significant difference in the SOD activity of clotted whole blood between premature infants with the idiopathic respiratory distress syndrome or infants with bronchopulmonary dysplasia and appropriate controls. These findings show some conflict with those of Bonta et al. (Ref. 103) who observed an inverse relation between erythrocyte SOD activity (expressed in units/mg nonhemoglobin protein) and gestational age, with a 36% decrease in activity in infants of over 36 weeks compared to infants of less than 29 weeks gestational age. Initial erythrocyte SOD levels were depressed (by 13%) in premature infants who developed the idiopathic respiratory distress syndrome and the survival of these infants, without development of bronchopulmonary dysplasia, was observed to correlate with augmentation of the erythrocyte SOD (in response to standard therapy).

It is not sufficiently clear to what extent erythrocyte SOD follows the variation of pulmonary SOD in response to oxygen stress. The data of Autor et al. (Ref. 86) indicate a correlation between mortality and failure to augment lung SOD in the idiopathic respiratory distress syndrome. These workers found an increase of total SOD activity from 17 ± 1 (SE) units/mg DNA in fetal lung (six 18- to 20-week old aborted fetuses) to 49 ± 6 (SE) units/mg DNA in infant lung (four autopsy specimens from 18-hour to 2-month old infants with normal lung histology) and 110 ± 15 (SE) units/mg DNA in adult lung (five autopsy specimens from 43 to 70-year old adults without lung disease). Lung SOD activity in three premature infants (26 to 32 weeks gestational age) who died of the idiopathic respiratory distress syndrome was 37 ± 4

(SE) units/mg DNA in autopsy specimens. These infants had received intensive oxygen therapy. The average birth weight of the infants was within normal limits for their average (midpoint of data) gestational age (29th week) in relation to standard data for fetal growth (Ref. 104). The survival time of the infants was 19 to 96 hours. Their mean lung SOD activity at autopsy (37 units/mg DNA) can be considered approximately normal for their gestational age, suggesting lack of response to the hyperoxic challenge of birth and oxygen therapy. (This can be seen by taking the autopsy lung SOD activities reported for aborted fetuses and neonates as representing the activities of the 19th and 38th (or 40th) week of gestation, respectively. Linear interpolation between these data points, with SOD activity expressed as a function of gestational age, indicates an SOD activity of about 32 units/mg DNA at the 29th week of gestation, with or without logarithmic transformation of both variables.)

Minced lung tissue from neonatal rats responds rapidly to hyperoxia with an increase in SOD activity when incubated in the presence of rat plasma (Ref. 86). When plasma (or serum) from premature infants is substituted for rat plasma an increase in SOD activity is seen more often with samples from infants without the idiopathic respiratory distress syndrome (88% of cases) than samples from infants with the syndrome (33% of cases). This suggests that in the idiopathic respiratory distress syndrome the plasma may lack a normal factor or possess an inhibitory factor for positive response of neonatal lung SOD to hyperoxia (Ref. 105). The plasma factor has been reported to have a protein component with a molecular weight exceeding 50,000 (see Ref. 106). In neonatal rat lung the cell which can rapidly increase its SOD in response to hyperoxia is the alveolar macrophage and the SOD involved is the mitochondrial Mn-SOD (Ref. 107-110).

In the data of Autor et al. (Ref. 86) adult autopsy lung shows on average an increase of 124% in SOD activity over neonatal autopsy lung. While this can be interpreted as an adaptation to continuing oxygen stress in adult life, during embryonic life lung SOD activity increases with gestational age under hypoxic conditions. A general interpretation which can be put on certain observations in the rat (Refs. 111-113) is that lung SOD can vary slowly in some compartment and cell type as a U-shaped function of the oxic stimulus, between 10 and 90% O_2, with the extremum at air breathing. In the adult rat lung it is conceivable that mitochondrial Mn-SOD of Type II cells (compare Refs. 112,113) behaves in this paradoxical fashion.

SUPEROXIDE DISMUTASE AND HEMOLYTIC ANEMIA

There is ample evidence for the production of superoxide by autoxidation of oxyhemoglobin (and oxymyoglobin) under certain conditions (Refs. 114-121) and this can be expected to occur in vivo, with increased rate in certain types of hemolytic anemia (Refs. 70,122). Current knowledge presupposes three intracellular anti-oxidant defence enzymes, namely, SOD, GSH-Px and catalase, together with vitamin E

as a nonspecific antioxidant (Ref. 123). The relationship of the defense systems
to the micro-environment of the pre-eminently oxidizable molecules of the erythrocy
namely, hemoglobin and the polyunsaturated fatty acids of the membrane lipid, is
known only in broad terms. CuZn-SOD is cytosolic as in other cells. GSH-Px, a
soluble enzyme by conventional criteria, may be partially bound or may have access
to the erythrocyte membrane (Ref. 73,124). Erythrocyte catalase may also be
membrane bound to a small extent (Ref. 124). Vitamin E is bound to the erythrocyte
membrane (Ref. 125). The interplay of the defense systems, in vitro and in vivo
is difficult to disentangle.

Evidence of hemolysis as a result of sufficient impairment of any of the
antioxidant defense systems is not clear except for the GSH-Px system. Erythrocyte
genetically deficient in GSH-Px are highly susceptible to oxidative drug-induced
hemolytic anemia (Ref. 126). In a general way the half-life of erythrocytes is
comparable to the half-life of glucose-6-phosphate dehydrogenase (G6PD) which (with
6-phosphogluconate dehydrogenase) provides NADPH for the GSH-Px system (Ref. 73).
It has been implied that superoxide might run down the reduced nucleotide in G6PD-
type hemolytic anemia (Ref. 127).

Deficiency of SOD, as an inborn error of metabolism, is not known and may not
be tolerated. Developmental or acquired deficiency of SOD is not clearly connected
with hemolytic anemia, as discussed below. Acatalasemia is well-tolerated with
only a mild increase in Heinz body formation. Erythrocyte SOD activity is significantly increased in acatalasemic subjects. GSH-Px activity is also high but the
normal range is not exceeded (Ref. 128). Vitamin E deficiency may be a cause of
hemolytic anemia in premature infants (see below). Vitamin E therapy decreases
the in vitro susceptibility of the erythrocytes to peroxidative hemolysis in some
cases of β-thalassemia (Ref. 129), but the average life-span of the erythrocytes
is not increased (Ref. 130).

Concetti et al. (Ref. 131) found no significant change in erythrocyte SOD
activity in 19 patients with β-thalassemia major (14 to 96 days after blood transfusion) and 5 patients with β-thalassaemia intermedia (30 to 400 days after
blood transfusion in 3 of the cases), with respect to normal controls. In
β-thalassemia major the serum iron concentration is increased with a saturated
binding capacity, unless the diet has been iron deficient. Iron overload occurs
as a complication of treatment by blood transfusion. There is in vitro evidence
that thalassemic erythrocytes are more sensitive to lipid peroxidation than normal
erythrocytes (Ref. 132), but to associate this with iron overload is unwarranted
since the typical biochemical marker of iron overload, i.e., ferritin, is practicall
absent in thalassemic erythrocytes (Ref. 133). However, as Winterhalter (Ref. 134)
has remarked, the circulating erythrocytes in thalassemia are those which have
survived the (presumptive) challenge by superoxide in the bone marrow. This is
an apt remark since the destruction of erythrocytes begins in the bone marrow

where lipid peroxidation promoted by iron is not excluded in thalassemia as sideronormoblasts can be found in the circulation (Ref. 135). In β-thalassemia major there is a variable synthesis of fetal hemoglobin which improves the form and life-span of the erythrocytes which contain it. This needs to be taken into consideration in the overall picture of hemolysis in this condition.

By means of polarographic assay of hemolysates, Rotilio et al (Ref. 136) found that the average level of erythrocyte SOD may be slightly lower in the newborn than in adults, irrespective of birth term. Erythrocyte GSH-Px activity was considered to be slightly decreased in premature neonates. Serum bilirubin was also measured in the neonates, several of whom had neonatal jaundice with serum bilirubin values in the range 8-21 mg/dl. Low erythrocyte SOD was associated with hyperbilirubinemia in two of three full-term infants showing maximal acetylphenylhydrazine-induced in vitro hemolysis. Erythrocyte GSH-Px activity was high in these two infants.

While it is clear that hemolysis is an important factor in neonatal hyper-bilirubinemia (Ref. 137), it should be noted that serum bilirubin can rise in the newborn because of immaturity of the UDP-glucuronyl transferase system in the liver. Thus about 40% of newborn infants have a serum bilirubin level of over 4 mg/dl during the first week (Ref. 138). Examination of the data of Rotilio et al. (Ref. 136) shows no correlation between serum bilirubin and erythrocyte SOD (or SOD/GSH-Px ratio) in the 17 neonates with bilirubin levels in the range 8-21 mg/dl. There is a low correlation between serum bilirubin and erythrocyte GSH-Px activity in the data for these neonates, but the coefficient of correlation ($r = 0.38$) is not significant. Rotilio et al. (Ref. 136) concluded that the absolute activity as well as the balance of the activities of erythrocyte SOD and GSH-Px are contributing factors in the nonimmune hemolytic anemia of the neonate, although their results scarcely support this view.

Any hypothesis of oxidative hemolysis has to take into account the degree (and nature) of the oxidative stress and the total antioxidant potential of the erythrocyte represented by the ability to scavenge active oxygen species and reduce hydroperoxides. Hemolysis in vitro can, with rare exceptions, be equated with shortening of the life-span of the erythrocytes, which are cleared from the circulation by the reticuloendothelial system following the development of some critical, prehemolytic lesion. Oxidative attack can occur on hemoglobin, leading to formation of Heinz bodies, and on the erythrocyte stroma, leading to as yet unspecified lipid peroxidation.

It is doubtful whether SOD deficiency plays a part in neonatal (oxidative) hemolysis (Ref. 139). The susceptibility of neonatal erythrocytes to oxidative hemolysis was shown by Gross et al. (Ref. 140) who reported a slight decrease in erythrocyte GSH-Px activity in premature infants. Infants, particularly premature babies, may have both lower serum vitamin E levels and decreased erythrocyte GSH-Px activities compared to adults (Ref. 141), and a hemolytic anemia which responds to treatment with vitamin E is known in newborn babies (Ref. 142).

Erythrocyte SOD activity is increased (by a factor of 1.7) while GSH-Px and catalase activities are decreased (by factors of 0.5 and 0.8, respectively) in sickle cell anemia. Together with these enzymatic changes sickled erythrocytes have given evidence of increased lipid peroxidation and formation of Heinz bodies (Ref. 143). Thus the erythrocytes appear to have a peroxidation potential greater than their total antioxidant potential. It is not known whether the rise in SOD activity is due to increased production or decreased elimination of superoxide. Decreased enzymatic dismutation of superoxide is a distinct possibility in sickled erythrocytes because of the diffusion-control of the SOD reaction (Ref. 144) and the rise in the microviscosity of the erythrocytes. The reason for the fall in GSH-Px and catalase activities is not clear. Erythrocyte GSH-Px activity can increase when SOD activity is increased, as in trisomy 21 (see above), but this type of linkage, which is favorable to the erythrocyte, is not operative in sickle cell patients.

In a case of hemolytic-uremic syncrome in an infant, Kobayashi et al. (Ref. 145) found a decrease of 32, 55 and 64% in erythrocyte SOD activity, with respect to an age control, 18, 39, and 45 days, respectively, after the onset of the disease. The second and third determinations were made during a period of symptomatic improvement, which preceeded fatal relapse, and suggest that the erythrocyte SOD may have some prognostic value in the disease. The hemolytic-uremic syndrome is characterized by microangiopathic hemolytic anemia, renal failure and platelet consumption. The primary event appears to be damage to the endothelial lining of the renal glomerular capillaries by a Schwartzman-like reaction (Refs. 146,147). The erythrocytes are probably damaged by the fibrin deposited on the vascular endothelium as a result of disseminated intravascular coagulation. Destruction of erythrocytes as a result of lipid peroxidation is another possibility (Refs. 145,148). The decrease in erythrocyte phospholipid content found by O'Regan et al. (Ref. 149) can be explained as a consequence of release or destruction of phospholipid, according to whether the erythrocytes are physically damaged by fibrin (an established mechanism in microangiopathic hemolytic anemia (see Ref. 146) or chemically damaged by lipid peroxidation. O'Regan et al. (Ref. 149) also observed low serum vitamin E levels in two children with the hemolytic-uremic syndrome. Despite this finding (vitamine E being a labile factor) and the decrease of erythrocyte SOD observed by Kobayashi et al. (Ref. 145), the hypothesis of lipid peroxidation needs further experimental support. The numerous bizarre and deformed erythrocytes observed, as was to be expected, by Kobayashi et al. (Ref. 145) might have lost SOD (and other components) as they seem to lose phospholipid (thromboplastin, see Ref. 147) after damage by fibrin, and lipid peroxidation may be a secondary phenomenon in the hemolytic anemia.

SUPEROXIDE DISMUTASE AND NERUOLOGICAL DISORDER

Loomis et al. (Ref. 150) observed that SOD, measured according to Misra and Fridovich (Ref. 95), is quite evenly distributed in human brain, including gray and white matter. The enzyme was found in all conventional cell fractions. The supernatant fraction contained 26% of the total activity but this could be increased to 80-85% by hypoosmotic treatment or brief sonication of the homogenate. The synaptosomal subfraction of the crude mitochondrial fraction is rich in the enzyme. This was shown for guinea pig gray matter. Two cases of Huntington's chorea had apparently normal specific activity (i.e., within the limits of mean ± 2 SD) in cerebral cortex, caudate nucleus and putamen. This finding has to be regarded with some caution because of glial cell infiltration and the likelihood that these cells are richer in SOD than neuron, as demonstrated for rat cortical cells (Ref. 151). (The regional and subcellular distribution of SOD in rat brain (Ref. 152) is quite similar to that found by Loomis et al. (Ref. 150) in human brain.) Furthermore, Loomis et al. (Ref. 150) alluded to the observation (Ref. 153) that neuronal enzymes involved in the synthesis of putative synaptic transmitters, notably, choline acetyl transferase and glutamic acid decarboxylase, are dramatically reduced in Huntington's chorea. On general grounds there should be awareness of the inadequacy of reporting brain SOD activity without probing the number and type of cells being studied.

The regional distribution of SOD in human brain reported by Loomis et al. (Ref. 150) is compared in Table 2 with that found by Koster et al. (Ref. 154). There is good agreement between the two sets of data, supporting the conclusion of fairly homogenous (though by no means equal) distribution of SOD (as measured) in human brain (Ref. 150). Koster et al. (Ref. 154) also reported the fraction of SOD activity insensitive to 1 mM cyanide as Mn-SOD activity, but this interpretation currently requires knowledge of the activity of human Mn-SOD at pH ≥ 10.0.

Erythrocyte SOD activity is essentially normal in Wilson's disease (hepatolenticular degeneration) even when serum ceruloplasmin is not measurable (Ref. 155). Wilson's disease is now recognized as a copper storage disorder apparently involving the mechanisms that regulate the passage of copper into the ceruloplasmin-synthesizing the biliary-excretion pathways in the liver. Long-term treatment of the disease with D-penicillamine causes a gradual decrease in erythrocyte SOD activity. Decrease of serum ceruloplasmin is much greater (Ref. 155). A similar trend was observed in copper-depleted rats (Refs. 156,157). In these animals plasma copper and ceruloplasmin activity decreased before erythrocyte copper and SOD activity. Whereas the decrease in plasma ceruloplasmin activity kept pace with the decrease in plasma copper, the decrease in erythrocyte (or brain) CuZn-SOD activity lagged behind the decrease in erythrocyte (or brain tissue) copper. This is understandable in terms of slow turnover of CuZn-SOD and the fractional contribution (about 60% for erythrocytes) of the enzyme to the total erythrocyte (or

222

TABLE 2

Regional distribution of superoxide dismutase in human brain[a]

Region	SOD (Ref. 150)	SOD (Ref. 154)
Frontal cortex:	-	0.71
Gray matter	0.80	-
White matter	1.23	-
Temporal cortex:	-	0.68
Gray matter	0.82	-
Parietal cortex:		
Gray matter	0.90	-
White matter	0.81	-
Occipital cortex	-	0.81
Hippocampus	1.08	0.93
Corpus callosum	-	1.11
Caudate nucleus	1.07	0.85
Putamen	1.01	-
Thalamus	1.14	1.11
Hypothalamus	1.13	-
Mammillary body	-	1.31
Midbrain	-	1.16
Midbrain without substantia nigra	1.12	-
Substantia nigra	1.30	-
Cerebellum:		
Cortex	1.31	1.12
White matter	-	1.12
Dentate nucleus	0.91	-
Pons	0.86	1.15
Medulla oblongata	0.90	0.95

[a]Values are reported specific activities (taking the midpoint of the range for three specimens in the case of the data of Ref. 150) normalized with respect to the overall mean (41 units SOD/mg protein for the data of Ref. 150 and 9.5 µg SOD/mg protein for the data of Ref. 154).

brain tissue) copper. Copper deficiency causes a decrease of CuZn-SOD activity in experimental animals, particularly in liver and erythrocytes (Refs. 158-161). Manganese deficiency markedly decreases the activity of mitochondrial SOD in liver and brain in experimental animals (Ref. 162). The effect of dietary zinc deficiency on CuZn-SOD (activity) is not dramatic (Ref. 159,163).

Copper-deficient neonatal rats show decreased CuZn-SOD activity as part of a global decrease of tissue copper and copper-containing enzymes in the brain, norepinephrine is decreased in these rats (Ref. 164). The sensitivity of the central nervous system to copper deficiency during development is emphasized by Menkes' syndrome (Ref. 165). In the mottled mutant mouse model of this genetic disorder of copper utilization, brain copper concentration and copper-enzyme (including CuZn-SOD) activities are decreased (Refs. 166,167). It is not known how deficiency (or excess) of copper leads to degenerative changes in the central nervous system (Ref. 168). Multiple copper-enzyme deficiencies obviously compound the problem of perceiving the role of decreased CuZn-SOD (if any) in neurological disorder due to copper deficiency.

There is as yet no clear evidence of association between altered levels of SOD and neurological or psychiatric disease (Ref. 169). It is difficult to ascribe a pathological effect to increased levels of CuZn-SOD activity (as measured in erythrocytes) in psychiatric cases (Refs. 15,16,170) without involving other factors (see above). A moderate increase (by a factor of 1.2) in erythrocyte and platelet CuZn-SOD activity has been reported in cases of childhood autism. Platelet Mn-SOD activity was not appreciably altered. GSH-Px activity was low in erythrocytes but not in platelets (Ref. 171). CuZn-SOD activity in erythrocytes and lymphocytes and Mn-SOD activity in lymphocytes are not altered in cases of juvenile neuronal ceroid-lipofuscinosis with respect to neurological controls (epileptics) or healthy adults (Ref. 172). Low GSH-Px levels are likely in this disease (Ref. 173).

Superoxide dismutase in the nervous system is of obvious interest in relation to protection of catecholamines and unsaturated lipids against autoxidation. In view of the high rate of oxygen consumption the most important source of superoxide in the brain is probably the respiratory chain. In contrast to heart and liver mitochondria, rat brain mitochondria do not generate superoxide and hydrogen peroxide with succinate as substrate (Ref. 174). This may explain why succinate can protect the brain against oxygen toxicity (Ref. 175). However, superoxide is generated when dihydro-orotate is oxidized by rat brain mitochondria (Ref. 176). Oxidation of dihydro-orotate in brain probably occurs at an appreciable rate (compared to liver) because of the magnitude of pyrimidine nucleotide biosynthesis, and can be considered as the most significant pathway of superoxide production (Ref. 169).

Evidence of mechanisms by which superoxide may be causally related to damage to nervous tissue has not been readily forthcoming, as in other tissues. Rat brain NaK-ATPase is partially inhibited (irreversibly) by superoxide generated by xanthine oxidase (Ref. 177). Both NaK-ATPase and p-nitrophenylphosphatase activity of the enzyme are affected. CuZn-SOD exerts a protective action in the reaction mixture. Since the enzyme is a lipoprotein entity, lipid peroxidation has been suggested as a likely mechanism of the inhibition (Ref. 177), but further evidence in support of this view is clearly needed.

The mechanism of depletion of nigro-striatal dopamine in Parkinson's disease has been of topical interest since this specific defect was reported in 1960 (Ref. 178). Oxygen radical toxicity is not excluded (see Ref. 16). Attention may here be drawn to a possible mechanism of dysfunction of the SOD protective system which has been relatively neglected, namely, that the substrate (superoxide) may escape the enzyme by reaction with positively charged species in a suitable environment (Ref. 179). Reaction with metal ions may produce destructive complexes which are not attacked by SOD. Although various metals are neurotoxic, copper and manganese are of particular interest because of copper deposition in the central nervous system (particularly in the basal ganglia) in Wilson's disease and the occurrence of (toxic) Parkinsonism in chronic manganese poisoning. In manganese intoxication in the squirrel monkey, toxic Parkinsonism is associated with selective depletion of dopamine (and serotonin) in the caudate nucleus (Ref. 180). Whatever the meaning of this observation, metal complexes of superoxide deserve consideration in relation to oxygen radical and metal toxicity in the nervous system.

SUPEROXIDE DISMUTASE IN INFLAMMATORY AND AUTOIMMUNE DISEASE

The role of superoxide in the inflammatory process came to the forefront with the demonstration by Babior et al. (Ref. 82) that polymorphonuclear leukocytes release superoxide into the surrounding medium during phagocytosis. This process is defective in chronic granulomatous disease (Ref. 181). The mechanism of superoxide generation by activated neutrophils (and other phagocytes) appears to involve an NADPH-oxidase system in the plasma membrane (Refs. 182,183).

Copper-zinc superoxide dismutase inhibits the inflammatory reaction, as judged by edema formation in two animal models, the reversed passive Arthus reaction (Ref. 184) and the prostaglandin phase of carrageenan-induced foot edema in the rat (Ref. 184,185). In both cases it suppresses the migration of neutrophils to the site of inflammatory challenge (Ref. 184). Catalase does not have this effect. A strongly chemotactic factor for neutrophils is formed in human plasma exposed in vitro to superoxide generated by xanthine oxidase. This response is abolished by CuZn-SOD, while catalase has no effect. The chemotactic effect is demonstrable in vitro and in vivo. The activity is associated with the albumin fraction of plasma. After lipid extraction, reconstitution of superoxide-dependent chemotactic activity is observed only in the presence of serum albumin. The chemotactic activity appears to follow the reduction by superoxide of a hydroperoxy fatty acid bound to serum albumin (Ref. 186). Binding to serum albumin may in fact stabilize the chemotactic product. These observations imply that neutrophils can amplify their initial response to an inflammatory stimulus via secretion of superoxide and activation of a neutrophil chemotactic factor of plasma, which helps to explain the anti-inflammatory action of exogenous CuZn-SOD. It would seem that superoxide-dependent generation of chemotactic activity occurs despite the presence of ceruloplasmin in plasma. This is consistent with the observation that ceruloplasmin (which is one of the acute phase proteins) does not have specific SOD activity (Ref. 187).

Other leukocyte chemotactic factors of fatty acid origin are known (Ref. 186). The lipoxygenase products of the arachidonic acid cascade, hydroperoxyicosatetrenoic acid (HPETE) and its reduction product, hydroxyicosatetrenoic acid (HETE), are chemotactic, HETE being more potent (Ref. 188). Superoxide-generating systems in vitro produce a potent neutrophil chemotactic factor from purified arachidonic acid by a process dependent upon oxygen activation beyond the stage of superoxide formation (Refs. 189,190). The significance of this type of reaction in vivo remains to be established. It is possible that this type of chemotactic factor and superoxide-dependent chemotactic factor of plasma are somehow related (Ref. 186).

The phagocytic cells are secretory organs of inflammation. Up to the stage of phagosome formation granulocytes liberate superoxide, products of the arachidonic acid cascade, and lysosomal enzymes particularly neutral proteinases (see Ref. 190). Superoxide promotes early death of granulocytes (Ref. 191), degradation of synovial fluid (Refs. 192,193), and breakdown of cartilage collagen (Ref. 194) in vitro. It is difficult, however, to assess the exact role of the radical in inflammatory injury in vivo.

This problem has been investigated by Del Maestro et al. (Ref. 195) in the microvasculature of the hamster cheek pouch utilizing exogenous superoxide generated by xanthine oxidase. Increased permeability to macromolecules (FITC-dextran 150), occasional petechial hemorrhages, and alterations of granulocyte behavior were observed in postcapillary veules. Macromolecular extravasation was decreased by CuZn-SOD, catalase, DMSO or L-methionine, indicating the participation of various active oxygen species in the endothelial injury. The alterations of granulocyte behavior included increased rolling frequency, decreased velocity, and increased adhesion to the endothelium. These phenomena were inhibited by CuZn-SOD, while catalase or L-methionine showed no effect. Petechial hemorrhages increased both macromolecular extravasation and granulocyte adhesion to the endothelium. Lipid peroxidation, consequent to hydroxyl radical formation from superoxide by a Haber-Weiss process, was evoked to explain the (initial) endothelial injury. The alterations of granulocyte behavior were attributed to a superoxide-dependent factor. In fact similar behavior was observed with plasma previously exposed to superoxide (generated by xanthine oxidase), and a parallel was drawn with the superoxide-dependent chemotactic factor of plasma (Ref. 186). The suggestion of lipid peroxidation, initiated by hydroxyl radical, as a mechanism of tissue (endothelial) injury in inflammation needs experimental verification. A metal-catalyzed Haber-Weiss reaction is feasible under the conditions of phagocyte-mediated inflammation, with transferrin (Ref. 196) or granulocyte lactoferrin (Refs. 197,198) as the catalyst. A role of SOD as an anti-inflammatory agent would then be to prevent hydroxyl radical production by interception of superoxide.

The therapeutic potential of SOD (bovine CuZn-SOD, orgotein) in inflammatory disease has begun to emerge, particularly in rheumatoid arthritis and osteoarthritis (Ref. 199). Rheumatoid arthritis is the clinical model, *par excellence*, of chronic phagocyte-mediated inflammation (Ref. 200). While cellular immune reactions predominate in rheumatoid synovial tissue (pannus) and participate in cartilage and bone erosion, in synovial fluid there is a continuous interaction of granulocytes with immune complexes which propagates the tissue injury. Scudder et al. (Ref. 201) found no consistent alteration in erythrocyte SOD activity in rheumatoid arthritis. However, Rister et al. (Ref. 202,203) found a decrease in polymorphonuclear leukocyte SOD in juvenile rheumatoid arthritis.

The therapeutic efficacy of CuZn-SOD in rheumatoid arthritis is supported by double-blind, placebo-controlled trials (Ref. 199) but, as yet, it is not known how far it meets the stringent criterion of radiological assessment over a long period, which is needed to show whether a drug favorably affects the course of rheumatoid arthritis (Ref. 204). The finding that corticosteroids suppress leukocyte superoxide production (Refs. 205,206) is of considerable interest in relation to initiation and progression of rheumatoid inflammation. There is evidence that prednisolone has a markedly favorable effect (not shown by cortisone) on the manifestations of early rheumatoid arthritis, which gives the impression of a drug able to prevent the initiation of an inflammation that it cannot suppress once started (Ref. 207). This is a point to be considered in relation to the anti-inflammatory action of CuZn-SOD. The enzyme appears to produce a polymorphonuclear leukocytosis when given systematically (Ref. 208). This would be an advantage if exogenous CuZn-SOD protects granulocytes against premature lysis or leakage *in situ* during phagocytosis in vivo. Interaction of CuZn-SOD with cell membranes (Refs. 209-211) may be invoked to explain its observed protective effect on human neutrophils (Ref. 191) and leaky Duchenne dystrophic muscle cells (Ref. 212) which show normal intracellular CuZn-SOD (Ref. 213), in vitro, but further studies with probing of the cell membrane and the stimulus-secretion mechanism of neutrophils (see Ref. 190), are desirable.

An interesting feature of rheumatoid arthritis is the consistently low serum histidine concentration, which appears to be related to the activity of the disease (Refs. 204,214). It is reasonable to inquire whether the low serum histidine is related to scavenging of active oxygen species at the sites of inflammation. Histidine is regarded as a (nonspecific) scavenger of singlet oxygen, a thermodynamically feasible product of the Haber-Weiss reaction. For the purposes of the present discussion, it is immaterial whether histidine scavenges singlet oxygen or hydroxyl radicals or both (Ref. 215). Among the commonly used drugs in rheumatoid arthritis (excluding CuZn-SOD) only D-penicillamine appears to have the ability to restore the serum histidine concentration to near normality with long term treatment (Ref. 204). It is desirable to know whether CuZn-SOD has a similar action since D-penicillamine may exert an SOD-mimetic action (Refs. 216,217) and, thereby, a histidine-sparing effect by intercepting superoxide and the formation of Haber-Weiss products.

Photochemically or enzymatically generated superoxide produces chromosome breaks and rearrangements in normal lymphocyte cultures which do not occur in the presence of SOD (Refs. 16,218). Exogenous SOD (and catalase) prevent radiation-induced chromosome breaks in lymphocyte cultures (Refs. 219,220) and spontaneously occurring chromosome breaks in cultures from patients with Fanconi's anemia (Ref. 221) or Werner's syndrome (Refs. 222). Erythrocytes (on a corpuscular basis) and fibroblasts have been found to have normal SOD levels in Fanconi's anemia and ataxia telangiectasia, another condition with spontaneous chromosome breakage (Refs. 223-225). Erythrocyte SOD per gram hemoglobin is decreased by a factor of about 0.7 in Fanconi's anemia (Ref. 226) but it is doubtful whether SOD deficiency plays an important role in this condition. The proportional effect of exogenous SOD in reducing the frequency of micronuclei is similar in normal and Fanconi fibroblasts for both spontaneous and mitomycin C-induced chromosomal breakage in tissue culture (Ref. 227).

Apart from the chromosome breakage syndromes, increased chromosome breakage is also a frequent finding in blood cultures from patients with progressive systematic sclerosis (scleroderma), systematic lupus erythematosus, rheumatoid arthritis, dermatomyositis, and periarteritis nodosa (Ref. 218). Emerit et al. (Ref. 228) discovered clastogenic activity in the serum of patients with progressive systematic sclerosis. So far sera from patients with systematic lupus erythematosus and rheumatoid arthritis have also been shown to possess clastogenic activity (Ref. 218). It is not clear whether the same clastogenic factor is present in these diseases. In rheumatoid arthritis the clastogenic activity can be higher in synovial fluid than in serum. Ultrafiltration indicates that the clastogenic activity is associated with a factor (or factors) in the molecular weight range 1000-10,000 daltons. The activity is destroyed by heating above 50°C and by ribonuclease but not by proteolytic enzymes (Ref. 218).

The chromosome aberration rate in blood cultures in the diseases under consideration appears to follow the order: systemic lupus erythematosus > progressive systemic sclerosis > rheumatoid arthritis. The abberation rate is higher in blood cultures than in lymphocyte cultures, and is consistently reduced by exogenous SOD. Other agents which reduce the aberration rate in blood cultures include D-penicillamine (tested in rheumatoid arthritis (Ref. 218)) and L-cysteine (tested in progressive systemic sclerosis (Ref. 219)). Exogenous SOD also reduces to nearly normal values the aberration rates produced in blood cultures of healthy subjects by clastogenic factor from patients. Lymphocyte extracts in systemic lupus erythematosus and rheumatoid arthritis have a clastogenic effect not found

with normal lymphocytes. The clastogenic factor is released into the culture
medium, since co-cultivation of clastogenic (systemic lupus erythematosus; female
patient) and normal lymphocytes (male subject) increases the chromosome aberration
rate (by 26-31%) in the normal cells. Sister chromatid exchanges (in the presence
of bromo-deoxyuridine) are higher than normal in blood cultures from patients with
progressive systemic sclerosis. Clastogenic factor from these patients and patients
with systemic lupus erythematosus increases the rate of sister chromatid exchanges
in normal blood cultures. SOD inhibits this effect (Ref. 218).

Normal lymphocytes show a very low basal production of superoxide (as measured
by NBT reduction), which is stimulated by phytohemagglutinin (used to stimulate
cell division in cultures) and further elevated by clastogenic factor. The maximal
rate over a thirty minute period is 2.1×10^4 molecules per cell per second (Ref.
16), which is only 0.4% of the rate for activated granulocytes. Michelson (Ref. 16)
has suggested that increased production of superoxide (or secondarily of hydroxyl
radicals) induced by clastogenic factor might cause chromosome damage.

Whole body gamma-irradiation has been found to result in the appearance of
clastogenic activity in the serum (together with decrease of erythrocyte SOD and
increase of GSH-Px activity) in cases of accidental overdosage (above 600 rads).
Gamma-irradiation (400-1200 rads) of whole blood (but not of plasma) in vitro
results in the appearance of clastogenic factor with molecular weight in the
range 1000-10,000 daltons (Ref. 16,218). This implicates blood cells as a
source of clastogenic factor.

In an animal model of immune-complex disease, the New Zealand black (NZB)
mouse, increased chromosome breakage in blood cultures is associated with the
presence of a clastogenic factor in serum (also present in the supernatant of
fibroblast cultures), which is active towards human lymphocytes. Treatment of
NZB mice with bovine CuZn-SOD by subcutaneous injection produces on average a
70% decrease in chromosome breakages in blood cultures (Ref. 16). Administration
of CuZn-SOD mitigates the immune-complex glomerulonephritis to which these animals
are genetically susceptible (Ref. 199). Intramuscular injections of bovine CuZn-SOD
also decreased the chromosome aberration rate in blood cultures in a case of
severe systemic lupus erythematosus (with symptomatic improvement) and in three
cases of rheumatoid arthritis (without symptomatic improvement although there
was diminished consumption of complement) (Ref. 230).

It is sufficiently clear that exogenous SOD inhibits the expression of clastogenic activity. It is difficult to understand the action of clastogenic factor
in terms of chromosome damage by oxygen-free radicals (Ref. 16), given a sufficient
degree of radical production, unless it is assumed (to take one difficulty) that
intracellular SOD exerts no protective function even in normal lymphocytes. Although
discordant values have been reported for leukocytes (see Ref. 231), SOD activity
in human blood cells would appear to follow the order: erythrocytes < granulocytes

< lymphocytes (non-T lymphocytes < T lymphocytes) (Refs. 101,232), so that significant scavenging of superoxide can be predicted for lymphocytes. It does not seem likely that the intracellular SOD is overwhelmed in view of the low rate of (extracellular) superoxide production associated with the conditions of chromosome breakage (Ref. 16). Pending observations to the contrary, it can be suggested that clastogenic factor enhances a surface (or subsurface) production of superoxide promoted by phyto-hemagglutinin (by themselves lectins trigger only weak superoxide production in granulocytes (Ref. 233)), which activates a clastogenic pathway involving the factor. This would explain the action of exogenous SOD without the need to invoke a transmembrane effect. Clastogenic activity is higher in blood cultures than in lymphocyte cultures (Ref. 218), suggesting that in blood cultures activation of a clastogenic pathway at the surface of lymphocytes may be facilitated by additional factors in blood.

SUPEROXIDE DISMUTASE AND MALIGNANCY

The current view that malignancy is associated with decrease or loss of mito-chondrial Mn-SOD activity (Ref. 234) arose from the observation that human lung fibroblast WI-38 cells transformed by SV-40 virus have very little or no Mn-SOD (cyanide-insensitive SOD) activity although their total SOD activity is somewhat elevated (Ref. 235). Subsequently Dionisi et al. (Ref. 236) showed that fast-growing experimental tumors of the rat and mouse (Ehrlich ascites tumor (Lettre) mutant and Morris hepatoma 3924A) lack mitochondrial SOD. Loss or decrease of Mn-SOD has been demonstrated in various animal tumors (with the possible exception of mouse neuroblastoma)(Ref. 234) and in human myelocytic, monocytic and lympho-cytic leukemia (Refs. 237-239). It remains to be seen to what extent the generalization that malignancy is associated with decrease or loss of Mn-SOD can be made. A preliminary report (Ref. 16) indicates that in human breast cancer Mn-SOD (and CuZn-SOD) can be high when tumor tissue is compared with normal tissue from the same patient (in one patient Mn-SOD was elevated by a factor of 4.2 and CuZn-SOD was elevated by a factor of 2.1). Overall, Mn-SOD values appear to show wide dispersion without clear tendency to lie outside the upper or lower limits of the normal range. CuZn-SOD values also appear to show wide dispersion but with a clear tendency to exceed the upper limit of the normal range. These findings indicate that in assessment of SOD activity in human cancer, which may be of value in relation to radiation sensitivity (Ref. 240), the normal tissue of the patient may provide the best base-line. Another factor to be taken into consideration is that SOD activity may be higher at the margin than at the center of a tumor, as found by Petkau et al. (Ref. 241) for experimental rat mammary carcinoma.

With regard to CuZn-SOD, the hypothesis that this enzyme is lowered in tumor cells (together with Mn-SOD) (Ref. 242) is supported by observations on various animal tumors (Ref. 234). However, this is not a universal feature of tumors since CuZn-SOD activity is increased in transformed WI-38 fibroblast cells (Ref. 23 mouse L1210 leukemia cells (Ref. 234), human leukemia cells (Refs. 237,238), and cases of human breast cancer (as already noted). The CuZn-SOD activity of squamous cell epithelioma is about 65% of that of normal human epidermis (Ref. 234). In human tumors the level of CuZn-SOD appears to be lower in those tumors which respond to radiation therapy than in those resistant to radiation (Ref. 240).

Deficiency of Mn-SOD has been proposed as a cancerous phenotype (Ref. 234). Certain syndromes, namely, trisomy 21 (Ref. 244) and the Dubin-Johnson-Sprinz syndrome (Ref. 245), are known to be associated with increased risk of malignancy. Deficiency of Mn-SOD has been demonstrated in platelets in trisomy 21 and in liver biopsy specimens in the Dubin-Johnson-Sprinz syndrome (Ref. 246), but it is not clear that this SOD deficiency predisposes to malignancy.

Oberley and Buettner (Ref. 234) have suggested that lowered CuZn-SOD activity, which is characteristic of many tumors, may be related to the potential of tumors for cell division. This view is supported by the observation of low CuZn-SOD activity in rapidly dividing cell systems whether normal (regenerating mouse liver) or malignant (mouse H6 hepatoma). Low rates of lipid peroxidation are observed in tumor mitochondrial and microsomal membranes (see Ref. 247). NADPH-dependent lipid peroxidation of microsomal membranes, microsomal generation of superoxide, and content of microsomal electron carriers are lower than normal in rat and mouse hepatomas, with rapidly diminishing values in the faster growing tumors. Microsomal lipid peroxidation induced by superoxide (generated by xanthine oxidase) or ascorbate follows a similar trend. In rapidly growing hepatoma microsomal lipid-to-protein ratio and degree of fatty acid unsaturation are decreased, and loss-of-freedom-of-motion parameters of spin labels incorporated in microsomal lipid are increased in value to a greater extent than in slowly growing hepatoma. Cytosolic SOD is lower in rapidly growing than in slowly growing hepatoma, and GSH-Px and catalase activity appear to follow the same trend. These observations predict a low availability of lipid peroxidase in tumor cells, which may contribute to the maintenance of uncontrolled mitotic activity (see Ref. 247). A comparative test of this hypothesis in normal, regenerating, and malignant liver cells is worthy of consideration.

ACKNOWLEDGMENT

The author is grateful to the Wellcome Trust for a Research Fellowship.

REFERENCES

1. Mann, T. and Keilin, D. (1939) Proc. Roy. Soc. B., 126, 305-315.
2. Markowitz, H., Cartwright, G.E., and Wintrobe, M.M. (1959) J. Biol. Chem., 234, 40-45.
3. Carrico, R.J. and Deutsch, H.F. (1969) J. Biol. Chem., 244, 6087-6093.
4. Carrico, R.J. and Deutsch, H.F. (1970) J. Biol. Chem., 245, 723-727.
5. McCord, J.M. and Fridovich, I. (1969) J. Biol. Chem., 244, 6049-6095.
6. Fridovich, I. (1975) Ann. Rev. Biochem., 44, 147-159.
7. Weisiger, R.A. and Fridovich, I. (1973) J. Biol. Chem., 248, 3582-3592.
8. Harris, J.I. and Steinman, H.M. (1977) in Superoxide and Superoxide Dismutases, Michelson, A.M., McCord, J.M., and Fridovich, I., eds., London: Academic Press, pp. 225-230.
9. McCord, J.M., Boyle, J.A., Day, E.D., Jr., Rizzolo, L.J., and Salin, M.L. (1977) in Superoxide and Superoxide Dismutases, Michelson, A.M., McCord, J.M., and Fridovich, I., eds., London: Academic Press, pp. 129-138.
10. Holme, E., Bankel, L., Lundberg, P.-A. and Waldenstron, J. (1980) in Biological and Clinical Aspects of Superoxide and Superoxide Dismutase, Bannister, W.H. and Bannister, J.V., eds., New York: Elsevier/North Holland, pp. 262-270.
11. Brewer, G.J. (1967) Am. J. Hum. Genet., 19, 674-680.
12. Baur, E.W. and Schoor, R.T. (1969) Science, 166; 1524-;525.
13. Fried, R., Fried, L.W., and Babin, D. (1970) Eur. J. Biochem., 16, 399-406.
14. Huber, W., Schulte, T., Carson, S., Goldhamer, R., and Vogin, E. (1968) Toxicol. Appl. Pharmacol., 12, 308-309.
15. Michelson, A.M., Puget, K., Durosay, P., and Bonneau, J.C. (1977) in Superoxide and Superoxide Dismutases, Michelson, A.M., McCord, J.M., and Fridovich, I., eds., London: Academic Press, pp. 467-499.
16. Michelson, A.M. (1979) in Metalloproteins, Weser, U., ed., Stuttgart: Georg Theime Verlag, pp. 88-116.
17. Beauchamp, C. and Fridovich, I. (1971) Anal. Biochem., 44, 276-287.
18. Lippitt, B. and Fridovich, I. (1973) Arch. Biochem. Biophys., 159, 738-741.
19. Beckman, G., Lundgren, E., and Tarnvik, A. (1973) Hum. Hered., 23, 338-343.
20. Kirjarinta, M., Fellman, J., Gustafson, C., Keisala, E., and Eriksson, A.W. (1969) Scand. J. Clin. Lab. Invest., 22, Suppl. 108, 46.
21. Ritter, H. and Wendt, G.G. (1971) Humangenetik, 14, 72.
22. Welch, S.G. and Mears, G.W. (1972) Hum. Hered., 22, 38-41
23. Beckman, G. (1973) Hereditas, 73, 305-310.
24. Beckman, G., Beckman, L., and Nilsson, L.-O. (1973) Hereditas, 75, 138-139.
25. Beckman, G. and Pakarinen, A. (1973) Humn. Hered. 23, 346-351.
26. Eriksson, A.W. (1974) in Genetic Polymorphisms and Diseases in Man, Ramot, B., Bonne, B., Goodman, R.M., and Szeinberg, A., eds., London: Academic Press, pp. 30-44.
27. Carter, N.D., Auton, J.A., Welch, S.G., Marshall, W.H., and Fraser, G.R. (1976) Hum. Hered., 26, 4-7.
28. Shinoda, T. (1970) Jap. J. Hum. Genet., 15, 144-152.
29. Harris, H., Hopkinson, D.A., and Robson, E.B. (1973) Ann. Hum. Genet., 37, 237-253.
30. Crosti, N., Serra, A., Cagiano-Malvezzi, D., and Tagliaferri, I. (1976) Ann. Hum. Biol., 3, 343-350.
31. Papiha, S.S. and Al-Agidi, S.K. (1976) Hum. Hered., 26, 394-400.
32. Teng, Y.B. and Lie-Injo, L.E. (1977) Hum. Genet., 36, 231-234.
33. Simeoni, E. and Gruener, O. (1979) Beitr. Gerichtl. Med., 37, 307-311.
34. Beckman, G., Beckman, L. and Nilsson, L.-O. (1975) Hereditas, 79, 43-46.
35. Marklund, S., Beckman, G. and Stigbrand, T. (1976) Eur. J. Biochem., 65, 415-422.
36. Shinoda, T., Matsunaga, E. and Koshinaga, J. (1974) Jap. J. Hum. Genet., 19, 243-250.
37. Tan, S.G. and Teng, Y.S. (1978) Jap. J. Hum. Genet., 23, 133-138.

38. Tan, Y.H., Tischfield, J. and Ruddle, F.H. (1973) J. Exp. Med., 137, 317-330.
39. Francke, U. and Taggart, R.T. (1979) Proc. Natl. Acad. Sci. USA, 76, 5230-5233.
40. Cox, D.R., Epstein, L.B., and Epstein, C.J. (1980) Proc. Natl. Acad. Sci. USA, 77, 2168-2172.
41. Creagan, R., Tischfield, J., Riciutti, F., and Ruddle, F.H. (1973) Humangenetik, 20-203-209.
42. Smith, M., Turner, B.M., Tanigaki, N., and Hirschhorn, K. (1978) Cytogenet. Cell, Genet., 22, 428-233.
43. Aula, P., Leisti, J. and Von Koskull, H. (1973) Clin. Genet., 4, 241-251.
44. Sichitiu, S., Sinet, P.M., Lejeune, J., and Frezal, J. (1974) Humangenetik, 23, 65-72.
45. Sinet, P.M., Allard, D., LeJeune, J., and Jerome, H. (1974) C.R. Acad. Sci., Ser. D., 278, 3276-3270.
46. Priscu, R. and Sichitiu, S. (1975) Humangenetik, 29, 79-83.
47. Gilles, L., Ferradini, C., Foos, J., Pucheault, J., Allard, D., Sinet, P.M. and Jerome, H. (1976) FEBS Lett., 69, 55-58.
48. Crosti, N., Serra, A., Rigo, A., and Viglino, P. (1976) Hum. Genet., 31, 197-202.
49. Frants, R.R., Eriksson, A.W., Jongbloet, P.H., and Hammers, A.J. (1975) Lancet, ii, 42-43.
50. Sinet, P.M., Lavelle, F., Michelson, A.M., and Jerome, H. (1975) Biochem. Biophys. Res. Commun., 67, 904-909.
51. Feaster, W.W., Kwok, L.W., and Epstein, C.J. (1977) Am. J. Hum. Genet., 29, 563-570.
52. Sinet, P.M., Couturier, J., Dutrillaux, B., Poissonnier, M., Raoul, O., Rethore, M.O., Allard, D., Lejeune, J., and Jerome, H. (1976) Exp. Cell. Res., 97, 47-55.
53. Sinet, P.M. (1977) in Superoxide and Superoxide Dismutases, Michelson, A.M., McCord, J.M. and Fridovich, I., eds., London: Academic Press, pp. 459-465.
54. Philip, T., Fraisse, J., Sinet, P.M., Lauras, B., Robert, J.M., and Freycon, F. (1978) Cytogenet. Cell. Genet., 22, 521-523.
55. Yamamoto, Y., Ogasawara, N., Gotoh, A., Komiya, H., Nakai, H., and Kuroki, Y. (1979) Hum. Genet., 48, 321-327.
56. Garber, P., Sinet, P.M., Jerome, H., and LeJeune, J. (1979) Lancet, ii; 914-915.
57. Kedziora, J., Bartosz, G., Leyko, W., and Rozynkowa, D. (1979) Lancent, i, 105.
58. Hagemeijer, A. and Smit, E.M.E. (1977) Hum. Genet., 38, 15-23.
59. Boveris, A. (1977) Adv. Exp. Med. Biol., 78, 67-82.
60. Boveris, A. and Turrens, J.F. (1980) in Chemical and Biochemical Aspects of Superoxide and Superoxide Dismutase, Bannister, J.V. and Hill, H.A.O., ed., New York: Elsevier/North Holland, pp. 84-91.
61. Harman, D. (1972) J. Am. Geriatr. Soc., 20, 145-147.
62. Owens, D., Dawson, J.C., and Losin, S. (1971) Am. J. Ment. Defic., 75, 602-612.
63. Burger, P.C. and Vogel, F.S. (1973) Am. J. Pathol., 73, 457-476.
64. Schneider, E.L. and Epstein, C.J. (1972) Proc. Soc. Exp. Biol. Med., 141, 1092-1094.
65. Segal, D.J. and McCoy, E.E. (1974) J. Cell. Physiol., 83, 85-90.
66. Martin, G.M., Sprague, C.A., and Epstein, C.J. (1970) Lab. Invest., 23, 86-92.
67. Orgel, L.E. (1963) Proc. Natl. Acad. Sci. USA, 49, 517-529.
68. Harley, C.B., Pollard, J.W., Chamberlain, J.W., Stanners, C.P., and Goldstein, S. (1980) Proc. Natl. Acad. Sci. USA, 77, 1885-1889.
69. Sinet, P.M., Jejeune, J. and Jerome, H. (1979) Life Sci., 24, 29-33.
70. Carrell, R.W., Winterbourn, C.C., and Rachmilewitz, E.A. (1975) Br. J. Haematol., 30, 259-264.
71. Cohen, G. and Hochstein, P. (1963) Biochemistry, 2, 1420-1428.
72. Oshino, N. and Chance, B. (1977) in Biochemical and Medical Aspects of Active Oxygen, Hayaishi, O. and Asada, K., eds., Tokyo: University of Tokyo Press, pp. 191-207.

73. Flohe, L. (1979) in Oxygen Free Radicals and Tissue Damage, Ciba Found. Symp. 65 (new ser.), Amsterdam: Excerpta Medica, 95-113.
74. Sinet, P.M., Michelson, A.M., Bazin, A., Lejeune, J., and Jerome, H. (1975) Biochem. Biophys. Res. Commun., 67, 910-915.
75. Pantelakis, S.N., Karaklis, A.G., Alexiou, D., Vardas, E., and Valaes, T. (1970) Am. J. Hum. Genet., 22, 184-193.
76. Sparkes, R.S. and Baughan, M.A. (1969) Am. J. Hum. Genet., 21, 430-439.
77. Layzer, R.B. and Epstein, C.J. (1972) Am. J. Hum. Genet., 24, 533-543.
78. Donald, L.J., Wang, H.S. and Hamerton, J.L. (1979) Cytogenet. Cell Genet., 23, 141-143.
79. Corberand, J., DeLarrard, B., Pris, J., and Colombies, P. (1974) Nouv. Rev. Fr. Hematol., 14, 298-301.
80. Humbert, J.R., Marks, M.I., Hathaway, W.E., and Thoren, Ch. H. (1971) Pediatrics, 48, 259-267.
81. Humbert, J.R., Kurtz, M.L., and Hathaway, W.E. (1970) Pediatrics, 45, 125-128.
82. Babior, B.M., Kipnes, R.S., and Curnutte, J.T. (1973) J. Clin. Invest., 52, 741-744.
83. Baehner, R.L., Boxer, L.A., and Davis, J. (1976) Blood, 48, 309-313.
84. Humbert, J.R., Solomons, C.C., and Ott, J.E. (1971) J. Pediatr., 78, 648-653.
85. Winterbourn, C.C., Hawkins, R.E., Brian, M., and Carrell, R.W. (1975) J. Lab. Clin. Med., 85, 337-341.
86. Autor, A.P., Frank, L., and Roberts, R.J. (1976) Pediatr. Res., 10, 154-158.
87. Legge, M., Brain, M., Winterbourn, C., and Carrell, R. (1977) Aust. Paediatr. J., 13, 25-28.
88. Del Villano, B.C., Tischfield, J.A., Schacter, L.P., Stilwill, D., and Miller, S.I. (1979) Alcohol. Clin. Exp. Res., 3, 291-296.
89. Del Villano, B.C., Miller, S.I., Schacter, L.P., and Tischfield, J.A. (1980) Science, 207, 991-993.
90. Dreosti, I.E. and Record, I.R. (1979) Br. J. Nutr., 41, 399-402.
91. Utsumi, K., Yoshioka, T., Yamanaka, N., and Nakazawa, T. (1977) FEBS Lett., 79, 1-3.
92. Ueda, K. and Ogata, M. (1978) Acta. Med. Okayama, 32, 393-397.
93. Stevens, C., Goldblatt, M.J., and Freedman, J.C. (1975) Mech. Ageing Dev., 4, 415-421.
94. Joenje, H., Frants, R.R., Arwert, F., and Eriksson, A.W. (1978) Mech. Ageing Dev., 8, 265-267.
95. Misra, H.P. and Fridovich, I. (1972) J. Biol. Chem., 247, 3170-3175.
96. Duncan, M.R., Dell'Orco, R.T., and Kirk, K.D. (1979) J. Cell. Physiol., 98, 437-441.
97. Somville, M. and Remacle, J. (1980) in Biological and Clinical Aspects of Superoxide and Superoxide Dismutase, Bannister, W.H. and Bannister, J.V., eds., New York: Elsevier/North Holland, pp. 292-293.
98. Van Hien, P., Kovacs, K., and Matkovics, B. (1974) Enzyme, 18, 341-347.
99. Sekiba, K. and Yoshioka, T. (1979) Am. J. Obstet. Gynecol., 135, 368-371.
100. Matkovics, B., Fodor, I. and Kovacs, K. (1975) Enzyme, 19, 285-293.
101. Kobayashi, Y., Ishigame, K., Ishigame, Y., and Usui, T. (1977) in Biochemical and Medical Aspects of Active Oxygen, Hayaishi, O. and Asada, K., eds., Tokyo: University of Tokyo Press, pp. 261-274.
102. Yoshioka, T., Sugiue, A., Shimada, T., and Utsumi, K. (1979) Biol. Neonate, 36, 173-180.
103. Bonta, B.W., Gawron, E.R., and Warshaw, J.B. (1977) Pediatr. Res., 11, 754-757.
104. Arey, L.B. (1965) Developmental Anatomy, Saunders, Philadelphia, 7th ed., p. 104.
105. Frank, L., Autor, A.P., and Roberts, R.J. (1977) J. Pediatr., 90, 105-110.
106. Roberts, R.J. (1979) J. Pediatr., 95, 904-909.
107. Stevens, J.B. and Autor, A.P. (1977) J. Biol. Chem., 252, 3509-3514.
108. Stevens, J.B. and Autor, A.P. (1977) Lab. Invest., 37, 470-478.
109. Autor, A.P. and Stevens, J.B. (1978) Photochem. Photobiol., 28, 775-780.

110. Autor, A.P. and Stevens, J.B. (1980) in Chemical and Biological Aspects of Superoxide and Superoxide Dismutase, Bannister, J.V. and Hill, H.A.O., eds., New York: Elsevier/North Holland, pp. 104-115.
111. Crapo, J.D. and Tierney, D.F. (1974) Am. J. Physiol., 226, 1401-1407.
112. Kimball, R.E., Reddy, K., Pierce, T.H., Schwartz, L.W., Mustafa, M.G., and Cross, C.E. (1976) Am. J. Physiol., 230, 1425-1431.
113. Sjostrom, K. and Crapo, J.D. (1978) The Physiologist, 21, 111.
114. Misra, H.P. and Fridovich, I. (1972) J. Biol. Chem., 247, 6960-6962.
115. Wever, R., Oudega, B. and Van Gelder, B.F. (1973) Biochim. Biophys. Acta, 302, 475-478.
116. Wallace, W.J., Maxwell, J.C. and Caughey, W.S. (1974) Biochem. Biophys. Res. Commun., 57, 1104-1110.
117. Brunori, M., Falcioni, G., Fioretti, E., Giardina, B. and Rotilio, G. (1975) Eur. J. Biochem., 53, 99-104.
118. Lynch, R.E., Lee, G.R., and Cartwright, G.E. (1976) J. Biol. Chem., 251, 1015-1019.
119. Winterbourn, C.C., McGrath, B.M., and Carrell, R.W. (1976) Biochem. J., 155, 493-502.
120. Miura, T., Ogawa, N., and Ogiso, T. (1978) Chem. Pharm. Bull., 26, 1261-1266.
121. Gotoh, T. and Shikama, K. (1976) J. Biochem., 80, 397-399.
122. Rotilio, G., Fioretti, E., Falcioni, G., and Brunori, M. (1977) in Superoxide and Superoxide Dismutases, Michelson, A.M., McCord, J.M. and Fridovich, I., eds., London: Academic Press, pp. 239-244.
123. Fridovich, I. (1979) in Oxygen Free Radicals and Tissue Damage, Ciba Found. Symp. 65 (new series), Amsterdam: Excerpta Medica, pp. 1-4.
124. Michelson, A.M. and Durosay, P. (1977) Photochem. Photobiol., 25, 55-63.
125. Chow, C.K. (1975) Am. J. Clin. Nutr., 28, 756-760.
126. Necheles, T.F. (1964) in Glutathione, Flohe, L., Benohr, H. Ch., Sies, H., Waller, H.D., and Wendenl, A., eds., Stuttgart: Georg Thieme Verlag, pp. 173-180.
127. Leipzig, R.M., Brewer, G.J., and Oelshlegel, F.J., Jr., (1975) in Isozymes, 3rd Int. Conf., Vol. 2, Markert, C., ed., London, Academic Press, pp. 667-679.
128. Takahara, S. and Ogata, M. (1977) in Biochemical and Medical Aspects of Active Oxygen, Hayaishi O and Asada, K., eds., Tokyo: University of Tokyo Press, pp. 275-297.
129. Zannos-Mariolea, L., Tzortzatou, F., Dendaki-Svolaki, K., Katerellos, Ch., Kavallari, M., and Matsaniotis, N. (1974) Br. J. Haematol., 26, 193-199.
130. Winterhalter, K.H. (1979) in Oxygen Free Radicals and Tissue Damage, Ciba Found. Symp. 65 (new ser.), Amsterdam: Excerpta Medica, p. 74 (discussion).
131. Concetti, A., Massei, P., Rotilio, G., Brunori, M., and Rachmilewitz, E.A. (1976) J. Lab. Clin. Med., 87, 1057-1064.
132. Stocks, J., Kemp, M., and Dormandy, T.L. (1971) Lancet, i, 266-269.
133. Goldstein, B.D. (1979) in Oxygen Free Radicals and Tissue Damage, Ciba Found. Symp. 65 (new series), Amsterdam: Excerpta Medica, p. 73 (discussion)
134. Winterhalter, K.H. (1979) in Oxygen Free Radicals and Tissue Damage, Ciba Found. Symp. 65 (new ser.), Amsterdam: Excerpta Medica, pp. 89-90 (discussion).
135. Sandoz Atlas of Haematology (1973) Undritz, E., ed., Basle: Sandoz Ltd., 2nd edition, Fig. 23 A, B.
136. Rotilio, G., Rigo, A., Bracci, R., Bagnoli, F., Sargentini, I., and Brunori, M. (1977) Clin. Chim. Acta, 81, 131-134.
137. Necheles, T.F., Rai, U.S. and Valaes, T. (1976) Acta Paediatr. Scand., 65, 361-367.
138. Claireaux, A.E. (1960) Br. Med. J., i, 1528-1534.
139. Bracci, R., Ciccoli, L., Falciani, G., De Donno, M., and Dettori, M. (1978) Boll. Soc. Ital. Biol. Sper., 54, 879-882.
140. Gross, R.T., Bracci, R., Rudolph, N., Schroeder, E., and Kochen, J.A. (1967) Blood, 29, 481-493.
141. Emerson, P.M., Mason, D.Y., and Cuthbert, J.E. (1972) Br. J. Haematol., 22, 667-680.

142. Oski, F.A. and Barness, L.A. (1967) J. Pediatr., 70, 211-220.
143. Das, S.K. and Nair, R.C. (1980) Br. J. Haematol., 44, 87-92.
144. Rotilio, G., Bray, R.C., and Fielden, E. M. (1972) Biochim. Biophys. Acta, 268, 605-609.
145. Kobayashi, Y., Okhata, S., Tanabe, K., Tanaka, Y., Ueda, K., and Usui, T. (1978) Hiroshima J. Med. Sci., 27, 181-183.
146. Goldstein, M.H., Churg, J., Strauss, L., and Gribetz, D. (1979) Nephron, 23, 263-272.
147. Gwyn Williams, D. (1979) Br. Med. J., ii, 183 (discussion).
148. O'Regan, S. and Fong, J.S.C. (1978) Med. Hypotheses, 4, 353-361.
149. O'Regan, S., Melhorn, D.K., Chesney, R.W., Kaplan, B.S., and Drummond, K.N. (1975) Pediatr., Res., 9, 377.
150. Loomis, T.C., Yee, G., and Stahl, W.L. (1976) Experientia, 32, 1374-1375.
151. Savolainen, H. (1978) Res. Commun. Chem. Pathol. Pharmacol., 21, 173-176.
152. Thomas, T.N., Priest, D.G., and Zemp, J.W. (1976) J. Neurochem., 27, 309-310.
153. Stahl, W.L. and Swanson, P.D. (1974) Neurology, 24, 813-819.
154. Koster, J.F., Slee, R.G., and Van Berkel, Th. J.C. (1980) in Biological and Clinical Aspects of Superoxide and Superoxide Dismutase, Bannister, W.H. and Bannister, J.V., eds., New York: Elsevier/North Holland, pp. 294-303.
155. Alexander, N.M. and Benson, G.D. (1975) Life Sci., 16, 1025-1032.
156. Bohnenkamp, W. and Weser, U. (1976) Biochim. Biophys. Acta, 444, 396-406.
157. Bohnenkamp, W. and Weser, U. (1977) in Superoxide and Superoxide Dismutases, Michelson, A.M., McCord, J.M., and Fridovich, I., eds., London: Academic Press, pp. 387-394.
158. Williams, D.M., Lynch, R.E., Lee, G.R., and Cartwright, G.E. (1975) Proc. Soc. Exp. Biol. Med., 149, 534-536.
159. Bettger, W.J., Fish, T.J., and O'Dell, B.L. (1978) Proc. Soc. Exp. Biol. Med., 158, 278-282.
160. Bettger, W.J., Savage, J.E., and O'Dell, B.L. (1979) Nurt. Repts. Int., 19, 893-900.
161. Paynter, D.I., Moir, R.J., and Underwood, E.J. (1979) J. Nutr., 109, 1570-1576.
162. DeRosa, G., Leach, R.M. and Hurley, L.S. (1978) Fed. Proc., 37, 594.
163. Dreosti, I.E. and Record, I.R. (1978) Br. J. Nutr., 40, 133-137.
164. Prohaska, J.R. and Wells, W.W. (1974) J. Neurochem., 23, 91-98.
165. Menkes, J.H., Alter, M., Steigleder, G.K., Weakley, D.R., and Sung, J.B. (1962) Pediatrics, 29, 764-779.
166. Hunt, D.M. (1974) Nature, 249, 852-854.
167. Hunt, D.M. (1977) Comp. Biochem. Physiol., 57C, 79-83.
168. Evans, G.W. (1977) Adv. Nutr. Res., 1, 167-187.
169. Fried, R. (1979) J. Neurosci. Res., 4, 435-441.
170. Golse, B., Debray, Q., Puget, K., and Michelson, A.M. (1978) Nouv. Press. Med., 7, 2070-2071.
171. Golse, B., Debray-Ritzen, P., Durosay, P., Puget, K., and Michelson, A.M. (1978) Rev. Neurol., 134, 699-705.
172. Marklund, S. and Plum, C.M. (1978) J. Neurochem., 31, 521-523.
173. Westermarck, T. (1977) Acta Pharmacol. Toxicol., 41, 121-128.
174. Sorgato, M.C., Sartorelli, L., Loschen, G., and Azzi, A. (1974) FEBS Lett., 45, 92-95.
175. Sanders, A.P., Hall, I.H., and Woodhall, B. (1965) Science, 150, 1830-1831.
176. Forman, H.J. and Kennedy, J. (1976) Arch. Biochem. Biophys., 173, 219-224.
177. Hexum, T.D. and Fried, R. (1979) Neurochem. Res., 4, 73-82.
178. Ehringer, H. and Hornykiewicz, O. (1960) Klin. Wochenschr., 38, 1236-1239.
179. Hill, H.A.O. (1979) in Oxygen Free Radicals and Tissue Damage, Ciba Found. Symp. 65 (new ser.), Amsterdam: Excerpta Medica, pp. 363-364 (discussion).
180. Neff, N.H., Barrett, R.E., and Costa, E. (1969) Experientia, 25, 1140-1141.
181. Curnutte, J.T., Kipnes, R.S., and Babior, B.M. (1975) N. Eng. J. Med., 293, 628-632.
182. Babior, B.M., Curnutte, J.T., and Kipnes, R.S. (1975) J. Clin. Invest., 56, 1035-1042.

236

183. Babior, B.M. (1979) Biochem. Biophys. Res. Commun., 91, 222-226.
184. McCord, J.M., Stokes, S.H., and Wong, K. (1979) Adv. Inflammation Res., 1, 278-280.
185. Oyanagui, Y. (1976) Biochem. Pharmacol., 25, 1465-1472.
186. Petrone, W.F., English, D.K., Wong, K., and McCord, J.M. (1980) Proc. Natl. Acad. Sci. USA, 77, 1159-1163.
187. Bannister, J.V., Bannister, W.H., Hill, H.A.O., Mahood, J.F., Willson, R.L., and Wolfenden, B.S. (1980) FEBS Lett., 118, 127-219.
188. Goetzl, E.J., Woods, J.M., and Gorman, R.R. (1977) J. Clin. Invest., 59, 179-183.
189. Perez, H.D. and Goldstein, I.M. (1979) Fed. Proc., 38, 1170.
190. Weissmann, G., Korchak, H.M., Perez, H.D., Smolen, J.E., Goldstein, I.M. and Hoffstein, S.T. (1979) Adv. Inflammation Res., 1, 95-112.
191. Salin, M.L. and McCord, J.M. (1975) J. Clin. Invest., 56, 1319-1323.
192. McCord, J.M. (1974) Science, 185, 529-531.
193. Puig-Parellada, P. and Planas, J.M. (1978) Biochem. Pharmacol., 27, 535-537.
194. Greenwald, R.A. and Moy, W.W. (1979) Arth. Rheum., 22, 251-259.
195. Del Maestro, R.F., Arfors, K.-E., Bjork, J., and Planker, M. (1980) in Biological and Clinical Aspects of Superoxide and Superoxide Dismutase Bannister, W.H. and Bannister, J.V., eds., Elsevier/North Holland, pp. 127-140.
196. McCord, J.M. and Day, E.D., Jr. (1978) FEBS Lett., 86, 139-142.
197. Ambruso, D.R. and Johnston, R.B., Jr. (1981) J. Clin. Invest., 67, 352-360.
198. Bannister, J.V., Bannister, W.H., Hill, H.A.O., and Thornally, P.J. (1982), Biochim. Biophys. Acta, 715, 116-120.
199. Huber, W. and Menander-Huber, K.B. (1980) in Clinics in Rheumatic Diseases, Anti-Rheumatic Drugs II, Huskisson, E.C., ed., London: Saunders, in press.
200. Bonta, I.L. and Parnham, M.J. (1978) Biochem. Pharmacol., 27, 1611-1623.
201. Scudder, P., Stocks, J. and Dormandy, T.L. (1976) Clin. Chim. Acta, 69, 397-403.
202. Rister, M., Bauermeister, K., Gravert, U., and Gladtke, E. (1978) Lancet, i, 1094.
203. Rister, M., Bauermeister, K., Gravert, U. and Gladtke, E. (1979) Eur. J. Pediatr., 130, 127-136.
204. Wright, V. and Amos, R. (1980) Br. Med. J., i, 964-966.
205. Nelson, D.H. and Ruhmann-Wennhold, A. (1978) J. Clin. Endocrinol. Metab., 46, 702-705.
206. Nelson, D.H., Meikle, A.W., Benowitz, B., Murray, D.K., and Ruhmann-Wennhold, A. (1978) Trans. Assoc. Am. Physicians, 91, 381-387.
207. West, H.F. (1980) Br. Med. J., i, 310.
208. Huber, W., Saifer, M.G.P., and Williams, I.D. (1980) in Biological and Clinical Aspects of Superoxide and Superoxide Dismutase, Bannister, W.H. and Bannister, J.V., eds., New York: Elsevier/North Holland, pp. 395-407.
209. Petkau, A. and Chelack, W.S. (1976) Biochim. Biophys. Acta, 433, 445-456.
210. Petkau, A., Kelly, K., and Lepock, J.R. (1980) in Biological and Clinical Aspects of Superoxide and Superoxide Dismutase, Bannister, W.H. and Bannister, J.V., eds., New York: Elsevier/North Holland, pp. 335-347.
211. Petkau, A., Chelack, W.S., Kelly, K., and Friesen, H.G. (1980) in Active Oxygen and Medicine, Autor, A.P., ed., New York: Raven Press, in press.
212. Ionasescu, V., Stern, L.Z., Ionasescu, R., and Rubenstein, P. (1979) Ann. Neurol., 5, 107-110.
213. Kar, N.C. and Pearson, C.M. (1979) Clin. Chim. Acta., 94, 277-280.
214. Gerber, D.A. and Gerber, H.G. (1977) J. Chronic Dis., 30, 115-127.
215. Michelson, A.M. (1979) in Oxygen Free Radicals and Tissue Damage, Ciba Found. Symp. 65 (new ser.), Amsterdam: Excerpta Medica, p. 277 (discussion).
216. Younes, M. and Weser, U. (1977) Biochem. Biophys. Res. Commun. 78, 1247-1253.
217. Robertson, P., Jr. and Fridovich, I. (1980) Arch. Biochem. Biophys., 203, 830-831.

218. Emerit, I. and Michelson, A.M. (1980) in Biological and Clinical Aspects of Superoxide and Superoxide Dismutase, Bannister, W.H. and Bannister, J.F., eds., New York: Elsevier/North Holland, pp. 384-394.
219. Nordenson, I., Beckman, G., and Beckman, L. (1976) Hereditas, 82, 125-126.
220. Nordenson, I. (1978) Hereditas, 89, 163-167.
221. Nordenson, I. (1977) Hereditas, 86, 147-150.
222. Nordenson, I. (1977) Hereditas, 87, 151-154.
223. Brown, K.W. and Harnden, D.G. (1978) Lancet, ii, 1260-1261.
224. Abeliovich, D. and Cohen, M.M. (1978) Isr. J. Med. Sci., 14, 284-287.
225. Sheridan, R.B. III and Huang, P.C. (1979) Mutat. Res., 61, 381-386.
226. Joenje, H., Frants, R.R., Arwert, F., De Bruin, G.J.M., Kostense, P.J., Van De Kamp, J.J.P., De Koning, J., and Eriksson, A.W. (1979) Scand. J. Clin. Lab. Invest., 39, 759-764.
227. Raj, A.S. and Heddle, J.A. (1980) Mutat. Res., 78, 59-66.
228. Emerit, I., Levy, A. and Housset, E. (1973) Ann. Genet., 16, 135-138.
229. Emerit, I., Levy, A. and Housset, E. (1974) Humangenetik, 25, 221-226.
230. Emerit, J., Camus, J.P., and Michelson, A.M. (1980) in Biological and Clinical Aspects of Superoxide and Superoxide Dismutase, Bannister, w.H. and Bannister, J.V., eds., New York: Elsevier/North Holland, pp. 381-383.
231. McCue, J.P. (1979) Exp. Haematol., 7, 361-368.
232. Kobayashi, Y., Okahata, S., Sakano, T., Tanabe, K., and Usui, T. (1979) FEBS Lett., 98, 391-393.
233. Minikami, S., Nakagawara, A., and Nakamura, M. (1977) in Biochemical and Medical Aspects of Active Oxygen, Hayaishi, O. and Asada, K., eds., Tokyo: University of Tokyo Press, pp. 229-246.
234. Oberley, L.W. and Buettner, G.R. (1979) Cancer Res., 39, 1141-1149.
235. Yamanaka, N.Y. and Deamer, D. (1974) Physiol. Chem. Phys., 6, 95-106.
236. Dionisi, O., Galeotti, T., Terranova, T., and Azzi, A. (1975) Biochim. Biophys. Acta, 403, 292-300.
237. Yamanaka, N., Ota, K. and Utsumi, K. (1977) in Biochemical and Medical Aspects of Active Oxygen, Hayaishi, O. and Asada, K., eds., Tokyo: University of Tokyo Press, pp. 183-190.
238. Yamanaka, N., Nishida, K., and Ota, K. (1979) Physiol. Chem. Phys., 11, 253-256.
239. Issels, R.D., Wilmanns, W. and Weser, U. (1980) in Biological and Clinical Aspects of Superoxide and Superoxide Dismutase, Bannister, W.H. and Bannister, J.V., eds., New York: Elsevier/North Holland, pp. 281-285.
240. Sykes, J.A., McCormack, F.X., Jr., and O'Brien, T.J. (1978) Cancer Res., 38, 2759-2762.
241. Petkau, A., Monasterski, L.G., Kelly, K., and Friesen, H.G. (1977) Res. Commun. Chem. Pathol. Pharmacol., 17, 125-132.
242. Peskin, A.V., Koen, Ya. M., and Zbarskii, I.B. (1977) FEBS Lett., 78, 41-45.
243. Galeotti, T., Borello, S., Seccia, A., Farallo, E., Bartoli, G.M., and Serri, F. (1980) Arch. Dermatol. Res., 267, 83-86.
244. Knudson, A.G., Jr., Strong, L.C., and Anderson, D.E. (1973) Progr. Med. Genet., 9, 113-158.
245. Edwards, R.H. (1975) Gastroenterology, 68, 734-749.
246. Peters, T.J. and Seymour, C.A. (1978) Clin. Sci. Mol. Med., 54, 549-553.
247. Galeotti, T., Bartoli, G.M., Bartoli, S., and Bertoli, E. (1980) in Biological and Clinical Aspects of Superoxide and Superoxide Dismutase, Bannister, W.H. and Bannister, J.V., eds., New York: Elsevier/North Holland, pp. 106-117.

CHAPTER 11 ILL-PLACED IRON, OXYGEN FREE RADICALS AND DISEASE: SOME RECENT
AND NOT SO RECENT RADIATION STUDIES

R. L. WILLSON
Biochemistry Department, Brunel University, Uxbridge, Middlesex, U.K.

INTRODUCTION

"A consideration of various isolated reports in the literature has led us to
the hypothesis that oxygen poisoning and radiation injury have at least one common
basis of action, possibly through the formation of oxidizing free radicals. This
article reviews the pertinent material that led to this hypothesis and also presents
the supporting evidence obtained from (i) experiments on the protective action
against oxygen poisoning by substances of varied chemical nature known to increase
resistance to irradiation and (ii) experiments on the survival in oxygen of mice
irradiated and exposed to high oxygen tensions simultaneously or at different
intervals.
Concerning free-radical formation, it is generally believed that the chemical
actions of ionizing radiation on aqueous solutions are mainly indirect (Ref. 1),
involving the primary formation of the free radicals H$\cdot$ and OH$\cdot$ with subsequent
formation of H_2O_2, atomic oxygen, and $OH_2^{\bullet}$ (Ref. 2). In the presence of oxygen,
increased amounts of the powerful and quantitatively important OH$\cdot$, as well as
the less reactive but more persistent $HO_2^{\bullet}$, would be expected.

Free-radical formation is also expected in normal oxidative metabolism. One
mechanism by which molecular oxygen can be reduced is the compulsory univalent
transfer of electrons described by Michaelis (Ref. 3), according to which, in the
presence of protons, one may expect the formation of OH$\cdot$, $HO_2^{\bullet}$, and H_2O_2. Daniels
et al. (Ref. 4) have discussed the possible occurrence of an oxidizing free radical
$RO_2^{\bullet}$ during the reduction of oxygen, and several other authors (Refs. 5-10) have
indicated the occurrence of free radicals as such or bound with enzymes in normal
metabolic reactions. As one of the reactants, it might be expected that increased
concentrations of oxygen would increase the formation of oxidizing free radicals."

So began an article entitled "Oxygen Poisoning and X-irradiation: A Mechanism
in Common" written in 1954 by Gerschman and colleagues of the University of
Rochester School of Medicine and Dentistry (Ref. 11).

Two years later a paper entitled "Aging: a theory based on free radical and
radiation chemistry" was published (Ref. 12). The paper by Harman of the Donner
Laboratory Berkeley ended:

"Aging and the degenerative diseases associated with it are attributed basically
to the deleterious side attacks of free radicals on cell constituents and on
connective tissues. The free radicals probably arise largely through reactions
involving molecular oxygen catalyzed in the cell by the oxidative tissues by
traces of metal such as iron, cobalt and manganese."

By 1954 considerable information concerning the chemical properties of OH$\cdot$,
$O_2^{\bullet-}$, its conjugate acid, $HO_2^{\bullet}$ and various organic free radicals in solution had
accumulated particularly from radiation studies (Refs. 13-18) and from experiments
with the Fenton iron-hydrogen peroxide system (Refs. 19-23). Many reactions involving
iron, free radicals, and oxygen had been documented, e.g.:

$$O_2^{\bullet -} + Fe^{3+} \rightarrow O_2 + Fe^{2+}$$
$$Fe^{2+} + H_2O_2 \rightarrow OH^{\bullet} + OH^- + Fe^{3+}$$
$$HO_2^{\bullet} + Fe^{2+} \rightarrow HO_2^- + Fe^{3+}$$
$$OH^{\bullet} + HCO_2H \rightarrow {}^{\bullet}CO_2H + H_2O$$
$${}^{\bullet}CO_2H + Fe^{3+} \rightarrow CO_2 + Fe^{2+} + H^+$$

Data concerning the role of free radicals in systems exposed to ionizing radiation had come mostly from conventional chemical analysis of the radiation products (Refs. 24-25). Since yields were generally small systems were consequently often exposed to high radiation doses and the kinetic and stoichiometric interpretation of results was often extremely complex. Although many of the concepts arising still hold true today it is not surprising that data was occasionally misinterpreted. For example during studies with aqueous solutions of methyl methacrylate it was found that thiourea offered no protection against radiation-induced polymerization (Ref. 26). From studies with Fenton's reagent it was known that hydroxyl radicals induced polymerization (Ref. 27). Alexander and Fox (Ref. 26) therefore inferred erroneously that hydroxyl radicals did not react rapidly with thiourea. This error was then compounded when it was concluded that $HO_2^{\bullet}$ was the damaging species in irradiated biological systems. On irradiation of aqueous solutions of polymethyacrylate as well as several biological systems, thiourea had been shown to have a protective effect.

The damaging effects were also greater when oxygen was present. Since thiourea was not supposed to react rapidly with $OH^{\bullet}$, $HO_2^{\bullet}$ was deemed responsible. This immediately aroused considerable interest in radiobiological circles. Radiation chemists, perhaps having more faith in the previously published literature concerning the in vitro reactions of $HO_2^{\bullet}$ and $OH^{\bullet}$ however, appear to have been more disdainful. A discussion contribution by Weiss at a meeting on the role of peroxidation in radiobiology in Paris in 1957 perhaps reflects some of the strong feelings engendered at the time (Ref. 28).

"With regard to the HO_2 radicals, I do not think that there can be any doubt that this radical exists; there are many quite independent proofs for its existence and it has also been clearly demonstrated by the mass spectrographic work of Robertson and others. However, it is a great pity that two or three years ago there was a tendency, by certain quarters, to make the HO_2 responsible for almost everything which happens in radiobiology. If we look at the reaction of HO_2 in vitro, it is obvious that this radical is relatively unreactive towards saturated organic systems, where it does not do anything or only very rarely, but on the other hand, it can act as an oxidizing agent towards strongly reducing substances such as ferrous ions and as a reducing agent, in the form of its anion O_2^-, towards e.g., ceric salts. However, there seems to be no justification to explain almost everything in radiobiology by the action of HO_2, as was done particularly by Alexander. It is unfortunate that as much time still has to be wasted now to point out that these views were really of very little consequence."

In spite of these occasional misinterpretations it seems to have been generally accepted by the late 1950s that although $HO_2^{\bullet}$ could react with strongly reducing species such as Fe^{2+}, ascorbate and cysteine, the hydroxyl radical was the much more potent oxidant. Experiments in which the presence of oxygen increased the extent of radiation damage did not necessarily imply reactions of $HO_2^{\bullet}$:oxygen could inhibit restitution reactions leading to the repair of damage induced by $OH^{\bullet}$ (Refs. 29-31).

With the advent of the pulse radiolysis technique in 1960 the rapid reactions of $OH^{\bullet}$ with a wide variety of organic molecules and inorganic ions was soon demonstrated unequivocally (Refs. 32-37). Both $HO_2^{\bullet}$ and $O_2^{\bullet-}$ were shown to be relatively unreactive: $HO_2^{\bullet}$ generally acting as a weak oxidant and $O_2^{\bullet-}$ a weak reductant. The absolute rates of reaction of $OH^{\bullet}$ with organic molecules were generally found to be very high, nucleic acid derivatives for example reacting at near diffusion controlled rates (Ref. 37). In contrast, no evidence appeared indicating any reactions between $O_2^{\bullet-}$ and nucleic acid derivatives (Refs. 38,39). Indeed pulse radiolysis and previous stationary state studies showed that the thymine electron adduct reacted rapidly with oxygen to form $O_2^{\bullet-}$ rather than the reverse (Refs. 40-42).

$$T^{\bullet-} + O_2 \rightarrow T + O_2^{\bullet-}$$

Fridovich and McCord's suggestion in 1969 that an enzyme existed to protect against the damaging effect of $O_2^{\bullet-}$, thus came as something of a surprise to radiation chemists (Ref. 43). What were these damaging actions? The superoxide radical had been shown to react rapidly with tetranitromethane (Refs. 44,45) but this was hardly biologically relevant. It might also react with ascorbate, with some -SH groups and with metal ions but could these be considered vital targets?

The subsequent suggestions that the reaction of $O_2^{\bullet-}$ and H_2O_2 lead directly to the formation of $OH^{\bullet}$ or that $O_2^{\bullet-}$ dismutation leads to the formation of singlet oxygen offered little comfort (Refs. 46-48). It was known that singlet oxygen could damage organic molecules and that in general both $O_2^{\bullet-}$ and H_2O_2 were formed in irradiated oxygenated systems. However, the possibilities that these might react together according to the mechanism of Haber and Weiss to produce $OH^{\bullet}$ or that singlet oxygen was involved had rarely if ever been invoked to explain radiation induced biological damage.

In retrospect the 1973 paper of Fong and colleages entitled "Evidence that peroxidation of lysosomal membranes is initiated by hydroxyl free radicals produced during flavin enzyme activity? seems to have heralded the beginning of the revival of interest of radiation chemists in oxygen toxicity (Ref. 49). The proposal of an involvement of iron in the formation on $OH^{\bullet}$ from $O_2^{\bullet-}$ by way of the Fenton reaction did seem as if it might account for the apparent contradiction that reactions of $O_2^{\cdot-}$ can lead to biological damage in spite of its low reactivity towards likely vital molecules.

$$O_2^{\cdot-} + Fe^{3+} \text{ (chelate)} \rightarrow O_2 + Fe^{2+} \text{ (chelate)}$$
$$H_2O_2 + Fe^{2+} \text{ (chelate)} \rightarrow OH^{\cdot} + OH^- + Fe^{3+} \text{ (chelate)}$$
$$\text{Net:} O_2^{\cdot-} + H_2O_2 \rightarrow O_2 + OH^{\cdot} + OH^-$$

The marked effect of trace iron contamination on the course of radiation induced reactions of organic compounds and vice versa had been common knowledge for half a century (Refs. 50-52). The radiation-induced dephosphorylation of nucleic acid components had been found to be stimulated by the presence of iron salts and the protective action of sulphydryl compounds had been suggested to be due in part to their ability to form complexes with transition metal ions (Refs. 53,54). Recently studies with pulmonary macrophages have provided further support for a role of iron in some forms of radiation injury (Ref. 55). Cell viability as measured by dye exclusion, was not significantly affected after exposure to 12 k. rads of X-rays but was reduced to 37% after 24-hours incubation. In the presence of not only superoxide dismutase and catalase but also the metal chelating agent diethylene-triamine penta acetic acid (DETAPAC) considerable protection was afforded. Unlike EDTA, which offered no significant protection, DETAPAC is thought to bind iron in a manner which inhibits its involvement in reactions involving $O_2^{\cdot-}$ and H_2O_2 (Refs. 56,57).

"ILL-PLACED IRON" NOT "OXYGEN" TOXICITY?

Involvement of iron in many of the biochemical and biological effects broadly attributed to oxygen toxicity now seems to be taken for granted in many quarters (Ref. 58-65). However, it does raise a number of questions particularly, "In what form is the iron?" "What is its origin?" Is is well known that iron in biology is carefully controlled to prevent it randomly catalyzing the oxidation of sensitive molecules such as thiols or lipids (Refs. 66,67). Macromolecules such as hemoglobin, transferin, ferritin, the cytochromes and the various iron-containing enzymes are designed for a specific purpose. If iron is able to react with $O_2^{\cdot-}$ and H_2O_2 it must no longer be present in such safe compartments, i.e., it must be "decompartmentalized." How has this occurred? Furthermore, if it has occurred this step may be critical and it may be more appropriate to consider relevant damage as due to "iron" rather than "oxygen" toxicity.

The possibility that "decompartmentalized" iron, perhaps better described as "ill-placed iron," may be involved in several forms of tissue injury was discussed at a recent Ciba Symposium on Iron Metabolism (Ref. 68). A natural or xenobiotic agent, perhaps even a virus, may under certain circumstances complex iron and

carry it to a site where it should not be normally and where it subsequently
catalyzes oxidation reactions. A similar cooperative effect has been proposed
for the bacteriocidal action of 8-hydroxyquinoline (oxine) and was recently used
to explain the chemotherapeutic action of bleomycin (Refs. 69,70). The toxic
action of the encephalomyelitis virus was ascribed as long ago as 1947 to it
having the ability to transport iron across the blood brain barrier, which is
normally impervious to the metal ion (Fig. 1)(Ref. 71).

Although any hydroxyl radicals generated in biological tissue through the
action of iron would inevitably differ in their distribution from those produced
radiolytically, their basic chemical properties would be the same. Their
subsequent fate would be determined only by their environment.

It is in this light that the technique of pulse radiolysis has been established
at Brunel to investigate the mechanisms of possible free radical reactions involved
in general tissue injury. Once the radiation pulse is finished the fact that the
radicals have been generated radiolytically can be forgotten. Information concerning reaction of $OH^\bullet$ and other free radical reactions in vitro can be readily
obtained. Whether such reactions occur in vivo, is of course, another matter.

PULSE RADIOLYSIS

The pulse radiolysis technique originally described in 1960 can be considered
as the high energy analogue of flash photolysis with the flash lamp replaced by
a pulsed source of ionizing reduction such as a linear accelerator (Refs. 72,73).
Many free radicals are highly colored and absorb at wavelengths different from
those of the molecules from which they are derived. This enables a wide variety
of free radical reactions initiated by the ionizing pulse to be followed by
conventional fixed wavelength UV/visible spectrophotometry. There are two
provisios however. First it is of course imperative that the whole analytical
system is designed so that the operator is not exposed to harmful radiation.
Second, because of the microsecond time response required, an oscilloscope or
transient recorder must be used rather than the usual mechanical pen and chart
recorder (Ref. 36).

When aqueous solutions are given a pulse of radiation, ionized water molecules
and electrons are formed but, within a nanosecond of the end of the pulse, these
will subsequently interact with other solvent molecules to form principally
hydroxyl radicals $OH^\bullet$, and solvated electrons, e^-_{aq}

$$H_2O \rightarrow H_2O^{\bullet +} + e$$
$$H_2O^{\bullet +} + H_2O \rightarrow OH^\bullet + H_3O^+$$
$$e + nH_2O \rightarrow e^-_{aq}$$

These species may react with themselves or with other substances present. Although

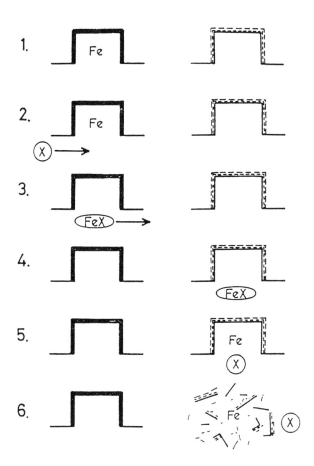

Fig. 1. "Ill-placed iron" leading to oxidative damage: iron decompartmentali-
zation by a chelating agent X.

OH˙ is a strong oxidizing agent and e^-_{aq} a strong reducing agent the reaction of each species can be studied individually by using selective free radical scavengers, solutes which react relatively rapidly with one species leaving the other free to undergo the reaction of interest. Alternatively both species may be converted to the same radical, for example as when using nitrous oxide.

It cannot be over-emphasized that although the radicals studied by pulse radiolysis are generated using electrons of 4 MeV energy and doses in the range 1-20 Joule per kg, the hydroxyl radicals and solvated electrons formed ca 3 uM of each per Joule absorbed are of thermal energy and are no different than those of similar structure generated chemically or biochemically.

FREE RADICALS, PROTEINS AND THE INITIAL SUSCEPTIBILITY OF TRYPTOPHAN

Proteins provide a wide variety of different sites for attack by electrophilic radicals such as OH˙. Although considerable information concerning free radical-induced damage to amino acids and proteins has been obtained from product analysis of irradiated systems little direct information was available concerning the initial events taking place until the advent of pulse radiolysis. Hydroxyl radical reactions can be conveniently studied by using aqueous solutions saturated with nitrous oxide. Solutions are designed so that e^-_{aq} react principally with nitrous oxide to form OH˙.

$$H_2O \rightsquigarrow OH˙ \quad + \quad e^-_{aq}$$

$$e^-_{aq} \quad + \quad N_2O \quad \rightarrow \quad N_2 \quad + \quad OH^- \quad + \quad OH˙$$

Although it is now known that OH˙ reacts rapidly with several amino acids the transient absorption observed on pulse radiolysis of nitrous oxide saturated solutions of lysozyme strongly resembles that observed with tryptophan alone (Fig. 2)(Ref. 74). Following pulse radiolysis studies with various methylated indole derivatives Armstrong and Swallow (Ref. 75) concluded that the fine structure of the spectrum obtained with tryptophan could be attributed to species formed from the attack of OH˙ on the aromatic ring as well as at C_2 and C_3 of the indole ring (Fig. 3).

Attack at C_2 had been previously proposed by Jayson, Scholes and Weiss following stationary state product analysis of irradiated solutions of the amino acid (Ref. 76). Studies with Fenton's reagent by Eich and Rochelmayer had also previously indicated attack at the aromatic ring (Ref. 77).

Recent pulse radiolysis studies have shown that the peroxy radical $CCl_3O_2˙$ also reacts with tryptophan but in this instance two other species are formed, one of which appears to be a peroxy radical adduct, the other the radical trp˙ with the radical center on the ring nitrogen (Refs. 78,79).

The radical $CCl_3O_2˙$ can be readily formed by pulse radiolysis of air saturated solutions containing carbon tetrachloride and either (a) excess isopropanol,

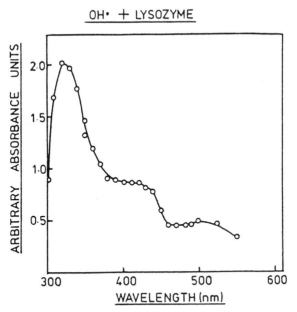

Fig. 2. Composite absorption spectrum of the radicals produced by attack of OH·
on lysozyme as measured by pulse radiolysis.

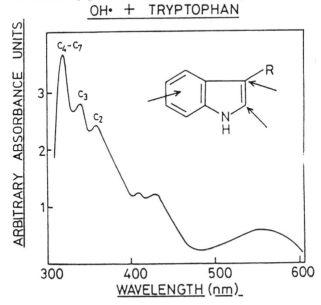

Fig. 3. Composite absorption spectrum of the radicals produced by reaction of
OH· with tryptophan as measured by pulse radiolysis.

(b) acetone and isopropanol or (c) t-butanol according to:

$$H_2O \rightsquigarrow OH^{\bullet} + e_{aq}^-$$

(a) $e_{aq}^- + CCl_4 \rightarrow CCl_3^{\bullet} + Cl^-$

$OH^{\bullet} + CH_3CHOHCH_3 \rightarrow CH_3^{\bullet}COHCH_3 + H_2O$

$CH_3^{\bullet}COHCH_3 + CCl_4 \rightarrow CCl_3^{\bullet} + CH_3COCH_3 + H^+ + Cl^-$

(b) $e_{aq}^- + CH_3COCH_3 \rightarrow CH_3^{\bullet}CO^-CH_3$

$CH_3^{\bullet}CO^-CH_3 + H_2O \rightarrow CH_3^{\bullet}COHCH_3 + OH^-$

$CH_3^{\bullet}COHCH_3 + CCl_4 \rightarrow CCl_3^{\bullet} + CH_3COCH_3 + H^+ + Cl^-$

(c) $e_{aq}^- + CCl_4 \rightarrow CCl_3^{\bullet} + Cl^-$

$OH^{\bullet} + CH_3(CH_3)_2COH \rightarrow {}^{\bullet}CH_2(CH_3)_2OH + H_2O$

Followed by:

$$CCl_3^{\bullet} + O_2 \rightarrow CCl_3O_2^{\bullet}$$

The t-butanol radical ${}^{\bullet}CH_2(CH_3)_2OH$ and its related peroxy radical have been found to be relatively unreactive in most systems studied. On pulse radiolysis of air saturated solutions containing 50% isopropanol and 0.1 M CCl_4 a transient absorption with a maximum at 470 nm and shoulder at 520 nm was observed (Fig. 4). The absorption appeared exponentially and first order in tryptophan corresponding to:

$$CCl_3O_2^{\bullet} + \text{tryptophan} \rightarrow \text{products} \quad k = 8.5 \times 10^7 \ M^{-1}s^{-1}$$

An absorption spectra with a maximum at 520 nm had been previously observed (Ref. 80) on pulse radiolysis of nitrous oxide saturated solutions of tryptophan containing excess thiocyanate or bromide and had been attributed to $trp^{\bullet}$ formed according to reactions such as:

$$e_{aq}^- + N_2O \rightarrow N_2 + OH^{\bullet} + OH^-$$

$$OH^{\bullet} + CNS^- \rightarrow CNS^{\bullet} + OH^-$$

$$CNS^{\bullet} + CNS^- \rightarrow (CNS)_2^{\bullet-}$$

$$(CNS)_2^{\bullet-} + trpH \rightarrow trpH^{\bullet+} + 2 CNS^-$$

$$trpH^{\bullet+} \rightarrow trp^{\bullet} + H^+$$

When the spectrum of $trp^{\bullet}$ was normalized to the spectra from CCl_3O_2 at 520 nm and a difference spectrum obtained (Fig. 5), this was assigned to another radical possibly the adduct formed with the radical center at C_3.

Support for at least two species being present and that at least one of the species was $trp^{\bullet}$ came from studies with the dipeptide tryptophanyltyrosine. Prutz

PULSE RADIOLYSIS OF TRYPTOPHAN

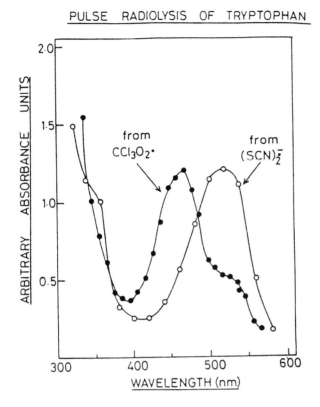

Fig. 4. Composite absorption spectrum of the radicals produced by the reaction of $CCl_3O_2^{\cdot}$ and $(SCN)_2^{\cdot -}$ with tryptophan.

and Land had previously shown by pulse radiolysis that when the azide radical $N_3^{\cdot}$ reacts with tryptophanyltyrosine attack takes place predominantly on the tryptophan moiety but this damage is quickly transferred to the tyrosine phenolic group by an intramolecular electron transfer process (Refs. 81,82). The absorption due to trp$^{\cdot}$ at 520 nm was observed initially but this subsequently decayed and absorption at 410 nm characteristic of a phenoxy radical grew in simultaneously.

$$OH^{\cdot} + N_3^{-} \rightarrow N_3^{\cdot} + OH^{-}$$
$$N_3^{\cdot} + trpH - tyrOH \rightarrow trpH^{\cdot +} - tryOH$$
$$trpH^{\cdot +} - tyrOH \rightarrow trp^{\cdot} - tyrOH + H^{+}$$
$$trp^{\cdot} - tyrOH \rightarrow trpH - tyrO^{\cdot}$$

On pulse radiolysis of tryptophanyltyrosine in the CCl_4-isopropanol system the absorption observed after 10 μs was the same as that seen with tryptophan with a maximum at 470 nm and shoulder at 520 nm. The absorption at 520 nm however subsequently decayed while the absorption at 410 nm increased. The absorption at 470 nm decreased only partially in agreement with it being due in part to a species other than trp˙ (Fig. 6). Further confirmation that this was the case came from studies with ascorbate. On pulse radiolysis of N_2O saturated solutions of tryptophan containing excess bromide and low concentrations of ascorbate (AH⁻), the trp˙ absorption at 520 nm was formed initially but decayed first order in ascorbate with the simultaneous formation of the ascorbate radical (A˙⁻) absorption at 360 nm.

$$OH^\bullet + Br^- \rightarrow Br^\bullet + OH^-$$
$$Br^\bullet + Br^- \rightarrow Br_2^{\bullet-}$$
$$Br_2^\bullet + trpH \rightarrow trpH^{\bullet+} + 2\ Br^-$$
$$trpH^{\bullet+} \rightarrow trp^\bullet + H^+$$
$$trp^\bullet + AH \rightarrow trpH + A^{\bullet-} \quad k = 1.1 \pm 0.1 \times 10^8\ M^{-1}s^{-1}$$

On pulse radiolysis of tryptophan in the presence of low concentrations of ascorbate in the CCl_4-isopropanol system the 470 nm absorption and shoulder at 520 nm were again observed initially (Fig. 7). Both absorptions, subsequently decayed first order in ascorbate concentration. The absorption at 470 nm again decayed only partially, however, and an increase at 360 nm occurred simultaneously. As a result of these experiments it was concluded that the reaction of $CCl_3O_2^\bullet$ with tryptophan yielded at least two species one trp˙ the other probably an adduct.

$$CCl_3O_2^\bullet + trpH \nearrow (CCl_3O_2 - trpH)^\bullet$$
$$\searrow CCl_3O_2^- + trpH^{\bullet+}$$
$$trp^\bullet + H^+$$

In order to determine whether similar reactions occurred with tryptophan incorporated in proteins, pulse radiolysis studies of lysozyme in the isoproponal-CCl_4 system were undertaken: an absorption very similar to that found with tryptophan was observed indicating that substantial attack took place at one or more of these residues (Fig. 8).

Related enzyme activity studies have recently shown that even in the presence of CCl_4 and 20% isopropanol or 10% isopropanol and 10% acetone, the viability of lysozyme is not affected. To test whether reaction of $CCl_3O_2^\bullet$ with the enzyme results in inactivation, stationary state irradiation studies have been undertaken using the Brunel 2,000 curie "cave-type" Co60 gamma source. Lysozyme activity was measured by determining the rate of decrease in turbidity when an aliquot of enzyme solution was added to a suspension of lyophilized *Micrococcus lysodeikticus* (Ref. 83).

It had been shown previously that when lysozyme is irradiated in phosphate buffered N_2O saturated solutions the enzyme is inactivated in agreement with the damaging action of OH˙ (Ref. 74).

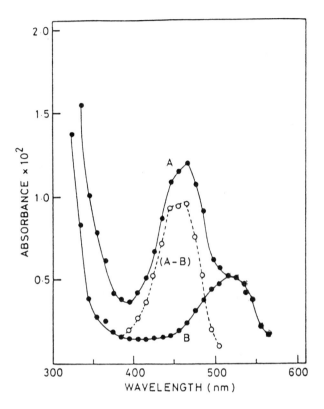

Fig. 5. Difference absorption spectrum (A-B) obtained by subtracting spectrum assigned to trp normalized at 520 nm from the composite absorption attributed to reactions of $CCl_3O_2^{\cdot}$.

$$H_2O \xrightsquigarrow{} OH^{\cdot} + e_{aq}^{-}$$

$$e_{aq}^{-} + N_2O \rightarrow N_2 + OH^{-} + OH^{\cdot}$$

$$OH^{\cdot} + lysozyme \rightarrow inactivation$$

When the enzyme is irradiated in air saturated solutions containing excess iso-propanol and acetone little inactivation is observed in agreement with $O_2^{\cdot-}$ being relatively unreactive (Fig. 9).

$$e_{aq}^{-} + CH_3COCH_3 \xrightarrow{H^+} CH_3^{\cdot} COHCH_3$$

$$OH^{\cdot} + CH_3CHOHCH_3 \longrightarrow CH_3^{\cdot} COHCH_3 + H_2O$$

$$CH_4^{\cdot}COHCH_3 + O_2 \xrightarrow{OH^-/HPO_4^{2-}} CH_3COCH_3 + O_2^{\cdot-} + H_2O/H_2PO_4^{-}$$

$$O_2^{\cdot-} + lysozyme \longrightarrow inactivation slow if at all.$$

In the additional presence of CCl_4 however considerable inactivation was observed plainly due to the action of $CCl_3O_2^{\cdot}$ (Fig. 9).

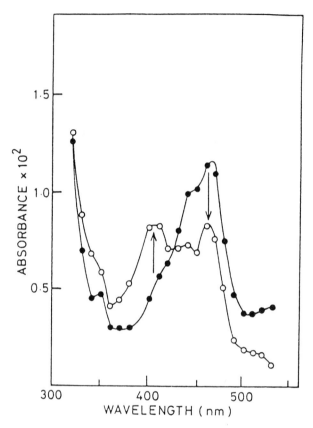

Fig. 6. Absorption spectra observed on pulse radiolysis of aqueous solutions containing carbon tetrachloride and tryptophanyltyrosine after (●) 10 and (○) 100 μs (see text).

Since ribonuclease does not contain any tryptophan residues it was of interest to see whether this enzyme could be inactivated by the action of $CCl_3O_2^{\bullet}$. Somewhat surprisingly inactivation again occurred in the isopropanol/CCl_4 system, indicating that $CCl_3O_2^{\bullet}$ also reacted readily with at least one amino acid other than tryptophan. Indeed inactivation by $CCl_3O_2^{\bullet}$ was greater than with OH$^{\bullet}$ (Fig. 10). At present the most likely candidate for attack by $CCl_3O_2^{\bullet}$ appears to be methionine. Of the common amino acids studied to date only cysteine and methionine react rapidly with the radical in neutral solution. In alkaline solution tyrosine also reacts rapidly in agreement with the phenol group being more sensitive to oxidation when ionized.

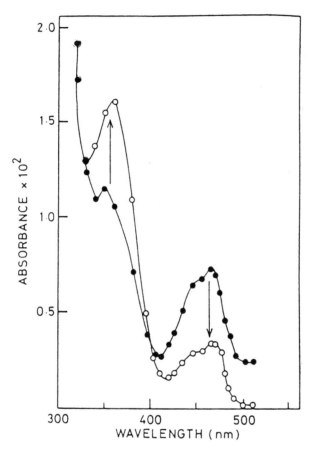

Fig. 7. Absorption spectra observed on pulse radiolysis of aqueous solution containing carbon tetrachloride, tryptophan and ascorbate after (●) 5 and (O) 100 μs (see text).

ELECTRON TRANSFER REACTIONS AND THE ULTIMATE SUSCEPTIBILITY OF ASCORBATE

In addition to the above amino acids, the reaction of $CCl_3O_2^{\bullet}$ and related peroxy radicals with a variety of organic compounds have recently been undertaken (Refs. 85-88). The absolute rates of reaction of phenol (pH = 12) and ascorbic acid (pH = 7) have been found to increase with increasing substitution of choline atoms, i.e.

$$CH_3O_2^{\bullet} \quad < \quad ClCH_2O_2^{\bullet} \quad < \quad Cl_2CHO_2^{\bullet} \quad < \quad CCl_3O_2^{\bullet}$$

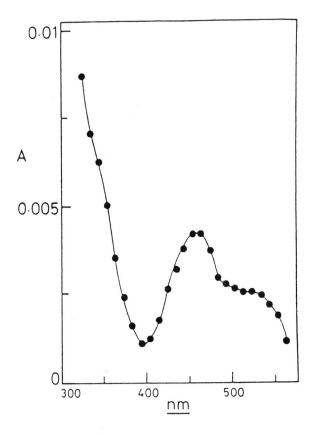

Fig. 8. Composite absorption spectrum of radicals produced by attack of $CCl_3O_2^{\cdot}$ on lysozyme as measured by pulse radiolysis.

In the case of $CH_3O_2^{\cdot}$ formed on pulse radiolysis solutions of dimethylsulphoxide saturated with nitrous oxide-oxygen mixture only the reaction with ascorbate has so far been observed (see Table 1).

$$(CH_3)_2SO + OH^{\cdot} \rightarrow CH_3SO_2H + CH_3^{\cdot}$$

$$CH_3^{\cdot} + O_2 \rightarrow CH_3O_2^{\cdot}$$

$$CH_3O_2^{\cdot} + AH^- \rightarrow CH_3O_2H + A^{\cdot -} \qquad k = 2.2 \pm 0.3 \times 10^6$$

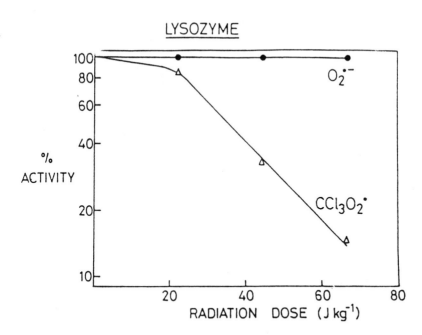

Fig. 9. Inactivation of lysozyme in aqueous solution by radicals generated by γ-irradiation.

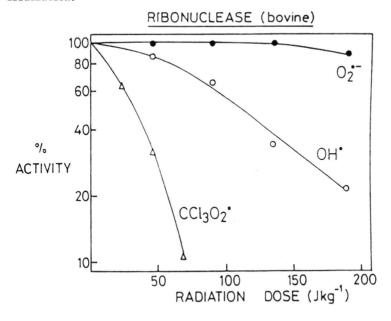

Fig. 10. Inactivation of ribonuclease in aqueous solution by radicals generated by γ-irradiation.

TABLE 1

Absolute rate constants ($M^{-1}s^{-1}$) for the reaction of aliphatic peroxy radicals with ascorbate and promethazine at pH 7.

	Ascorbate	Promethazine
$Cl_3CO_2^{\cdot}$	$1.8 \pm 0.4 \times 10^8$	$6.0 \pm 0.4 \times 10^8$
$Cl_3CHO_2^{\cdot}$	$2.2 \pm 0.6 \times 10^8$	$1.4 \pm 0.1 \times 10^8$
$ClCH_2O_2^{\cdot}$	$9.2 \pm 1.5 \times 10^7$	$3.3 \pm 0.2 \times 10^7$
$CH_3O_2^{\cdot}$	$2.2 \pm 0.3 \times 10^6$	$-$

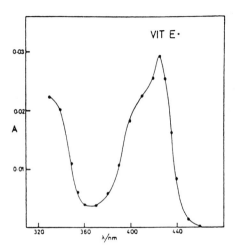

Fig. 11. Absorption spectrum of the phenoxyl radical of vitamin E measured by pulse radiolysis.

Other compounds found to react rapidly with $CCl_3O_2^{\cdot}$ include various phenols (RO^-) such as propylgallate and vitamin E, phenothiazines such as promethazine and chlorpromaxine (CZ) as well as the so-called "singlet oxygen scavengers," diphenyl furan, DABCO and β-carotene.

$$CCl_3O_2^{\cdot} + RO^- \rightarrow CCl_3O_2^- + RO^{\cdot}$$

$$CCl_3O_2^{\cdot} + CZ \rightarrow CCl_3O_2^- + CZ^{\cdot+}$$

$$CCl_3O_2^{\cdot} + \beta\text{-carotene} \rightarrow CCl_3O_2^- \quad \beta\text{-carotene}^{\cdot+}$$

The above findings are in agreement with previous observations that compounds such as promethazine, propylgallate and vitamine E offer some protection against certain aspects of carbon tetrachloride induced liver damage (Ref. 89). Clearly they can only exhibit such an effect if the free radical resulting from vital molecules. For example the chlorpromazine radical has been reported to react with the enzyme uridine diphosphate glucose oxido-reductase and with ATPase causing inactivation (Refs. 91-94).

It is therefore of interest that the radical cation of chlorpromazine $CZ^{\cdot+}$ has been found (Ref. 95) to react rapidly with adrenaline and dihydroxyphenylala-nine (DOPA), reactions which may have some relevance to the reported side effect of melanin deposition in the skin of patients treated with the phenothiazine (Refs. 96,97).

$$CZ^{\cdot+} + \text{adrenaline} \rightarrow \text{products} \quad k = 0.8 \times 10^8 \ M^{-1}s^{-1}$$

$$CZ^{\cdot+} + \text{DOPA} \rightarrow \text{products} \quad k = 1.2 \times 10^8 \ M^{-1}s^{-1}$$

The phenothiazine radical-cations also react rapidly with α-tocopherol (vit EH) and with ascorbate (AH^-) either directly or indirectly--reactions which may be of relevance to the nutrition of patients undergoing long-term therapy with drugs such as chlorpromazine (Ref. 95).

$$CZ^{\cdot+} + \text{vit EH} \rightarrow CZ + \text{vit E}^{\cdot} + H^+$$

$$CZ^{\cdot+} + AH \rightarrow CZ + A^{\cdot-} + H^+$$

$$\text{vit E}^{\cdot} + AH^- \rightarrow \text{vit EH} + A^{\cdot-}$$

To date no reaction of $A^{\cdot-}$ with other molecules has been observed by pulse radiolysis. In the cell however there is evidence that NADH dependent enzyme systems can reduce $A^{\cdot-}$ back to the parent molecule (Refs. 98-101). If vitamin E acts as a primary antioxidant and repairs a potentially damaging organic free radical clearly these reactions can allow the repair to be linked to NADH oxidation and a wide range of biochemical processes.

CONCLUSION

Hopefully the above examples illustrate how, with careful experimental design, radiation studies can provide useful information concerning free radical reaction of relevance to other forms of tissue injury. In particular the pulse radiolysis technique is providing valuable mechanistic information. The above experiments with halogenated peroxy radicals, for example, give some indication of the type of reactions simple aliphatic peroxy radicals may undergo, although more slowly. Furthermore, the results with ribonuclease showing $OH^{\cdot}$ to be less damaging than $CCl_3O_2^{\cdot}$ point to the possibility that, in some in vivo situations on a simple numerical basis, OH· may be less efficient in causing biological damage than a less electrophilic peroxy radical.

A return to the heated discussions of the 1950s seems imminent.

ACKNOWLEDGMENTS

The installation of the pulse radiolysis equipment at Brunel would not have been possible without the generous support of the Cancer Research Campaign, the technical support of Mr. A. J. Searle, the electronic assistance of Mr. Brian Wolfenden, and the computer programming expertise of Mr. Jeff Mahood. The computer facility and Cobalt 60 radiation unit were kindly provided by the Medical Research Council.

REFERENCES

1. Rajewsky, B. (1952) Brit. J. Radiol., 25, 550-552.
2. 6th Int. Cong. Radiol. (1951) Brit. J. Radiol., 24, 416, 422, 428.
3. Michaelis, L. (1946) Am. Scientist, 34, 573-596.
4. Daniels, M., Scholes, G. and Weiss, J. (1953) Nature, 171, 1153-1154.
5. Barron, E.S.G. and Levine, S. (1952) Arch. Biochem. Biophys., 41, 175-187.
6. Polonovski, M. (1953) Produits Pharm., 8, 181.
7. Swallow, A.J. (1953) Biochem. J., 54, 253-257.
8. Mosher, W.A. (1951) J. Franklin Inst., 251, 665.
9. LuValle, J.E. and Goddard, D.R. (1948) Quart. Rev. Biol., 23, 197.
10. Tappel, A.L., Boyer, P.D., and Lundberg, W.O. (1952) J. Biol. Chem., 199, 267-281.
11. Gerschman, R., Gilbert, D.L., Nye, S.W., Dwyer, P., and Fenn, W.D. (1954) Science, 119, 623-626.
12. Harman, D. (1956) J. Gerentol., 11, 298-300.
13. Risse, O. (1929) Strahlentherapie, 34, 578-581.
14. Weiss, J. (1944) Nature, 153, 748-750.
15. Weiss, J. (1946) Trans. Farad. Soc., 43, 314-324.
16. Dainton, F.S. (1947) Nature, 160, 268-269.
17. Allen, A.O. (1953) Disc. Farad. Soc., 12, 79-87.
18. Barron, E.S.G. (1954) Radiat. Res., 1, 109-124 and ref. cited.
19. Haber, F. and Weiss, J. (1934) Proc. Roy. Soc. A, 147, 332-351.
20. Baxendale, J.H., Evans, M.G., and Park, G.S. (1946) Trans. Farad. Soc., 42, 155-169.
21. Merz, J.H. and Waters, W.A. (1949) J. Chem. Soc., 49, 2427-2433.
22. Collinson, E., Dainton, F.S. and Holmes, B. (1950) Nature, 165, 267-269.
23. Udenfriend, S., Clark, C.T., Axelrod, J., and Brodie, B.B. (1954) J. Biol. Chem., 208, 731-739.
24. Hart, E.J. (1952) J. Am. Chem. Soc., 74, 4174-4178.
25. Allen, A.O. (1954) Radiat. Res., 1, 85-96.
26. Alexander, P. and Fox, M. (1952) Nature, 170, 1022-1023.
27. Evans, M.G. (1947) Trans. Fard. Soc., 43, 266-274.
28. Weiss, J. (1958) in Organic Peroxides in Radiobiology, Haissinsky, M., ed., London and NY: Pergamon Press, p. 140.
29. Alexander, P. and Charlesby, A. (1955) Proc. Radiobiology Symp. Liege, Bacq, Z.M. and Alexander, P., eds., London: Butterworths Scientific Publications, pp. 49-60.
30. Alper, T. (1956) Radiat. Res., 5, 573-586.
31. Howard Flanders, P. (1960) Nature, 186, 485-487.
32. Dorfman, L.M., Taub, I.A., and Buhler, R.E. (1962) J. Chem. Phys., 36, 3051-3061.

33. Adams, G.E., Boag, J.W., Currant, J., and Michael, B.D. (1965) in Pulse Radiolysis, Ebert, M., Keene, J.P., Swallow, A.J., and Baxendale, J.H., eds., New York and London: Academic Press, pp. 131-143.
34. Scholes, G., Shaw, P., Willson, R.L., and Ebert, M. (1965) in Pulse Radiolysis, Ebert, M., Keene, J.P., Swallow, A.J., and Baxendale, J.H., eds., New York and London: Academic Press, pp. 151-164.
35. Dorfman, L.M. and Adams, G.E. (1973) NSRDS-NBS No. 46, U.S. Department of Commerce, National Bureau of Standards, Bethesda.
36. Willson, R.L. (1979) in Biochemical Mechanisms of Liver Injury, Slater, T.F., ed., London and New York: Academic Press, pp. 123-224.
37. Willson, R.L. (1979) in Oxygen Free Radicals and Tissue Damage, Ciba Foundation Symp. 65 (new series), Amsterdam: Excerpta Medica, pp. 19-35.
38. Blok, J., Luthjens, L.H., and Roos, A.L.M. (1967) Radiat. Res., 30, 468-482.
39. Blok, J. and Verhey, W.S.D. (1968) Radiat. Res., 34, 689-703.
40. Scholes, G. and Willson, R.L., Trans. Farad. Soc., 63, 2983-2993.
41. Theard, L.M., Peterson, F.C., and Myers, L.S. (1968) Adv. Chem. Ser. J. Am. Chem. Soc., 81, 603.
42. Loman, H. and Ebert, M. (1970) Int. J. Radiat. Biol., 18, 369-379.
43. McCord, J.M. and Fridovich, I. (1969) J. Biol. Chem., 244, 6049-6055.
44. Asmus, K.D. and Henglein, A. (1964) Ber. Bunsenges, Phys. Chem., 68, 348-352.
45. Rabani, J., Mulac, W.A., and Matheson, M.S. (1965) J. Phys. Chem., 69, 53-80.
46. Kahn, A.V. (1970) Science 168, 476-477.
47. Paschen, W. and Weser, U. (1973) Biochim. Biophys. Acta, 327, 217-222.
48. Kellogg, E.F. and Fridovich, I. (1975) J. Biol. Chem., 258, 8812-8817.
49. Fong, K., McCay, P.B., Poyer, J.L., Keele, B.B., and Misra, H. (1973) J. Biol. Chem., 248, 7792-7797.
50. Fricke, H. and Brownscombe, E.R. (1933) J. Am. Chem. Soc., 55, 2358-2363.
51. Hart, E. J. (1952) J. Am. Chem. Soc., 74, 4174-4178.
52. Dewhurst, H.A. (1951) J. Chem. Phys., 19, 1329.
53. Ward, J.F. (1971) Int. J. Radiat. Phys. Chem., 3, 239-249.
54. Lohman, W. (1965) Prog. Biochem. Pharmacol., 1, 118-136.
55. Autor, A.P., McLennan, G., and Fox, A.W. (1980) Molecular Basis of Environmental Toxicity, Bhatnagar, R.S., ed., Ann Arbor Science Publ. Inc., pp. 51-67.
56. Buettner, G.R., Oberley, L.W., and Leuthauser, S.W.H.C. (1978) Photochem. Photobiol., 28, 693-695.
57. Halliwell, B. (1978) FEBS Lett., 92, 321-326.
58. Halliwell, B. (1975) FEBS Lett., 56, 34-38.
59. Fong, K., McCay, P.B., Poyer, J.L., Misra, H., and Keele, B.B. (1976) Chem. Biol. Interact., 15, 77-89.
60. Ilan, Y.A. and Czapski, G. (1977) Biochim. Biophys. Acta, 498, 386-394.
61. Van Hemmen, J.J. and Meuling, W.J.A. (1977) Arch. Biochem. Biophys., 182, 743-748.
62. McCord, J.M. and Day, E.D. (1978) FEBS Lett., 86, 139-142.
63. Halliwell, B. (1978) FEBS Lett., 96, 238-242.
64. Gutteridge, J.M.C., Richmond, R. and Halliwell, B. (1979) FEBS Lett., 184, 469-472.
65. Grankvist, K., Marklund, S., and Taljedal, I.-B. (1979) FEBS Lett., 105, 15-18.
66. Mathews, A.P. and Walker, S. (1909) J. Biol. Chem., 6, 299-312.
67. Wills, E.D. (1965) Biochem. Biophys. Acta, 98, 238-251.
68. Willson, R.L. (1977) Ciba Symp. 51, Exsevier Excerpta Medica, North-Holland, pp. 331-354.
69. Albert, A. (1973) Selective Toxicity, London: Chapman and Hall.
70. Lown, J.W. and Sim, S. (1977) Biochem. Biophys. Res. Commun., 77, 1150-1157.
71. Racker, E. and Krimsky, I. (1947) J. Exp. Med., 85, 715-727.
72. McCarthy, R.L. and Machlachlan, A. (1960) Trans. Farad. Soc., 56, 1187-1200.
73. Dorfman, L.M. (1974) in Techniques of Chemistry, Vol. VI, Part II, New York: Wiley Interscience, pp. 436.
74. Adams, G.E., Willson, R.L., Aldrich, J.G., and Cundall, R.B. (1969) Int. J. Radiat. Biol., 16, 333-342.

75. Armstrong, R.G. and Swallow, A.J. (1969) Radiat. Res., 40, 563-579.
76. Jayson, G.G., Scholes, G. and Weiss, J. (1954) Biochem. J., 57, 386.
77. Eich, E. and Rochelmayer, H. (1966) Pharm. Acta Helv., 41, 109.
78. Willson, R.L. and Slater, T.F. (1975) in Fast Processes in Radiation Chemistry and Biology, Adams, G.E., Fielden, E.M., and Michael, B.D., eds., The Institute of Physics, John Wiley, pp. 147-161.
79. Packer, J.E., Mahood, J.S., Willson, R.L., and Wolfenden, B.S. (1981) Int. J. Radiat. Biol., 39, 135-141.
80. Adams, G.E., Aldrich, J.E., Bisby, R.H., Cundall, R.B., Redpath, J.L., and Willson, R.L. (1972) Radiat. Res., 49, 278-289.
81. Posener, M.L., Adams, G.E., Wardman, P., and Cundall, R.B. (1976) J. Chem. Soc. Farad. Trans., 72, 2231-2239.
82. Prutz, W.A. and Land, E.J. (1979) Int. J. Radiat. Biol., 36, 513-520.
83. Prutz, W.A., Butler, J., Land, E.J., and Swallow, A.J. (1980) Biochem. Biophys. Acta, 96, 408-414.
84. Searle, A.J.F., Taylor, J., and Willson, R.L. (1981) in publication
85. Packer, J.E., Slater, T.F., and Willson, R.L. (1978) Life Sci., 23, 2617-2620.
86. Packer, J.E., Slater, T.F., and Willson, R.L. (1979) Nature, 278, 737-738.
87. Packer, J.E., Willson, R.L., Bahnemann, D., and Asmus, K.-D. (1980) J. Chem. Soc. Perkin II, 296-299.
88. Packer, J.E., Mahood, J.S., Mora-Arellano, V., Slater, T.F., Willson, R.L., Wolfenden, B.S. (1981) Biochem. Biophys. Res. Comm., 98, 901-906.
89. Slater, T.F., ed. (1978) Biochemical Mechanisms of Liver Injury, London: Academic Press, 745-801.
90. Akera, T. and Brody, T.M. (1968) Mol. Pharmacol., 4, 600-612.
91. Akera, T. and Brody, T.M. (1969) Mol. Pharmacol., 5, 605-614.
92. Akera, T. and Brody, T.M. (1970) Mol. Pharmacol., 6, 557.
93. Akera, T. and Brody, T.M. (1972) Biochem. Pharmacol., 21, 1403-1411.
94. Mahood, J.S., Packer, J.E., Searle, A.J.F., Willson, R.L., and Wolfenden, B.S. (1980) in Phenothiazines and Structurally Related Drugs: Basic and Clinical Studies, Eckert, U. and Forrest, A., eds., Elsevier/North Holland, pp. 103-106.
95. Zelickson, A.S. and Zeller, A.C. (1964) J. Am. Med. Ass., 188, 3941.
96. Blois, M.S. (1965) J. Invest. Dermatol., 45, 475.
97. Staudinger, H., Krisch, K., and Leonhäuser, S. (1961) Ann. N.Y. Acad. Sci., 92, 195-207.
98. Schneider, W. and Staudinger, H. (1965) Biochim. Biophys. Acta., 96, 157-159.
99. Lumper, V.L., Schneider, W., and Staudinger, H. (1967) Hoppe-Seyler's Z. Physiol. Chem., 352, 1659-1674.
100. Ito, A., Hayashi, S., and Yoshida, K. (1981) Biochem. Biophys. Res. Comm., 101, 591-598.

INDEX